Immunological Mechanisms in Asthma and Allergic Diseases

Chemical Immunology

Vol. 78

Series Editors

Luciano Adorini, Milan
Ken-ichi Arai, Tokyo
Claudia Berek, Berlin
J. Donald Capra, Oklahoma City, Okla.
Anne-Marie Schmitt-Verhulst, Marseille
Byron H. Waksman, New York, N.Y.

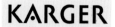 Basel · Freiburg · Paris · London · New York ·
New Delhi · Bangkok · Singapore · Tokyo · Sydney

Symposium held on the occasion of Prof. A. Barry Kay's 60th Birthday
and 20th year as Head of Department, London, June 24–25, 1999

··························

Immunological Mechanisms in Asthma and Allergic Diseases

Volume Editor   *Douglas S. Robinson*, London

26 figures, 2000

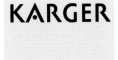

Basel · Freiburg · Paris · London · New York ·
New Delhi · Bangkok · Singapore · Tokyo · Sydney

Chemical Immunology

Formerly published as 'Progress in Allergy'
Founded 1939 by Paul Kallos

••••••••••••••••••••••••

Douglas S. Robinson, M.A., M.D.

Senior Lecturer, Allergy and Clinical Immunology, Imperial College School of Medicine,
National Heart and Lung Institute, London

Bibliographic Indices. This publication is listed in bibliographic services, including Current Contents® and Index Medicus.

Drug Dosage. The authors and the publisher have exerted every effort to ensure that drug selection and dosage set forth in this text are in accord with current recommendations and practice at the time of publication. However, in view of ongoing research, changes in government regulations, and the constant flow of information relating to drug therapy and drug reactions, the reader is urged to check the package insert for each drug for any change in indications and dosage and for added warnings and precautions. This is particularly important when the recommended agent is a new and/or infrequently employed drug.

© Copyright 2000 by S. Karger AG, P.O. Box, CH–4009 Basel (Switzerland)
www.karger.com
Printed in Switzerland on acid-free paper by Reinhardt Druck, Basel
ISSN 1015–0145
ISBN 3–8055–7112–7

Contents

Contents

Contents

Foreword

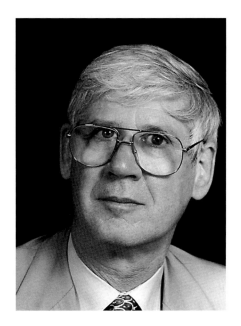

It is a great pleasure to write the foreword for this volume on 'Immunological Mechanisms in Asthma and Allergic Diseases' which arises out of a symposium organized on the occasion of Barry Kay's 60th birthday. The impact of Barry Kay's leadership in research directed to the understanding of allergic inflammation is not limited to his own laboratory but has profoundly influenced the field in general, and a laboratory such as my own in particular. As a result of his superb training with Robin Coombs in eosinophil biology, Barry Kay joined our laboratory in the early 1970s as a postdoctoral fellow and immediately directed our attention to the possible interactions between the eosinophil and the mast cell. He appreciated that mast cell activation was associated with eosinophil accumulation in experimental allergic reactions mediated by the IgG1 class antibody in the guinea pig based upon studies at skin sites. Accordingly, he with others in our laboratory used guinea pig lung slices sensitized with IgG1 and challenged with specific antigen to demonstrate the release of preform histamine and the associated generation of slow-reacting substance of anaphylaxis (SRS-A/cysteinyl leukotrienes) and a factor (factors) capable of attracting eosinophils by a chemotactic mechanism as assessed in a Boyden chamber. The shared release of these three mediators was observed in kinetic experiments as well as in dose-response analyses of the sensitizing immunoglobulin or the challenging antigen. Furthermore, by size discrimination as well as by target cell specificity, he established that the eosinophilotactic activity was distinct from the previously recognized cleavage fragment of the 5th guinea pig complement component. Finally, he turned to human lung fragments sensitized with allergen-specific IgE to once again demonstrate the associated release of histamine, SRS-A, and eosinophil chemotactic activity with appropriate allergen challenge. These studies represented an initial collaboration between a visiting postdoctoral fellow who quickly became a peer at the host laboratory.

Subsequently, in his own programme in Great Britain, Barry Kay and his colleagues demonstrated a number of unique biological properties of the eosinophil including VLA-4-dependent interaction with fibronectin and the consequent autocrine generation of granulocyte/macrophage-colony stimulating factor which provided cytoprotection. These and other studies of the eosinophil prompted his group's focus on the possible pathobiologic significance of the eosinophil in allergic disease in general, and bronchial asthma in particular, with the recognition that a key control cell of eosinophil function in that setting was of the T-cell lineage. Elegant studies using in situ hybridization and immunohistochemistry established that the Th2 phenotype was the key subset for the inflammatory process in which the eosinophil participated so prominently. More recently, he and his colleagues have provided compelling experiments to reveal a direct role of the T-cell lineage in the asthmatic reaction, that is, a pathobiologic function derived directly from the Th2 cell phenotype possibly without the intermediate role of IgE or an additional cell type.

His studies, after a 30-year interval during which we continued to discuss the pathobiology of bronchial asthma, have once again impacted on our laboratory, at this time at a distance. The appreciation of the role of the Th2 cell in bronchial asthma has prompted our own group to increase its focus on the role of that cell in the pathobiology of the human mast cell. Interestingly, we now find that reactive mast cell hyperplasia of human mast cells in a culture system is stem cell factor-dependent but readily driven by interleukin-5. Furthermore, the mast cell like the eosinophil and the Th2 cell expresses CCR-3 implying accumulation at an inflammatory site through the action of a chemokine such as eotaxin. The seminal work of Barry Kay and his colleagues in identifying the Th2 cell as central to allergic and asthmatic inflammation has provided an integrated and coherent basis for appreciating not only its direct role but the indirect contribution of this cell through its regulation of the two cells that complete the inflammatory triad, the mast cell and the eosinophil.

The work of Barry Kay and his colleagues is consistently innovative, uninfluenced by existing dogma, technically elegant, and always reproducible.

K. Frank Austen, Boston, Mass.

Robinson DS (ed): Immunological Mechanisms in Asthma and Allergic Diseases.
Chem Immunol. Basel, Karger, 2000, vol 78, pp 1–15

....

Scientific Overview of 20 Years' Work in the Department of Allergy and Clinical Immunology Under the Guidance of Professor A.B. Kay

Douglas S. Robinson

Allergy and Clinical Immunology, Imperial College School of Medicine,
National Heart and Lung Institute, London, UK

At the very end of 1979, Prof. Barry Kay succeeded as Head of Department in the Department of Clinical Immunology at the then Cardiothoracic Institute. The department had been founded as the first department of clinical immunology in the UK by Prof. Jack Pepys. Prof. Pepys had done much of the work establishing the clinical and laboratory background to the early- and late-phase response to allergen challenge and Barry Kay initially turned his interests in cell biology and factors released from mast cells recruiting other inflammatory cells to the late-phase response to allergen. In particular, early work from the laboratory focused on the elaboration of mast cell-derived chemotactic factors attracting neutrophils and eosinophils to the sites of allergic inflammation. Early observations included the detection of neutrophil chemotactic activity in serum during both early- and late-phase responses to inhaled allergen challenge in sensitized individuals [1]. Similar activity could be isolated in exercise-induced asthma in laboratory and HPLC analysis of this activity showed that the neutrophil chemotactic factor evoked by both exercise and allergen challenge eluted in a high molecular weight fraction [2]. The application of rosetting techniques showed evidence of neutrophil complement rosette formation, again during both early- and late-phase responses to antigen challenge by inhalation. This work was one of the first descriptions of cellular activation during the late-phase response to allergen [3]. The application of fibreoptic bronchoscopy to allow direct sampling of the airways in the mid-1980s allowed confirmation that there were indeed increased neutrophil numbers during the late-phase response to allergen in the airway. In a collaborative study with Diaz et al. [4] there were also increases in both eosinophils and lymphocytes in response to allergen challenge when compared to diluent control. Fibreoptic bronchoscopic sampling of the airways was also used to examine further the role of the eosinophil following on from the observations by Gleich and co-workers [5] that evidence of eosinophil degranulation could be obtained in patients dying of asthma, where immuno-fluorescence of lung samples showed extensive deposition of the eosinophil major basic protein (MBP). Analysis of bronchoalveolar lavage (BAL) fluid from asthmatic and control subjects showed increased concentrations of MBP in lavage fluid from asthmatics compared to control groups, and furthermore higher levels of MBP were detected in those with hyperactive airways compared to subjects with a methacholine PC_{20} >4 mg/ml. In addition, there was a correlation between MBP concentration in BAL and the methacholine PC_{20}, eosinophils in the lavage and PC_{20} and epithelial cell numbers in lavage and PC_{20} [6]. All of this led support to the hypothesis that eosinophil degranulation through release of basic protein such as MBP might damage the epithelium contributing to airway hyperresponsiveness in asthma.

With the description of T-cell-derived factors acting on eosinophils, attention at this time turned to the CD4 lymphocyte in asthma. Examination of peripheral blood lymphocytes by flow cytometry and increased expression of the activation marker CD25 by CD4 but not by CD8 lymphocytes in those admitted to hospital with acute severe asthma compared to mild asthma or nonasthmatic controls. Furthermore, during the patients' stay in hospital, and as lung function improved, the degree of expression of activation markers receded [7]. Bronchoscopic studies of lymphocyte activation in asthma included the elegant ultrastructural study by Jeffery et al. [8] which showed marked abnormalities in the airway mucosa and epithelium even in very mild asthmatics. Biopsies showed disruption of the normal epithelial lining, sub-basement membrane, hyaline thickening, and lymphocytes with atypical morphology compatible with activation. Application of immunohistochemistry to bronchial biopsies obtained from mild asthmatics showed again increased expression of the interleukin (IL)-2 receptor CD25 in asthmatic subjects compared to controls and this was accompanied by increased numbers of activated eosinophils [9].

In the 1980s, Sanderson [10] and others [11] described IL-5 as a T-cell-derived cytokine acting selectively on eosinophil differentiation and survival, and in 1991 Qutayba Hamid [12] in the group applied in situ hybridization to show increased numbers of cells expressing messenger RNA for IL-5 in bronchial biopsies from patients with asthma compared with control subjects and furthermore an increase in those with current symptoms. Extending the cytokines examined, Robinson et al. [13] showed increased numbers of BAL cells expressing cytokine mRNA of the Th2 profile, namely IL-4 and IL-5 in asthma but no difference between asthma and control subjects in the Th1 cytokine, interferon-γ (IFN-γ). Further work showed evidence of an increase in expression of the Th2 cytokines IL-4 and IL-5 by T cells in the BAL during the late-phase response to allergen [14, 15]. More recently, Sun Ying [16] has applied the technique of simultaneous in situ hybridization and immunohisto-chemistry to phenotype cells expressing messenger RNA for cytokines in biopsies and has confirmed that the predominant source of IL-4 and IL-5 messenger RNA is in fact CD3+ T cells with small contributions from both eosinophils and tryptase-positive mast cells. This work also confirms very low levels of expression of the Th1 cytokines IFN-γ and IL-2 in the airway mucosa of atopic asthmatics. The question of the allergen specificity of activated T cells and cytokine-producing T cells in the airway mucosa was addressed by work from Christopher Corrigan and Stephen Till in the department. Together with Stephen Durham [17] they performed segmental allergen challenge in sensitized asthmatic subjects and were able to show increased proliferative responses in cells obtained from BAL to the allergen used for challenge in asthmatic subjects compared with controls. Furthermore, by derivation of T-cell lines from BAL cells it was possible to show increased production of IL-5 from both CD4- and CD8- derived lines upon allergen stimulation [18].

Allergen-Induced Changes in the Skin

The cutaneous response to allergen has been an extremely useful model allowing initial studies such as those by Frew and Kay [19] which showed infiltration of eosinophils and CD4 T cells bearing activation markers and memory phenotypic markers into the late-phase response evoked by allergen. Further examination of cutaneous late responses again showed induction of Th2-type cytokines with increased numbers of cells expressing IL-4 and IL-5, GM-CSF and IL-3 in skin biopsies from allergen-challenged sites compared with diluent control sites but no increase in Th1 cytokines such as IFN-γ [20]. An advantage of using the cutaneous model for late-phase studies is that it allows repeated sampling and therefore time course studies can be performed. An example of this is the recent study by Sun Ying et al. [21] in collaboration with Andrew Walls and others in Southampton which has allowed detailed mapping of the time course of appearance of both inflammatory cells including eosinophils, neutrophils and, applying the novel antibody BB1, basophil infil-tration into the skin during late-phase response (fig. 1). This study has been extended out to 7 days allowing further study of the resolution of the late-

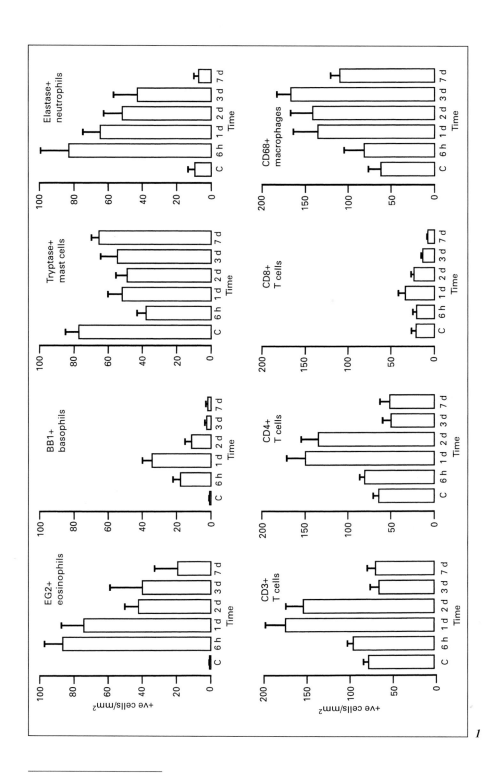

phase response and work in the department has also described resolution of the late-phase response by apoptosis [22]. Examination of the time course of cytokine elaboration also confirms an increase in both IL-4 and IL-5 mirroring the time course of cell infiltration into the cutaneous late-phase response [23] and more recently has allowed examination of the differential time course of expression of the CC chemokines, eotaxin and eotaxin-2, MCP-3, MCP-4 and RANTES [21].

The delineation of cellular and molecular changes during the late-phase response allowed dissection of the mechanisms of allergen immunotherapy. Initially, Varney et al. [24] carried out a double-blind placebo-controlled study which established dramatic improvements in symptoms and medication requirements in patients randomized to receive allergen injection immunotherapy compared with those receiving matched placebo injections. Examination of the effect of immunotherapy on the allergen-induced late-phase response showed a change both in the cellular infiltration and cytokine profile such that in skin biopsies there was an apparent increase in Th1 cytokines as well as Th2 cytokines in those patients who had been treated with immunotherapy, whereas those receiving placebo showed predominant Th2 profile as was seen prior to immunotherapy in all patients [25]. Similar work examining the cytokine expression in the nose in response to allergen before and after immunotherapy showed a diminution in the Th2 response and an increase in Th1 cytokines IL-2 and IFN-γ in those treated with immunotherapy [26]. These observations together with those of others in the field allowed the suggestion that immunotherapy may induce immune deviation with a reduction in the Th2 response and possible switch towards a Th1 response reducing IgE and eosinophilic inflammation in response to allergen (fig. 2).

Selective Eosinophil Accumulation

One of the major strands of research in the department has been mechanisms by which eosinophils selectively accumulate at sites of allergic inflammation. This work formed a logical conclusion of Prof. Kay's PhD thesis with Prof. Robin Coombs in Cambridge which was entitled 'Eosinophil leucocytes and allergic tissue reactions'. The work has addressed three main features

Fig. 1. Accumulation of inflammatory cells at the site of the allergen-induced late cutaneous reactions. Skin biopsies were obtained at different time points after intradermal injection of 30 biological units of allergen extract (ALK, Copenhagen, Denmark) or diluent control, and analysed by immunohistochemistry for eosinophils, basophils, mast cells, neutrophils, T-cell subsets and macrophages, as described in Ying et al. [21].

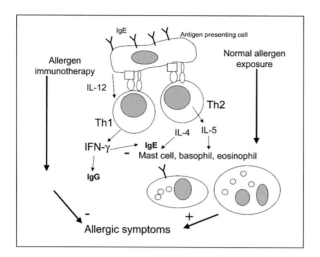

Fig. 2. Immune deviation after allergen injection immunotherapy. At sites of allergen challenge in the skin or nose, after allergen immunotherapy there was increased expression of the Th1 cytokine IFN-γ, and IL-12, which favours Th1 expansion, with concomitant decreases in numbers of IL-4 and IL-5 mRNA expressing cells. This leads to the suggestion that AII alters T-cell responsiveness away from a predominant Th2 pattern, towards a more Th1 cytokine profile.

leading to selective accumulation, namely adhesion, prolonged tissue survival and chemotaxis.

Adhesion

Garry Walsh who worked with Andy Wardlaw in the laboratory was among a series of workers who showed that eosinophils but not neutrophils expressed the adhesion molecule VLA-1 and went on to show that this was functionally relevant in terms of adhesion to the counter receptor VCAM-1 [27]. Further work in the department has shown increased expression of VCAM-1 in the airway after allergen challenge [28] and increased expression of both IL-4 and IL-13 which induce upregulation of VCAM in the late-phase cutaneous response to allergen. Furthermore, this work showed correlation between IL-13 expression and increased expression and increased expression of VCAM in the allergen-induced late-phase response [29]. As a functional consequence of eosinophil adhesion, Anwar et al. [30], working in the department, were able to show that eosinophil adhesion to fibronectin through the VLA-1-dependent pathways caused enhanced eosinophil survival and that furthermore this was due to the elaboration of GM-CSF in an autocrine manner from eosinophils.

Eosinophil Survival

The work showing increased GM-CSF expression by eosinophils themselves after fibronectin adhesion built on previous observations from this department and collaborators that eosinophils are capable of generating cytokines [31, 32]. Initial observations showed that eosinophils were a potential source of both IL-3 and GM-CSF and that these might thus act in an autocrine fashion to increased tissue survival. Subsequent work has gone on to show that eosinophils are a potential source of a wide variety of cytokines including IL-2, IL-3, IL-4, IL-5, IL-6, IL-8, GM-CSF and TGF-β amongst others [33–39]. Further work including subcellular fractionation of eosinophils allowed the demonstration that these cytokines were stored within different compartments of eosinophil granules and that both preformed mediators may be released and that there was the potential for differential release at different cytokines from eosinophils [40].

Chemotaxis

Following on from work during his stay as a postdoctoral fellow in Boston with Dr. Frank Austen, Prof. Kay has an interest in eosinophil chemotactic factors [41]. It was therefore gratifying to be able to identify some 20 years after the initial observation that eosinophil chemotactic factor of anaphylaxis in guinea pigs could largely be accounted by activity of leukotriene B_4 and 18S,15S-di-HETE [42] (fig. 3). Further work from the department had highlighted the potent activities in terms of eosinophil chemotaxis of platelet activating factor [43] and had also shown that leukotrienes could indeed be released from eosinophils following physiological stimuli such as IgG crosslinking [44]. Current attention in eosinophil chemotaxis has been focused by the elegant work of Prof. Tim Williams and his group [45] who describe the specific eosinophil chemoattractant CC chemokine, eotaxin. Application of in situ hybridization and immunohistochemistry confirmed increased expression of both message and protein product for eotaxin in the airways of atopic asthmatics compared with control subjects and furthermore showed correlations between the numbers of cells expressing eotaxin and airways hyperresponsiveness and that there were also increased numbers of cells expressing the ligand for eotaxin CCR3 [46]. Further work is continuing in the group to examine the role of a variety of CC chemokines in recruitment of both eosinophils, T cells and basophils to the sites of allergic inflammation [47, 48].

Severe Asthma

Recognizing that much of the study of immunopathology of asthma has been in very mild patients who can be studied by fibreoptic bronchoscopy,

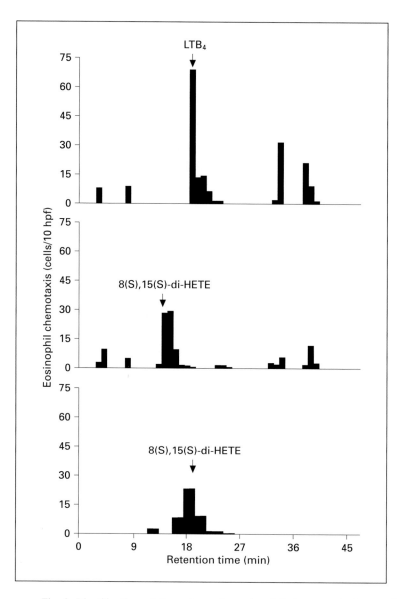

Fig. 3. Identification of the guinea pig eosinophil chemotactic factor of anaphylaxis (ECFA) as 8,15-di-HETE. RP- and SP-HPLC analysis of ECA showed coelution of the chemotactic activity with leukotriene B_4 and with 8,15-di-HETE [from 42].

the group has nonetheless recognized that the clinical need is larger in more severe patients who are difficult to manage and often require oral corticosteroids. In a series of collaborative studies with Dr. Neil Barnes, the department has studied other approaches to direct anti-T-cell therapy in severe steroid-dependent asthma. In a 12-week placebo-controlled double-blind study of cyclosporin there was a marked improvement in lung function in those patients receiving cyclosporin compared with control and further work went on to show in a 44-week study that cyclosporin could have a marked steroid-sparing effect in such severe steroid-dependent patients [49, 50]. The mechanisms of action of cyclosporin were further investigated following reports that in addition to inhibiting T-cell proliferation of cytokine production, cyclosporin might also act on mast cell degranulation. However, Sihra et al. [51] were able to show that cyclosporin inhibited the late-phase response to allergen challenge in the airway but did not affect the early response suggesting selective activity on those factors involved in the late-phase response.

Intrinsic Asthma

As a clinical problem and intriguing dilemma for mechanisms of asthma, the group has been involved in the study of intrinsic asthma in collaboration with Günter Menz and others at the Hochgebirgsklinik in Davos. Intrinsic asthma was defined by Rackeman [52] in the 1940s and is characterized by patients who are generally somewhat older than those with atopic asthma at the time of onset and who have no clinical history suggestive of allergen sensitization borne out by negative skin prick tests and no evidence of specific IgE by RAST to common aeroallergens. A series of studies from the department has shown initially that airway biopsies from intrinsic asthmatic compared with those with atopic allergic disease show common features, namely activation of T cells and eosinophil infiltration [15]. Furthermore that there is a common Th2 cytokine profile with increased numbers of cells expressing mRNA and protein product for both IL-4 and IL-5 in both types of asthma [53]. The role of IL-4 in intrinsic asthma is uncertain but studies from the group have also shown evidence of local IgE synthesis and increased infiltration of high-affinity IgE receptor-bearing cells in intrinsic asthma [54, 55], thus raising the possibility that IgE mechanisms to antigens as yet unknown contribute to the pathology of intrinsic asthma. The only clear difference between intrinsic and atopic asthma at the cellular level appears to be an increased signal in intrinsic asthma for macrophage infiltration with several studies showing increased numbers of CD68 macrophages together with increased expression of the GM-CSF receptor in the intrinsic variant of the disease

[15, 56, 57]. The functional significance of this is currently under investigation in the department.

Corticosteroid-Resistant Asthma

Following on from work in Edinburgh where Prof. Kay was involved in describing the phenotype of corticosteroid-resistant asthma [58–60], work in the department defined that those with no clinical response to oral prednisolone also showed abnormalities in T-cell proliferation and cytokine elaboration in the laboratory. Corrigan et al. [61] showed corticosteroid-resistant patients to show a lack of steroid-induced inhibition of both PHA-driven proliferation and cytokine production in vitro. Cytokine production from T cells is normally exquisitely sensitive to steroid inhibition. In particular, both in vitro production of IL-4 and IL-5 is inhibited by corticosteroids [62]. That this might be relevant to clinical asthma was confirmed in studies showing a reduction in the numbers of cells expressing IL-5 and IL-4 messenger RNA in bronchial biopsies and lavage obtained after a 2-week course of oral prednisolone in a double-blind placebo-controlled study. In this study, patients showed improvement in PC_{20} when treated with prednisolone and this was not seen in the parallel placebo-controlled group [63, 64]. Taking this work into the field of steroid resistance in collaboration with Qutayba Hamid in Montreal and Donald Leung in Denver, it was possible to show that steroid-resistant asthmatics did not show reduction in IL-5 expression in the airway following oral steroid treatment whereas this was seen in a parallel group of steroid-sensitive patients [65]. This again supports the hypothesis that IL-5 elaboration plays a role in the direct symptoms of asthma and both steroid-resistant asthma and the milder forms previously studied. Direct targetting of the T cell has been taken further in a recent study published in 1998 where nondepleting monoclonal antibodies against the CD4 co-receptor were used to reduce T-cell activation. In this study steroid-dependent asthmatics receiving a single dose of anti-CD4 showed an improvement in lung function over a 2-week period when compared with those receiving the matched placebo [66].

Conclusions

Much of the work over the last 10 years in the department has focused on T-cell activation and IL-5 elaboration as a major driving force for eosinophilic inflammation in allergic disease. This is borne out by observed correlations between levels of IL-5 expression and clinical manifestations of asthma such as airway narrowing and PC_{20} [67, 68]. Results of clinical studies using anti-IL-5 are eagerly awaited. The current work of the department focuses on dissociation of T-cell-mediated events in response to allergen from those that are IgE-dependent and in more recent work it has been possible to show induction of isolated late-phase responses in the airway following intradermal injection of allergen-derived peptides from the major cat allergen Fel d 1 that activate T cells but do not cross-link IgE [69]. Furthermore, this response was HLA-restricted. Subsequent injections of peptide did not evoke such responses and this approach may be of therapeutic use in inducing T-cell hyperresponsiveness and therefore have applications in immunotherapy [see Larché et al., in this book]. Further work continues to examine the factors driving eosinophil differentiation and release from the bone marrow together with recruitment into sites of allergic inflammation [70, 71].

References

1   Nagy L, Lee TH, Kay AB: Neutrophil chemotactic activity in antigen-induced late asthmatic reactions. N Engl J Med 1982;306:497–501.
2   Lee TH, Nagy L, Nagakura T, Walport MJ, Kay AB: The identification and partial characterisation of an exercise-induced neutrophil chemotactic factor in bronchial asthma. J Clin Invest 1982;69: 889–899.
3   Durham SR, Carroll M, Walsh GM, Kay AB: Leukocyte activation in allergen-induced late-phase asthmatic reactions. N Engl J Med 1984;311:1398–1402.
4   Diaz P, Gonzalez MC, Galleguillos FR, Ancic P, Cromwell O, Shepherd D, Durham SR, Gleich GJ, Kay AB: Leukocytes and mediators in bronchoalveolar lavage during late-phase asthmatic reactions. Am Rev Respir Dis 1989;139:1383–1389.
5   Filley WV, Holley KE, Kephart GM, Gleich GJ: Identification by immunofluorescence of eosinophil granule major basic protein in lung tissues of patients with bronchial asthma. Lancet 1982;ii:11–16.
6   Wardlaw AJ, Dunnette S, Gleich GJ, Collins JV, Kay AB: Eosinophils and mast cells in bronchoalveolar lavage in mild asthma: Relationship to bronchial hyperreactivity. Am Rev Respir Dis 1988;137:62–69.
7   Corrigan CJ, Hartnell A, Kay AB: T lymphocyte activation in acute severe asthma. Lancet 1988; i:1129–1132.
8   Jeffery PK, Wardlaw AJ, Nelson FC, Collins JV, Kay AB: Bronchial biopsies in asthma: An ultrastructural, quantitative study and correlation with hyperreactivity. Am Rev Respir Dis 1989; 140:1745–1753.
9   Azzawi M, Bradley B, Jeffery PK, Frew A, Wardlaw AJ, Knowles G, Assoufi B, Collins JV, Durham S, Kay AB: Identification of activated T lymphocytes and eosinophils in bronchial biopsies in stable atopic asthma. Am Rev Respir Dis 1990;142:1407–1413.
10   Campbell HD, Tucker WQJ, Hort Y, Martinson ME, Mayo G, Clutterbuck EJ, Sanderson CJ, Young IG: Molecular cloning, nucleotide sequence and expression of the gene encoding human eosinophil differentiation factor (interleukin-5). Proc Natl Acad Sci USA 1987;84:6629–6631.
11   Kinashi T, Harada N, Severinson E, Tanabe T, Sideras P, Konishi M, Azuma C, Tominaga A, Bergstedt-Lindqvist S, Takahashi M, Matsuda F, Yaoita Y, Takatsu K, Honjo T: Cloning of complementary DNA encoding T cell replacement factor and identity with B cell factor II. Nature 1986;324:70–72.
12   Hamid Q, Azzawi M, Ying S, Moqbel R, Wardlaw AJ, Corrigan CJ, Bradley B, Durham SR, Collins JV, Jeffery PK, Quint DJ, Kay AB: Expression of mRNA for interleukin-5 in mucosal bronchial biopsies from asthma. J Clin Invest 1991;87:1541–1546.

13 Robinson DS, Hamid Q, Ying S, Tsicopoulos A, Barkans J, Bentley AM, Corrigan CJ, Durham SR, Kay AB: Predominant T_{H2}-type bronchoalveolar lavage T-lymphocyte population in atopic asthma. N Engl J Med 1992;326:298–304.

14 Robinson DS, Hamid Q, Bentley A, Ying S, Kay AB, Durham SR: Activation of CD4+ T cells, increased Th2-type cytokine mRNA expression, and eosinophil recruitment in bronchoalveolar lavage after allergen inhalation challenge in atopic asthmatics. J Allergy Clin Immunol 1993;92: 313–324.

15 Bentley AM, Menz G, Storz C, Robinson DS, Bradley B, Jeffery PK, Durham SR, Kay AB: Identification of T-lymphocytes, macrophages and activated eosinophils in the bronchial mucosa in intrinsic asthma: Relationship to symptoms and bronchial responsiveness. Am Rev Respir Dis 1992;146:500–506.

16 Ying S, Humbert M, Barkans J, Corrigan CJ, Pfister R, Menz G, Robinson DS, Larché M, Durham SR, Kay AB: Expression of IL-4 and IL-5 mRNA and protein product by CD4+ and CD8+ T cells, eosinophils and mast cells in bronchial biopsies obtained from atopic and non-atopic (intrinsic) asthmatics. J Immunol 1997; 158:3539–3544.

17 Till SJ, Durham SR, Rajakulasingam K, Humbert M, Huston D, Dickason R, Kay AB Corrigan CJ: Allergen-induced proliferation and interleukin-5 production by bronchoalveolar lavage and blood T cells after segmental allergen challenge. Am J Respir Crit Care Med 1998;158:404–411.

18 Till SJ, Li B, Durham S, Humbert M, Assoufi B, Huston D, Dickason R, Jeannin P, Kay AB, Corrigan C: Secretion of the eosinophil-active cytokines interleukin-5, granulocyte/macrophage colony-stimulating factor and interleukin-3 by bronchoalveolar lavage CD4+ and CD8+ T cell lines in atopic asthmatics, and atopic and non-atopic controls. Eur J Immunol 1995;25:2727–2731.

19 Frew AJ, Kay AB: The relationship between infiltrating CD4+ lymphocytes, activated eosinophils and the magnitude of the allergen-induced late phase cutaneous reaction in man. J Immunol 1988; 141:4158–4164.

20 Kay AB, Ying S, Varney V, Gaga M, Durham SR, Moqbel R, Wardlaw AJ, Hamid Q: Messenger RNA expression of the cytokine gene cluster, IL-3, IL-4, IL-5 and GM-CSF in allergen-induced late-phase cutaneous reactions in atopic subjects. J Exp Med 1991;173:775–778.

21 Ying S, Robinson DS, Meng Q, Barata LT, McEuen AR, Buckley MG, Walls AF, Askenase PW, Kay AB: C-C chemokines in allergen-induced late-phase cutaneous responses in atopic subjects: Association of eotaxin with early 6-hour eosinophils, and eotaxin-2 and MCP-4 with the later 24-hour tissue eosinophilia, and relationship to basophils and other C-C chemokines (MCP-3 and RANTES). J Immunol 1999;163:3976–3984.

22 Ying S, Meng Q, Taborda-Barata L, Kay AB: Apoptosis of neutrophils and eosinophils and their ingestion by macrophages is associated with resolution of the allergen-induced cutaneous late-phase response in human atopic subjects. Proc Assoc of Am Physicians 1997;109:42–50.

23 Barata LT, Ying S, Grant JA, Humbert M, Barkans J, Meng Q, Durham SR, Kay AB: Allergen-induced recruitment of Fc(RI+ eosinophils in human atopic skin. Eur J Immunol 1997;27:1236–1241.

24 Varney V, Gaga M, Frew AJ, Aber VA, Kay AB, Durham SR: Usefulness of immunotherapy in patients with severe summer hayfever uncontrolled by antiallergic drugs. Br Med J 1991;302:265–269.

25 Varney VA, Hamid QA, Gaga M, Ying S, Jacobson M, Frew AJ, Kay AB, Durham SR: Influence of grass pollen immunotherapy on cellular infiltration and cytokine mRNA expression during allergen-induced late-phase cutaneous responses. J Clin Invest 1993;92:644–651.

26 Durham SR, Ying S, Varney VA, Jacobson MR, Sudderick RM, Mackay IS, Kay AB, Hamid QA: Grass pollen immunotherapy inhibits allergen-induced infiltration of CD4+ T lymphocytes and eosinophils in the nasal mucosa and increases the number of cells expressing messenger RNA for interferon-γ. J Allergy Clin Immunol 1996;97:1356–1365.

27 Walsh GM, Mermod JJ, Hartnell A, Kay AB, Wardlaw AJ: Human eosinophil, but not neutrophil, adherence to IL-1 stimulated HUVEC is $\alpha_4\beta_1$ (VLA-4) dependent. J Immunol 1991;146:3419–3423.

28 Bentley AM, Durham SR, Robinson DS, Menz G, Storz C, Cromwell O, Kay AB, Wardlaw AJ: Expression of the endothelial and leukocyte adhesion molecules, ICAM-1, E-selectin and VCAM-1 in the bronchial mucosa in steady state and allergen-induced asthma. J Allergy Clin Immunol 1993; 92:857–868.

29   Ying S, Meng Q, Barata LT, Robinson DS, Durham SR, Kay AB: Associations between IL-13 and IL-4 (mRNA and protein), VCAM-1 expression and the infiltration of eosinophils, macrophages and T cells in allergen-induced late-phase cutaneous reactions in atopic subjects. J Immunol 1997; 158:5050–5057.

30   Anwar ARE, Moqbel R, Walsh GM, Kay AB, Wardlaw AJ: Adhesion to fibronectin prolongs eosinophil survival. J Exp Med 1993;177:839–843.

31   Moqbel R, Hamid Q, Ying S, Barkans J, Hartnell A, Tsicopoulos A, Wardlaw AJ, Kay AB: Expression of mRNA and immunoreactivity for the granulocyte/macrophage colony-stimulating factor in activated human eosinophils. J Exp Med 1991;174:749–752.

32   Kita H, Ohnishi T, Okubo Y, Weller D, Abrams JS, Gleich GJ: Granulocyte-macrophage colony-stimulating factor and interleukin-3 release from human peripheral blood eosinophils and neutrophils. J Exp Med 1991; 174: 743.

33   Nakajima H, Gleich GJ, Kita H: Constitutive production of IL-4 and IL-10 and stimulated production of IL-8 by normal peripheral blood eosinophils. J Immunol 1996;156:4859–4866.

34   Lacy P, Moqbel R: Eokines: synthesis, storage and release from human eosinophils. Mem Inst Oswaldo Cruz 1997; 92 Suppl 2: 125–33.

35   Moqbel R, Ying S, Barkans J, Newman TM, Kimmitt P, Wakelin M, Taborda-Barata L, Meng Q, Corrigan CJ, Durham SR, et al: Identification of messenger RNA for IL-4 in human eosinophils with granule localization and release of the translated product. J Immunol 1995;155:4939–4947.

36   Dubucquoi S, Desreumaux P, Janin A, Klein O, Goldman M, Tavernier J, Capron A, Capron M: Interleukin-5 synthesis by eosinophils: Association with granules and immunoglobulin-dependent secretion. J Exp Med 1994;179:703–708.

37   Lacy P, Levi-Schaffer F, Mahmudi-Azer S, Bablitz B, Hagen SC, Velazquez J, Kay AB, Moqbel R: Intracellular localization of interleukin-6 in eosinophils from atopic asthmatics and effects of interferon-γ. Blood 1998;91:2508–2516.

38   Nakajima H, Gleich GJ, Fukuda T, Makino S, Kita H: Production of IL-8 and release of eosinophil-derived neurotoxin by normal peripheral blood eosinophils. Int Arch Allergy Immunol 1997; 114(suppl 1):36–39.

39   Elovic A, Wong DT, Weller PF, Matossian K, Galli SJ: Expression of transforming growth factors-α and -β₁ messenger RNA and product by eosinophils in nasal polyps. J Allergy Clin Immunol 1994;93:864–869.

40   Levi-Schaffer F, Barkans J, Newman TM, Ying S, Wakelin M, Hohenstein R, Barak V, Lacy P, Kay AB, Moqbel R: Identification of interleukin-2 in human peripheral blood eosinophils. Immunology 1996;87:155–161.

41   Kay AB, Stechschulte DJ, Austen KF: An eosinophil leukocyte chemotactic factor of anaphylaxis. J Exp Med 1971;133:602–619.

42   Sehmi R, Cromwell O, Taylor GW, Kay AB: The identification of guinea pig eosinophil chemotactic factor of anaphylaxis as leukotriene B₄ and 8(S),15(S)-di-HETE. J Immunol 1991;147:2276–2283.

43   Wardlaw AJ, Moqbel R, Cromwell O, Kay AB: Platelet activating factor: A potent chemotactic and chemokinetic factor for human eosinophils. J Clin Invest 1986;78:1701–1706.

44   Shaw RJ, Walsh GM, Cromwell O, Moqbel R, Spry CJF, Kay AB: Activated human eosinophils generate SRS-A leukotrienes following physiological (IgG-dependent) stimulation. Nature 1985; 316:150–152.

45   Jose PJ, Griffiths-Johnson DA, Collins PD, Walsh DT, Moqbel R, Totty NF, Truong O, Hsuan JJ, Williams TJ: Eotaxin: A potent eosinophil chemoattractant cytokine detected in a guinea pig model of allergic airways inflammation. J Exp Med 1994;179:881–887.

46   Ying S, Robinson DS, Meng Q, Rottman J, Kennedy R, Ringler DJ, Mackay CR, Daugherty BL, Springer MS, Durham SR, Williams TJ, Kay AB: Enhanced expression of eotaxin and CCR3 mRNA and protein in atopic asthma. Association with airway hyperresponsiveness and predominant co-localization of eotaxin mRNA to bronchial epithelial and endothelial cells. Eur J Immunol 1997;27:3507–3516.

47   Humbert M, Ying S, Corrigan CJ, Menz G, Barkans J, Pfister R, Meng Q, Van Damme J, Opdenakker G, Durham SR, Kay AB: Bronchial mucosal expression of the CC chemokine genes RANTES and MCP-3 in symptomatic atopic and non-atopic asthmatics: Relationship to EG2 + eosinophils and the eosinophil-active cytokines IL-5, GM-CSF and IL-3. Am J Respir Cell Mol Biol 1997;16:1–8.

48   Ying S, Taborda-Barata L, Meng Q, Humbert M, Kay AB: The kinetics of allergen-induced transcription of messenger RNA for monocyte chemotactic protein-3 (MCP-3) and RANTES in the skin of human atopic subjects: Relationship to eosinophil, T-cell and macrophage recruitment. J Exp Med 1995;181:2153–2159.

49   Alexander AG, Barnes NC, Kay AB: Trial of cyclosporin A in corticosteroid-dependent chronic severe asthma. Lancet 1992;339:324–328.

50   Lock SH, Kay AB, Barnes NC: Double-blind, placebo-controlled study of cyclosporin A as a corticosteroid-sparing agent in corticosteroid-dependent asthma. Am J Respir Crit Care Med 1996; 153:509–514.

51   Sihra BS, Durham SR, Walker S, Kon OM, Barnes NC, Kay AB: Effect of cyclosporin A on the allergen-induced late asthmatic reaction. Thorax 1997;52:447–452.

52   Rackeman FM: A working classification of asthma. Am J Med 1947;3:601–606.

53   Humbert M, Durham SR, Ying S, Kimmitt P, Barkans J, Assoufi B, Pfister R, Menz G, Robinson DS, Kay AB, Corrigan CJ: IL-4 and IL-5 mRNA and protein in bronchial biopsies from atopic and non-atopic asthmatics: Evidence against 'intrinsic' asthma being a distinct immunopathological entity. Am J Respir Crit Care Med 1996;154:1497–1504.

54   Humbert M, Grant JA, Taborda-Barata L, Durham SR, Pfister R, Menz G, Barkans J, Ying S, Kay AB: High affinity IgE receptor (FcεRI)-bearing cells in bronchial biopsies from atopic and non-atopic asthma. Am J Respir Crit Care Med 1996;153:1931–1937.

55   Durham SR, Ying S, Meng Q, Humbert M, Gould H, Kay AB: Local expression of ε germ-line gene transcripts (Iε) and RNA for the ε heavy chain of IgE (Cε) in the bronchial mucosa in atopic and non-atopic asthma, in press.

56   Kotsimbos AT, Humbert M, Minshall E, Durham S, Pfister R, Menz G, Tavernier J, Kay AB, Hamid Q: Upregulation of α GM-CSF receptor in non-atopic but not in atopic asthma. J Allergy Clin Immunol 1997;99:666–672.

57   Kotsimbos AT, Ghaffar O, Minshall E, Humbert M, Durham SR, Pfister R, Menz G, Kay AB, Hamid QA: Expression of the IL-4 receptor α-subunit is increased in bronchial biopsy specimens from atopic and nonatopic asthmatic subjects. J Allergy Clin Immunol 1998;102:859–866.

58   Carmichael J, Paterson IC, Diaz P, Crompton GK, Kay AB, Grant IWB: Corticosteroid resistance in chronic asthma. Br Med J 1981;282:1419–1422.

59   Poznansky MC, Gordon ACH, Douglas JG, Krajewski AS, Syllie AH, Grant IWB: Resistance to methylprednisolone in cultures of blood mononuclear cells from glucocorticoid-resistant asthmatic patients. Clin Sci 1984;67:639–645.

60   Poznansky MC, Gordon ACH, Grant IWB, Wyllie AH: A cellular abnormality in glucocorticoid-resistant asthma. Clin Exp Immunol 1985;61:135–142.

61   Corrigan CJ, Brown PH, Barnes NC, Szefler SJ, Tsai JJ, Frew AJ, Kay AB: Glucocorticoid resistance in chronic asthma. Glucocorticoid pharmacokinetics, glucocorticoid receptor characteristics and inhibition of peripheral blood T cell proliferation by glucocorticoids in vitro. Am Rev Respir Dis 1991;144:1016–1025.

62   Rolfe FG, Hughes JM, Armour CL, Sewell WA: Inhibition of interleukin-5 gene expression by dexamethasone. Immunology 1992;77:494–499.

63   Robinson DS, Hamid Q, Ying S, Bentley AM, Assoufi B, North J, Meng Q, Durham SR, Kay AB: Prednisolone treatment in asthma is associated with modulation of bronchoalveolar lavage cell interleukin-4, interleukin-5 and interferon-γ cytokine gene expression. Am Rev Respir Dis 1993;148:401–406.

64   Bentley AM, Hamid Q, Robinson DS, Schotman E, Meng Q, Assoufi B, Kay AB, Durham SR: Prednisolone treatment in asthma: Reduction in the numbers of eosinophils, T cells, tryptase-only positive mast cells (MCT) and modulation of interleukin-4, interleukin-5 and interferon-γ cytokine gene expression within the bronchial mucosa. Am J Respir Crit Care Med 1996;153:551–556.

65   Leung DYM, Martin RJ, Szefler SJ, Sher ER, Ying S, Kay AB, Hamid Q: Dysregulation of interleukin-4, interleukin-5 and interferon-γ gene expression in steroid-resistant asthma. J Exp Med 1995;181:33–40.

66   Kon OM, Sihra BS, Compton CH, Leonard T, Kay AB, Barnes NC: Randomised, dose-ranging, placebo-controlled study of a chimeric antibody to CD4 (keliximab) in chronic severe asthma. Lancet 1998;352:1109–1113.

67   Robinson DS, Ying S, Bentley AM, Meng Q, North J, Durham SR, Kay AB, Hamid Q: Relationships among numbers of bronchoalveolar lavage cells expressing messenger ribonucleic acid for cytokines, asthma symptoms, and airway methacholine responsiveness in atopic asthma. J Allergy Clin Immunol 1993;92:397–403.

68   Humbert M, Corrigan CJ, Kimmitt P, Till SJ, Kay AB, Durham SR: Relationship between bronchial mucosal interleukin-4 and interleukin-5 mRNA expression and disease severity in atopic asthma. Am J Respir Crit Care Med 1997;156:704–708.

69   Haselden BM, Kay AB, Larché M: IgE-independent MHC-restricted T cell peptide epitope-induced late asthmatic reactions. J Exp Med 1999;189:1885–1894.

70   Robinson DS, Damia R, Zeibecoglou K, Molet S, North J, Yamada T, Kay AB, Hamid Q: CD34 +/ IL-5Rα mRNA + cells in the bronchial mucosa in asthma: Evidence for airway eosinophil progenitors. Am J Respir Cell Mol Biol 1999;20:9–13.

71   Zeibecoglou K, Ying S, Yamada T, North J, Burman J, Bungre J, Meng Q, Kay AB, Robinson DS: Increased mature and immature CCR3 messenger RNA + eosinophils in bone marrow from atopic asthmatics compared to atopic and non-atopic control subjects. J Allergy Clin Immunol 1999;103: 99–106.

Douglas S. Robinson, MA, MD, FRCP, Senior Lecturer, Allergy and Clinical Immunology,
Imperial College School of Medicine, National Heart and Lung Institute,
Dovehouse Street, London SW3 6LY (UK)
Tel. +44 171 351 8116, Fax +44 171 376 3138, E-Mail d.s.robinson@ic.ac.uk

Robinson DS (ed): Immunological Mechanisms in Asthma and Allergic Diseases.
Chem Immunol. Basel, Karger, 2000, vol 78, pp 16–29

··························

Regulation of Th2 Cytokine Gene Transcription

Paul Lavender, David Cousins, Tak Lee

Department of Respiratory Medicine and Allergy, Kings College London, UK

Introduction

Differentiation of haematopoietic stem cells to yield the different lymphoid cell lineages is one of the better understood mammalian developmental pathways. Reverse genetics and the generation of mutant mouse strains have yielded a wealth of information on molecules playing important roles in the production of individual cell types. Once T lymphocytes are generated they may undergo further lineage determination to derive either Th1 cells, which play an important role in the cell-mediated immune response to intracellular pathogens, or Th2 cells, which are involved in humoral immunity and allergic responses. Determination of factors controlling this event has been an important goal. In this chapter we assess the influence of some of the major candidates for phenotypic determination culminating in the Th2 lineage.

The earliest stages of T-cell development take place within the thymus. Bone marrow-derived stem cells, which lack expression of both CD3/T-cell receptor (TCR) complex and CD4 and CD8 co-receptors (double negative) are stimulated to express recombinase-activating genes 1 and 2 (Rag1 and Rag2). These proteins act to rearrange the TCR loci by V(D)J recombination thereby generating T cells with ligand specificity. The TCR-β locus is the first to be rearranged, CD4 and 8 are subsequently expressed on the cell surface to yield double positive T cells. These cells then rearrange the TCR-α chain and undergo both positive and negative selection through interaction with MHC molecules on thymic epithelium to form single positive CD4+ or CD8+ cells. Expression of sterile TCR transcripts by double negative cells indicates that the cell is competent for differentiative decisions prior to expression of recombination factors. It is likely that some of the earliest differentiative events will include expression of transcription factors either involved in TCR expression or regulating chromatin structure at these loci such that they are competent for transcription. Subsequent lineage development follows the naïve T cells encountering antigen in the peripheral lymphoid organs, although generation of effector proteins and cytokines from these naïve cells usually requires a number of cycles of cell division.

Essential Transcription Factors in T-Cell Development

Gene targeting experiments have been used to analyse the role of numerous transcription factors, identified by means of reverse genetics, in establishment of the T-cell lineage. For some proteins, analysis of null mutant mice has been hindered by the fact that functional knockout results in embryonic lethality. To circumvent this, a number of strategies have been employed, amongst which is the generation of chimaeric animals in which embryonic stem (ES) cells bearing a homozygous mutation in the gene of interest (–/–), are injected into Rag (–/–) blastocysts. The contribution of the mutant ES cells to haemato-poietic lineages can then be assessed. Because of the lack of recombination capacity, Rag –/– cells cannot differentiate to become mature lymphocytes. Many of the knockout strains generated have had complex phenotypes indicating the mutated factors are not solely involved in haematopoietic differentiation. Despite this, a number of candidates have been shown to have a critical role in lineage determination [Reviewed in 1–4]. Amongst the proteins playing an essential role in T-cell generation are PU1, Ikaros and GATA3.

PU1 is an Ets family transcription factor expressed within, and essential for, the lymphoid and myeloid cell lineages in the foetus. Two PU1 disruption experiments have been carried out, both of which targeted the DNA binding domain. The first experiment resulted in embryonic lethality preventing analysis of the adult haematopoietic system [5]. In the second, the mice survive despite lack of a foetal T-cell compartment, other cell types absent were B cells, granulocytes and monocytes. T-cell precursors were detectable in the postnatal thymus after 2 or 3 days [6]. Recent data have suggested that PU1 is only necessary for terminal myeloid differentiation but not for lineage commitment.

Ikaros is a zinc finger protein which is expressed in the foetal liver and thymus. Ikaros –/– foetal mice lack T, B and NK lineages while erythroid and myeloid cells remain unaffected. As in PU1 –/– animals, T-cell precursors become detectable within the thymus of Ikaros –/– mice following birth, displaying a similar timing to T-cell generation in PU1 –/– mice [7]. Double negative thymocyte precursor numbers are, however, greatly reduced and display skewed differentiation to the CD4+ lineage. These cells undergo a rapid transition to a neoplastic state. Ikaros is involved in T-cell proliferation, inactivation of a single allele leads to lymphoproliferation, lymphoma or leukaemia associated with a shortened G1 phase of the cell cycle [8]. In mice harbouring a dominant negative mutant of Ikaros, neither B nor T cells develop postnatally, suggesting that Ikaros acts together with a second factor, whose activity is abrogated by the dominant negative Ikaros protein. In Ikaros null mice this factor may complement some of the Ikaros functions to allow the limited generation of T-cell precursors. Recently, two novel Ikaros family members, Aiolos [9] and Helios [10, 11], have been described. Aiolos appears to play similar roles to Ikaros within the B-cell lineage. Lack of Aiolos causes deregulation of B-cell maturation and proliferation and the development of B-cell lymphomas [12]. Ikaros has an important role outside transcriptional activation; Fisher and co-workers [13] have demonstrated that it plays a role in lineage restriction. In the nuclei of B cells, Ikaros is localized to centromeric heterochromatin where it complexes with transcriptionally inactive genes, such as the T-cell surface molecules CD4 and CD8.

GATA3 is a member of a zinc finger transcription factor family which to date has six members. GATAs 1–3 are involved in haematopoietic cell differentiation whilst 4–6 are involved in heart and gut differentiation. In addition to the haematopoietic system, GATA3 is expressed in the CNS, kidney, adrenal and foetal liver. Generation of GATA3 –/– ES cells and chimaeric Rag 2 –/–, GATA3 –/– mice has exposed a pivotal role in T-cell development. Lack of GATA3 causes an arrest at, or before, the earliest stages of double negative selection and an absence of GATA3 –/– cells within double negative thymocytes. Normal populations of mature B cells are present within these animals suggesting that GATA3 –/– ES cells are able to rescue the defect in B-cell development seen in Rag 2 –/– mice [14]. GATA3 +/– mice are fertile and appear normal, in contrast, GATA3 –/– mice have a complex phenotype, mutant embryos survive until days 11 and 12 postcoitum but display internal bleeding, marked growth retardation, severe deformities of the brain and spinal cord and aberrant foetal liver haematopoiesis [15]. GATA3 has been shown to be involved in transcription of the TCRα [16], β [17] and δ [18] chains, whose expression precedes CD4 and CD8 production and single positive T-cell selection. It is also involved in transcription of the CD8α chain [19].

Th1/Th2 Cell Differentiation

Naïve CD4+ T-helper cells undergo divergent differentiation pathways to generate either Th1 or Th2 cell types dependent upon the nature of the

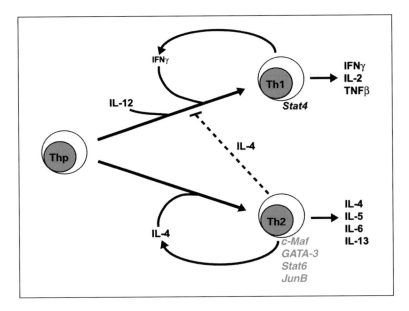

Fig. 1. Factors influencing Th1/Th2 differentiation. Cytokines are shown in black, transcription factors are shown in grey.

stimulus to which they are exposed (fig. 1). The two subtypes are classified by the pattern of cytokines that they produce [20, 21]. The cytokines generated by Th1 cells are IFN-γ and IL-2, whilst Th2 cells produce IL-4, IL-5, IL-6, IL-9, IL-10 and IL-13. Both subtypes express GM-CSF, IL-3 and TNF-α. Differentiation of Th2 cells is potentiated by IL-4, and TCR, CD4 and CD28 ligation. IL-4-mediated signals are of particular importance, when IL-4 is added to naïve T-cell cultures, a Th2 phenotype ensues. Although Th2 responses are significantly reduced in IL-4 –/– mice, the lineage is still generated, suggesting that IL-4-independent mechanisms exist for Th2 propagation [22]. The most critical effector of IL-4 is Stat6. Lymphocytes from Stat6-deficient mice fail to proliferate in the presence of IL-4 and fail to induce expression of the IL-4 receptor on the cell surface. Additionally, the Th2 lineage is not generated in the presence of either IL-4 or IL-13 [23]. Stat6 –/– mice also display defective immunoglobulin switching to IgE [24]. Th1 differentiation depends upon IL-12 and Stat4. In Th2 cells, IL-4 initiates a powerful positive feedback effect thereby potentiating its own production. Since IL-4 has been thought to be central to Th2 subtype determination, the ability to control its expression is of great clinical significance. The polarizing effects of IL-4 are enhanced due to repressive effects on other cytokines which results in inhibition of inappropriate cytokine expression. IL-4 downregulates IFN-γ expression by repressing transcription of the β subunit of the IL-12 receptor.

Numerous recent reports have suggested that IL-13 may play an important role within the Th2 lineage. IL-13 appears to act in concert with IL-4, both cytokines are expressed by Th2 cells and mast cells and are able to induce B cells to undergo isotype switching to IgE. IL-4 and IL-13 cross-compete for the IL-4 receptor α chain (IL-4Rα), although IL-13 does not bind directly, but recruits IL-4Rα into a receptor complex once it has interacted with its own primary binding chain, the IL-13 receptor α1 (IL-13Rα1) [25]. These data provide an explanation to the observation that IL-4 receptor disruption has a more severe phenotype than IL-4 knockout [26]. Both cytokines induce Stat6 expression. IL-13, rather than IL-4, has been proposed to be the central mediator of allergic asthma in mice since selective neutralization of IL-13 resulted in reversal of the pathophysiological features of the disease, airway hyperresponsiveness, eosinophil recruitment and mucus overproduction [27, 28]. IL-13 –/– mice have impaired development of Th2 cells and have significantly lower levels of IL-4 [29].

Studies in mutant mice have further identified individual roles for the two cytokines. In both IL-4 –/– and IL-13 –/– mice infected with *Schistosoma mansoni* eggs, a Th2 response is mounted with expression of IL-5 and eosinophil infiltration, as is production of IgE. In IL-4 –/–, IL-13 –/– double-deficient mice, no Th2 cell-mediated response is generated, and only very low levels of IL-5, which is a primary determinant of eosinophil differentiation, are produced. These mice also fail to produce IgE, instead there is increased production of IFN-γ and IgG2α indicative of a developing Th1 phenotype [30]. That these animals can produce IL-5, albeit at reduced levels, suggests alternative mechanisms for development of some Th2 characteristics. Despite the emerging importance of IL-13 in the Th2 phenotype, little work has been carried out on the analysis of factors required for its transcription.

A number of proteins have been postulated as controlling the differentiation of naïve T cells into the Th2 lineage. Analysis has centred on the IL-4 proximal promoter, which controls Th2-specific expression and cell proliferation. Proteins implicated in Th2-specific expression of IL-4 are GATA3, c-Maf, JunB and C/EBPβ.

GATA3

Numerous data support a role for GATA3 in Th2 specification. Zheng and Flavell [31] have demonstrated that GATA3 is expressed in both naïve and Th2 lineage cells but expression is extinguished in Th1 cells. GATA3 has been shown to have a role in transcriptional regulation of the IL-5 gene through direct interaction with sites within the proximal promoter [32, 33]. Conflicting data exists for regulation of the IL-4 promoter. Whilst Zheng and Flavell postulate an effect mediating transcription activation through the proximal 157bp of the IL-4 promoter, other groups have been unable to reproduce these data [33, 34], and there has been no demonstration of GATA3 protein binding to the IL-4 proximal promoter. It has been suggested that GATA3 might influence IL-4 transcription by acting through more distal enhancers [34]. In addition to its role in induction of the Th2 lineage, Murphy and co-workers [35] have recently suggested that GATA3 plays a role in inhibition of Th1 development which does not require IL-4. GATA3 represses IL-12 receptor β2 mRNA expression thereby preventing IL-12 signalling and consequently the positive effect of IL-12 in propagation of the Th1 lineage. High-level GATA3 expression induced by IL-4 is Stat6-dependent. Although GATA3 expression leads to augmentation of IL-4 expression in Th2 cells, re-expression of GATA3 in cells developed in Th1-inducing conditions does not lead to IL-4 expression, thus, GATA3 either functions in a time-restricted fashion and/or co-operates with other Th2-restricted factors. Moreover, it is suggested that loss of GATA3 expression in Th1 cells requires IL-12 signalling through Stat4.

c-Maf

c-Maf is a basic domain/leucine zipper family transcription factor, its involvement in IL-4 transcription was demonstrated when it was isolated from a yeast two hybrid screen for proteins that interact with NFATp. In combination with NFATp, c-Maf was shown to transcriptionally activate the IL-4 promoter [36]. Whereas the data supporting a role for GATA3 in transcriptional regulation of IL-4 in T cells is inconsistent, c-Maf has been shown to bind directly to the IL-4 promoter through a Maf response element (MARE) located in the proximal promoter [36, 37]. This region is known to be important for the Th2-specific expression of IL-4. c-Maf is expressed in numerous tissues including kidney, testis, placenta and skeletal muscle, but within the lymphoid system it is not expressed in Th1 cells and is upregulated during Th2 differentiation. Ectopic expression in B cells in conjunction with NFATp transactivates the endogenous IL-4 promoter. c-Maf, NFATp and the NFAT-interacting protein NIP45 are sufficient to activate the IL-4 promoter in HepG2 liver cells [37]. c-Maf (–/–) mice have recently been generated; Maf disruption affects both intrauterine and postnatal survival, with death occurring at E 17.5–18.5. c-Maf –/– mice also develop microphthalmia beginning approximately 2 weeks after birth [38]. Cultured spleen cells from c-Maf –/– mice produce virtually no IL-4, but other cytokines including IL-5, IL-6 and IL-10 are present, albeit at reduced levels. In contrast, IL-13 levels are normal, as are IgE levels [39]. Recent data from Brown and co-workers [40] have demonstrated that mast cells, which, along with basophils, can also generate IL-4, do not express c-Maf. It is suggested that the MARE located in the IL-4 proximal promoter is not critical for promoter function in these cells. How c-Maf plays a role in Th2 differentiation is unclear, since by the time it is upregulated following naïve T-cell activation (at day 8), differentiation has been completed for some days [36]. As disruption experiments implicate c-Maf in transcriptional activation of IL-4, it is possible that the source of IL-4 necessary to initiate Th2 lineage development from the naïve precursor is generated from a different cell type, and only subsequently is c-Maf activated to generate sufficient cytokine to cause Th2 proliferation.

JunB
A potential role for AP-1 proteins during T-helper cell differentiation was suggested by Flavell and co-workers [41], who demonstrated that a high level of AP-1 activity was induced upon stimulation of Th2 but not Th1 cells. This activity correlated with accumulation of JunB in Th2 cells but not Th1 or Th0 cells. It has been demonstrated that the P1 site within the proximal IL-4 promoter, which binds NFAT/AP1 complexes, drives Th2-restricted expression. JunB has been postulated as providing the specificity. In transgenic mice, JunB overexpression causes upregulation of IL-4, IL-5, IL-6 and IL-10, although it is unclear whether the effects on IL-5, IL-6 and IL-10 is direct or secondary to IL-4. JunB synergizes with c-Maf to activate IL-4 expression, and its activity is stimulated following phosphorylation by Jun N-terminal kinase [42].

C/EBPβ
C/EBPβ (NF-IL-6) has been shown to transcriptionally activate the IL-4 promoter [43], but its expression is not limited to Th2 cells. C/EBPβ binds to a number of sites within the IL-4 promoter, including sites within the proximal promoter where it binds weakly to an NFAT/AP1 site, and a MARE. Mutation of these sites within the IL-4 promoter abrogates transactivation in response to numerous stimuli. Krammer and co-workers [44] have additionally suggested that C/EBPβ may not be expressed in Th1 clones.

Chromatin Status and the Cytokine Locus
Human chromosome 5q contains a locus in which a number of Th2 cytokines genes are located (fig. 2), those for IL-4, IL-5 and IL-13 are in relatively close proximity, with IL-10 and nonlineage-restricted GM-CSF and IL-3 located more distally [45]. Also within this locus are KIF3A, encoding a microtubule motor and RAD50 which is involved in DNA repair. A locus at mouse chromosome 11q region appears to be similarly organized. The

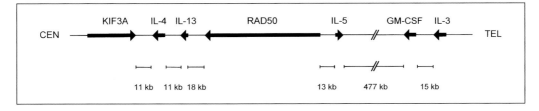

Fig. 2. Cytokine gene cluster on human chromosome 5q. Black boxes represent the gene position and size of primary transcript. Arrows indicate the direction of transcription. CEN indicates the direction of the centromere and TEL the direction of the telomere.

human 5q locus provides a useful tool to analyse potential co-ordinate regulation of cytokine expression and the chromatin boundaries that are permissive or inhibitory for gene expression. Numerous pieces of evidence suggest however, that regulation of the locus is complex.

Generation of a Th2-type phenotype is an inefficient process, and is regulated by the cell cycle. Naïve T cells differentiated in vitro require at least three cycles of cell division before they produce IL-4, however, once this status is achieved, daughter cells retain the productive capacity [46]. These data suggest that in naïve T cells the IL-4 locus is epigenetically repressed and that cell cycle progression provides an opportunity to stably alter this situation in the presence of differentiative signals. As a consequence, differentiated Th2 cells exposed to a second stimulus no longer require cell cycle progression in order to express IL-4. Two groups have demonstrated that IL-4 is expressed monoallelically, albeit not in an imprinted manner, with the probability of expression being regulated by the strength of the signal through the TCR [47, 48]. These data suggest a probabilistic mechanism in which transcription involves limiting components within the cell, which may either be induced or activated upon stimulation. This raises a number of questions related to the organization of transcription on a given allele: whether the cytokine genes are expressed from one allele and RAD50 and KIF3A from the other, and whether the cytokines are co-ordinately expressed. We have recently reported that intergenic transcription occurs around the IL-4 and IL-13 genes [49] in a similar fashion to that observed at the globin locus [50] thereby providing another possible mechanism for transcriptional regulation.

Recent data from Agarwal and Rao [51] working on the mouse 11q cytokine locus, have suggested that differentiation of naïve T cells to the Th2 lineage is accompanied by chromatin remodelling and change in methylation status. In experiments using DNase I hypersensitivity and RNase protection assays, they suggest that the IL-4 and IL-13 genes are remodelled in order to

---

generate an open chromatin structure, and in contrast, the IFN-γ gene is in a closed chromatin configuration. In Th1 cells the reverse is true, IFN-γ is in a DNase-I-sensitive configuration whilst the IL-4 gene is not. Furthermore, it was suggested that Th1 cells have a hypermethylated IL-4 locus, whilst in Th2 cells it is hypomethylated. It is suggested that the IL-4-responsive transcription factor Stat6 is essential for remodelling and also for the production of IL-4, IL-5, IL-10 and IL-13. Stat6 –/– naïve T cells differentiated to form Th2 cells, not only do not remodel the IL-4 gene, but perhaps more surprisingly, do not produce Th2-type cytokines, instead expressing IL-2 and IFN-γ in a similar manner to naïve T cells differentiated to become Th1 cells. These data imply that a factor or factors acting downstream of Stat6 acts pivotally in the establishment of a given status of chromatin conformation, and also in generation of a specific cytokine expression profile. Since it is likely that chromatin conformation is permissive or inhibitory for transcriptional activation, the most important step may be the induction of remodelling, which generates a stable chromatin context. In support of this, data from Glimcher and co-workers [36] has demonstrated that fusion of a Th1 cell with a Th2 cell does not lead to extinction of either IL-2 or IL-4. Additionally, Murphy and co-workers [35] have shown that expression of GATA3 in differentiated Th1 lymphocytes does not inhibit IFN-γ production, which is in direct contrast to the inhibition observed during the establishment of a differentiated lineage.

Factors mediating chromatin remodelling at the cytokine locus may be of critical importance in propagation of the Th2 cell. Amongst the candidates for this function is GATA3, firstly because of its central role in generation of the T-cell lineage, but also due to analogy and sequence conservation with GATA1. While there have been no reports of direct interactions between GATA3 and co-activators with inherent histone acetyltransferase (HAT) activity, GATA1 has recently been shown to interact with, and be acetylated by p300 and CBP [52, 53]; this acetylation stimulates GATA1-dependent transcription. Additionally, in *Aspergillus nidulans*, the GATA factor AreA has been shown to be essential for chromatin remodelling [54]. GATA1 has been shown to interact with the Friend of GATA (FOG) family of co-activators [55–57]. Data arguing against GATA3 mediating chromatin remodelling in the generation of Th2 cells, is the fact that it is present in naive Th0 cells, in which the IL-4 locus is not in a DNase-I-sensitive configuration. Th0 cells, however, express TCRs on the cell surface, and it is known that TCR-α, -β and -δ promoters are transcriptionally activated by GATA3. The data in favour of c-Maf playing a role in remodelling is much weaker since it is expressed after induction of the Th2 lineage. However, c-Maf in conjunction with NFAT and NIP45 is sufficient to permit expression of IL-4 from the endogenous locus in B cells, where GATA and other T-cell-restricted proteins are absent. Ectopic expression presumably also causes remodelling at this locus. NFATc has recently been shown to recruit the co-activator and HAT, CBP [58]. In contrast to c-Maf, JunB is an immediate early gene, which also has been shown to be able to recruit CBP/p300 to promoters [59]. JunB is widely expressed and it is not clear how ubiquitous factors might be able to mediate cell-type-specific gene expression unless as part of a complex requisite of lineage-restricted components.

Co-Ordinate Gene Regulation

Using single cell analysis by RT-PCR, Kelso et al. [60] have suggested that in a mixed cell population polarized to either a Th1 or Th2 phenotype, few, if any, cells displayed a cytokine expression profile fitting the Th1/Th2 paradigm. Many expressed none of the characteristic cytokines. This indicates that polarization at a population level can mask intercellular heterogeneity. Significant numbers of cells express mRNAs from both categories, e.g. IFN-γ and IL-4, although it appears that further polarization continues with repeated exposure to a stimulus. These data question whether co-ordinate regulation of the 5q cytokines takes place, since in only 12% of cells differentiated to form the Th2 lineage was IL-4 and IL-5 mRNA detected in the same cell. Since the analysis is limited by the fact that only a single time point can be assayed per cell, the capacity of that cell to express a different cytokine repertoire at a different time has not been assessed.

Summary and Conclusions

Because of the different functions of IL-4, IL-13 and IL-5, it would perhaps be surprising if common transcriptional mechanisms occur. However, because of the physical proximity of their genes within the human 5q locus, chromatin remodelling during T-cell differentiation may make transcription of all the genes permissible. If co-ordinate regulation were to take place, it might be argued that similar factors might be involved in expression of all of the cytokines. Emerging data on c-Maf and GATA3 regulation of IL-4 and IL-5 respectively argues that diverse proteins may be required for transcriptional activation. Alternatively, these factors may be responsible for regulating transcriptional competence, allowing fine control over generation of particular cytokines depending upon recognition of physiological cues. If competent for transcription, common factors, such as members of the NFAT and/or AP-1 families, may operate to regulate cytokine levels. To support this, we have recently identified a conserved palindrome located within the promoters of the different Th2-type cytokines, which acts as an enhancer of transcription [61]. Central to the capacity to express Th2 cytokines is likely to be the ability to remodel chromatin at the locus. It remains to be determined whether a single factor, or combination of factors acts to regulate this event. It is also unclear what the boundaries of remodelling within the locus are, i.e. whether IL-4 and IL-13 may be within open chromatin and IL-5 in a closed environment, and whether there is a hierarchy which determines whether particular cytokines are preferentially expressed irrespective of competence.

References

1   Clevers HC, Grosschedl R: Transcriptional control of lymphoid development: Lessons from gene targeting. Immunol Today 1996;17:336–343.
2   Georgopoulos K: Transcription factors required for lymphoid lineage commitment. Curr Opin Immunol 1997;9:222–227.
3   Glimcher LH, Singh H: Transcription factors in lymphocyte development – T and B cells get together. Cell 1999;96:13–23.
4   Kuo CT, Leiden JM: Transcriptional regulation of T lymphocyte development and function. Annu Rev Immunol 1999;17:149–187.
5   Scott EW, Simon MC, Anastasi J, Singh H: Requirement of transcription factor PU.1 in the development of multiple hematopoietic lineages. Science 1994;265:1573–1577.
6   McKercher SR, Torbett BE, Anderson KL, Henkel GW, Vestal DJ, Baribault H, Klemsz M, Feeney AJ, Wu GE, Paige CJ, Maki RA: Targeted disruption of the PU.1 gene results in multiple hematopoietic abnormalities. EMBO J 1996;15:5647–5658.
7   Wang JH, Nichogiannopoulou A, Wu L, Sun L, Sharpe AH, Bigby M, Georgopoulos K: Selective defects in the development of the fetal and adult lymphoid system in mice with an Ikaros null mutation. Immunity 1996;5:537–549.
8   Winandy S, Wu P, Georgopoulos K: A dominant mutation in the Ikaros gene leads to rapid development of leukemia and lymphoma. Cell 1995;83:289–299.
9   Morgan B, Sun L, Avitahl N, Andrikopoulos K, Ikeda T, Gonzales E, Wu P, Neben S, Georgopoulos K: Aiolos, a lymphoid-restricted transcription factor that interacts with Ikaros to regulate lymphocyte differentiation. EMBO J 1997;16:2004–2013.
10 Hahm K, Cobb BS, McCarty AS, Brown KE, Klug CA, Lee R, Akashi K, Weissman IL, Fisher AG, Smale ST: Helios, a T-cell-restricted Ikaros family member that quantitatively associates with Ikaros at centromeric heterochromatin. Genes Dev 1998;12:782–796.
11 Kelley CM, Ikeda T, Koipally J, Avitahl N, Wu L, Georgopoulos K, Morgan BA: Helios, a novel dimerization partner of Ikaros expressed in the earliest hematopoietic progenitors. Curr Biol 1998; 8:508–515.
12 Wang JH, Avitahl N, Cariappa A, Friedrich C, Ikeda T, Renold A, Andrikopoulos K, Liang L, Pillai S, Morgan BA, Georgopoulos K: Aiolos regulates B cell activation and maturation to effector state. Immunity 1998;9:543–553.
13 Brown KE, Guest SS, Smale ST, Hahm K, Merkenschlager M, Fisher AG: Association of transcriptionally silent genes with Ikaros complexes at centromeric heterochromatin. Cell 1997;91:845–854.
14 Ting CN, Olson MC, Barton KP, Leiden JM: Transcription factor GATA-3 is required for development of the T-cell lineage. Nature 1996;384:474–478.
15 Pandolfi PP, Roth ME, Karis A, Leonard MW, Dzierzak E, Grosveld FG, Engel JD, Lindenbaum MH: Targeted disruption of the GATA3 gene causes severe abnormalities in the nervous system and in fetal liver haematopoiesis. Nat Genet 1995;11:40–44.

16 Ho IC, Vorhees P, Marin N, Oakley BK, Tsai SF, Orkin SH, Leiden JM: Human GATA-3: A lineage-restricted transcription factor that regulates the expression of the T cell receptor alpha gene. EMBO J 1991;10:1187–1192.

17 Marine J, Winoto A: The human enhancer-binding protein GATA3 binds to several T-cell receptor regulatory elements. Proc Natl Acad Sci USA 1991;88:7284–7288.

18 Ko LJ, Yamamoto M, Leonard MW, George KM, Ting P, Engel JD: Murine and human T-lymphocyte GATA-3 factors mediate transcription through a *cis*-regulatory element within the human T-cell receptor delta gene enhancer. Mol Cell Biol 1991;11:2778–2784.

19 Hambor JE, Mennone J, Coon ME, Hanke JH, Kavathas P: Identification and characterization of an Alu-containing, T-cell-specific enhancer located in the last intron of the human CD8 alpha gene. Mol Cell Biol 1993;13:7056–7070.

20 Abbas AK., Murphy KM, Sher A: Functional diversity of helper T lymphocytes. Nature 1996;383: 787–793.

21 Fitch FW, McKisic MD, Lancki DW, Gajewski TF: Differential regulation of murine T lymphocyte subsets. Annu Rev Immunol 1993;11:29–48.

22 Kopf M, Le Gros G, Bachmann M, Lamers MC, Bluethmann H, Kohler G: Disruption of the murine IL-4 gene blocks Th2 cytokine responses. Nature 1993;362:245–248.

23 Kaplan MH, Schindler U, Smiley ST, Grusby MJ: Stat6 is required for mediating responses to IL-4 and for development of Th2 cells. Immunity 1996;4:313–319.

24 Shimoda K, van Deursen J, Sangster MY, Sarawar SR, Carson RT, Tripp RA, Chu C, Quelle FW, Nosaka T, Vignali DA, Doherty PC, Grosveld G, Paul WE, Ihle JN: Lack of IL-4-induced Th2 response and IgE class switching in mice with disrupted Stat6 gene. Nature 1996;380:630–633.

25 Hilton DJ, Zhang JG, Metcalf D, Alexander WS, Nicola NA, Willson TA: Cloning and characterization of a binding subunit of the interleukin-13 receptor that is also a component of the interleukin-4 receptor. Proc Natl Acad Sci USA 1996;93:497–501.

26 Barner M, Mohrs M, Brombacher F, Kopf M: Differences between IL-4R alpha-deficient and IL-4-deficient mice reveal a role for IL-13 in the regulation of Th2 responses. Curr Biol 1998;8: 669–672.

27 Wills-Karp M, Luyimbazi J, Xu X, Schofield B, Neben TY, Karp CL, Donaldson DD: Interleukin-13: Central mediator of allergic asthma. Science 1998;282:2258–2261.

28 Grunig G, Warnock M, Wakil AE, Venkayya R, Brombacher F, Rennick DM, Sheppard D, Mohrs M, Donaldson DD, Locksley RM, Corry DB: Requirement for IL-13 independently of IL-4 in experimental asthma. Science 1998;282:2261–2263.

29 McKenzie GJ, Emson CL, Bell SE, Anderson S, Fallon P, Zurawski G, Murray R, Grencis R, McKenzie AN: Impaired development of Th2 cells in IL-13-deficient mice. Immunity 1998;9:423–432.

30 McKenzie GJ, Fallon PG, Emson CL, Grencis RK, McKenzie AN: Simultaneous disruption of interleukin (IL)-4 and IL-13 defines individual roles in T helper cell type 2-mediated responses. J Exp Med 1999;189:1565–1572.

31 Zheng W, Flavell RA: The transcription factor GATA-3 is necessary and sufficient for Th2 cytokine gene expression in CD4 T cells. Cell 1997;89:587–596.

32 Zhang DH, Cohn L, Ray P, Bottomly K, Ray A: Transcription factor GATA-3 is differentially expressed in murine Th1 and Th2 cells and controls Th2-specific expression of the interleukin-5 gene. J Biol Chem 1997;272:21597–21603.

33 Zhang DH, Yang L, Ray A: Differential responsiveness of the IL-5 and IL-4 genes to transcription factor GATA-3. J Immunol 1998;161:3817–3821.

34 Ranganath S, Ouyang W, Bhattarcharya D, Sha WC, Grupe A, Peltz G, Murphy KM: GATA-3-dependent enhancer activity in IL-4 gene regulation. J Immunol 1998;161:3822–3826.

35 Ouyang W, Ranganath SH, Weindel K, Bhattacharya D, Murphy TL, Sha WC, Murphy KM: Inhibition of Th1 development mediated by GATA-3 through an IL-4-independent mechanism. Immunity 1998;9:745–755.

36 Ho IC, Hodge MR, Rooney JW, Glimcher LH: The proto-oncogene c-maf is responsible for tissue-specific expression of interleukin-4. Cell 1996;85:973–983.

37   Hodge MR, Chun HJ, Rengarajan J, Alt A, Lieberson R, Glimcher LH: NF-AT-driven interleukin-4 transcription potentiated by NIP45. Science 1996;274:1903–1905.

38   Kim JI, Li T, Ho IC, Grusby MJ, Glimcher LH: Requirement for the c-Maf transcription factor in crystallin gene regulation and lens development. Proc Natl Acad Sci USA 1999;96:3781–3785.

39   Kim JI, Ho IC, Grusby MJ, Glimcher LH: The transcription factor c-Maf controls the production of interleukin-4 but not other Th2 cytokines. Immunity 1999;10:745–751.

40   Sherman MA, Nachman TY, Brown MA: IL-4 production by mast cells does not require c-maf. J Immunol 1999;163:1733–1736.

41   Rincon M, Derijard B, Chow CW, Davis RJ, Flavell RA: Reprogramming the signalling requirement for AP-1 (activator protein-1) activation during differentiation of precursor CD4 + T-cells into effector Th1 and Th2 cells. Genes Funct 1997;1:51–68.

42   Li B, Tournier C, Davis RJ, Flavell RA: Regulation of IL-4 expression by the transcription factor JunB during T helper cell differentiation. EMBO J 1999;18:420–432.

43   Li-Weber M, Salgame P, Hu C, Davydov IV, Krammer PH: Differential interaction of nuclear factors with the PRE-I enhancer element of the human IL-4 promoter in different T cell subsets. J Immunol 1997;158:1194–1200.

44   Davydov IV, Krammer PH, Li-Weber M: Nuclear factor-IL-6 activates the human IL-4 promoter in T cells. J Immunol 1995;155:5273–5279.

45   Frazer KA, Ueda Y, Zhu Y, Gifford VR, Garofalo MR, Mohandas N, Martin CH, Palazzolo MJ, Cheng JF, Rubin EM: Computational and biological analysis of 680 kb of DNA sequence from the human 5q31 cytokine gene cluster region. Genome Res 1997;7:495–512.

46   Bird JJ, Brown DR, Mullen AC, Moskowitz NH, Mahowald MA, Sider JR, Gajewski TF, Wang CR, Reiner SL: Helper T cell differentiation is controlled by the cell cycle. Immunity 1998;9:229–237.

47   Riviere I, Sunshine MJ, Littman DR: Regulation of IL-4 expression by activation of individual alleles. Immunity 1998;9:217–228.

48   Bix M, Locksley RM: Independent and epigenetic regulation of the interleukin-4 alleles in CD4 + T cells. Science 1998;281:1352–1354.

49   Rogan DF, Cousins DJ, Staynov DZ: Intergenic transcription occurs throughout the human IL-4/IL-13 gene cluster. Biochem Biophys Res Commun 1999;255:556–561.

50   Ashe HL, Monks J, Wijgerde M, Fraser P, Proudfoot NJ: Intergenic transcription and transinduction of the human beta-globin locus. Genes Dev 1997;11:2494–2509.

51   Agarwal S, Rao A: Modulation of chromatin structure regulates cytokine gene expression during T cell differentiation. Immunity 1998;9:765–775.

52   Boyes J, Byfield P, Nakatani Y, Ogryzko V: Regulation of activity of the transcription factor GATA-1 by acetylation. Nature 1998;396:594–598.

53   Blobel GA, Nakajima T, Eckner R, Montminy M, Orkin SH: CREB-binding protein cooperates with transcription factor GATA-1 and is required for erythroid differentiation. Proc Natl Acad Sci USA 1998;95:2061–2066.

54   Muro-Pastor MI, Gonzalez R, Strauss J, Narendja F, Scazzocchio C: The GATA factor AreA is essential for chromatin remodelling in a eukaryotic bidirectional promoter. EMBO J 1999;18: 1584–1597.

55   Tsang AP, Visvader JE, Turner CA, Fujiwara Y, Yu C, Weiss MJ, Crossley M, Orkin SH: FOG, a multitype zinc finger protein, acts as a cofactor for transcription factor GATA-1 in erythroid and megakaryocytic differentiation. Cell 1997;90:109–119.

56   Tevosian SG, Deconinck AE, Cantor AB, Rieff HI, Fujiwara Y, Corfas G, Orkin SH: FOG-2: A novel GATA-family cofactor related to multitype zinc-finger proteins Friend of GATA-1 and U-shaped. Proc Natl Acad Sci USA 1999;96:950–955.

57   Svensson EC, Tufts RL, Polk CE, Leiden JM: Molecular cloning of FOG-2: A modulator of transcription factor GATA-4 in cardiomyocytes. Proc Natl Acad Sci USA 1999;96:956–961.

58   Avots A, Buttmann M, Chuvpilo S, Escher C, Smola U, Bannister AJ, Rapp UR, Kouzarides T, Serfling E: CBP/p300 integrates Raf/Rac-signaling pathways in the transcriptional induction of NF-ATc during T cell activation. Immunity 1999;10:515–524.

59   Lee JS, See RH, Deng T, Shi Y: Adenovirus E1A downregulates cJun- and JunB-mediated transcription by targeting their coactivator p300. Mol Cell Biol 1996;16:4312–4326.

60   Kelso A, Groves P, Ramm L, Doyle AG: Single-cell analysis by RT-PCR reveals differential expression of multiple type 1 and 2 cytokine genes among cells within polarized CD4+ T cell populations. Int Immunol 1999;11:617–621.

61   Staynov DZ, Cousins DJ, Lee TH: A regulatory element in the promoter of the human granulocyte-macrophage colony-stimulating factor gene that has related sequences in other T-cell-expressed cytokine genes. Proc Natl Acad Sci USA 1995;92:3606–3610.

Dr. Paul Lavender, Department of Respiratory Medicine and Allergy,
5th Floor Thomas Guy House, Kings College London, Guy's Campus,
London SE1 9RT (UK)
Tel. +44 20 7955 5000/ext3697, Fax +44 20 7403 8640, E-Mail paul.lavender@kcl.ac.uk

Robinson DS (ed): Immunological Mechanisms in Asthma and Allergic Diseases.
Chem Immunol. Basel, Karger, 2000, vol 78, pp 30–38

....

MHC-Restricted, IgE-Independent, Allergen Peptide-Induced Late Asthmatic Reactions

Mark Larché

Allergy and Clinical Immunology, Imperial College School of Medicine,
National Heart and Lung Institute, London, UK

Introduction

In recent decades the prevalence of allergic diseases has risen markedly, particularly in developed countries. Many factors have been implicated in the observed increase including more sedentary lifestyles, increased use of antibiotics, vaccination against infectious diseases, poor ventilation, increased use of carpets in the home, increased levels of pollution and genetic susceptibility. Whilst multiple genetic factors are likely to play a role in disease susceptibility, the absence of substantial changes in the human genome during this period make it unlikely that genetic polymorphisms alone are responsible. Analysis of each of these parameters has led to the conclusion that interactions between both genetic and environmental elements are most likely to account for the recent changes in disease prevalence.

To investigate the mechanisms underlying allergic inflammation, many investigators have employed allergen challenge, under controlled consitions, in both the skin (by intradermal injection) and the lung (by inhalation), followed by sampling of the target organ. Allergen inhalation challenge of allergic asthmatic subjects results in a bimodal reduction in airway calibre. The early asthmatic reaction (EAR) is rapid (peaking at approximately 15 min) and dependent upon IgE-mediated release of mast-cell-derived mediators such as histamine and leukotrienes [1–3]. Degranulation of mast cells occurs following the cross-linking of allergen-specific IgE molecules bound to the surface of mast cells via IgE receptors. In contrast, the late asthmatic reaction (LAR) is characterized by a progressive reduction in lung function which begins 2–4 h after challenge, reaches a plateau at 6–9 h and has generally resolved by 24 h. The associated decrease in airway function appears to represent the influence of a number of processes occurring within the airways and associated mucosal tissue. These include cellular infiltration and resultant inflammation, in addition to oedema resulting from vascular leakage following smooth muscle contraction. The LAR is characterized by infiltration of the mucosa with activated eosinophils and CD4+/CD25+ T cells. Analysis of infiltrating cells by in situ hybridization has demonstrated increased numbers of cells expressing mRNA for the Th2-type (interleukin (IL)-4 and IL-5) and eosinophil-active cytokines (IL-3, IL-5 and GM-CSF) [4, 5]. Expression of the eosinophil chemoattractant cytokine (chemokine) eotaxin has also been shown to be elevated in mucosal biopsies from baseline asthma [6].

The role of the various cell types and the inflammatory mediators which they produce in the initiation and maintenance of the LAR is only partially elucidated and is likely to involve multiple mechanisms occurring simultaneously. For example, treatment of allergic asthmatic individuals with a monoclonal antibody to IgE has been shown to reduce the magnitude of both the EAR and LAR following allergen challenge [7]. These results suggest that IgE plays a role not only in the EAR, but also in the LAR, perhaps constituting one of the components of the allergen-induced late reaction. The role of IgE in the LAR is currently unclear but the effect of the anti-IgE therapy may result from blockade of IgE-mediated allergen focusing by dendritic cells and other antigen presenting cells (APC), thereby reducing the magnitude of T-cell activation. A perennial problem in studying the LAR is the potential for persistent effects of components (both cellular and soluble) of the EAR. Leukotriene antagonists [8] have also been shown to reduce the magnitude of both the EAR and the LAR. Identification of the cellular source(s) of leukotrienes present during the reaction is difficult, although eosinophils would be prominent figures in any debate. Corticosteroids are effective in asthma through multiple modes of action. For example, corticosteroids inhibit CD4 T-cell activation and production of IL-4 and IL-5 in the airway. Furthermore, the clinical efficacy of cyclosporin A in severe steroid-dependent asthma has also been demonstrated [9] and a single infusion of monoclonal antibodies to CD4 improved lung function in chronic corticosteroid-dependent asthmatics [10]. Thus, a pivotal role for allergen-specific CD4+ Th2-type T cells in baseline asthma and in allergen-induced LAR has been established.

Activation of CD4+ T cells is dependent upon presentation of peptide fragments of processed antigen to specific T-cell receptors (TcR) by MHC class II on APC [11]. Productive T-cell responses also require co-stimulation through such pathways as CD28–CD80/CD86 [12, 13]. TcR engagement with a specific peptide-MHC complex in the absence of co-stimulation has been shown to result in a failure to respond to re-challenge [14, 15]. Recently, attention has focused on functional inactivation of T-cell responses leading to antigen-specific hyporesponsiveness or 'tolerance'. A number of different phenomena may give rise to demonstrable peripheral T-cell tolerance including deletion, inhibition of migration, active suppression and the induction of 'anergy'. In murine models, injection of peptides has been employed to induce T-cell anergy or nonresponsiveness, through as yet unexplained mechanisms [16, 17]. Additionally, there is good evidence for peptide-induced nonresponsiveness of human CD4 cells in vitro [18, 19].

Recently, Norman et al. [20] and Simons et al. [21] attempted to induce antigen-specific T-cell hyporesponsiveness in cat-allergic individuals by subcutaneous injection of two 27 amino acid peptides (termed IPC1 and IPC2). The relatively large size of the peptides may have been partly responsible for immediate-type (presumed IgE-mediated) hypersensitivity reactions observed in some patients [20]. Although the peptides gave limited protection against natural exposure to cats, large doses (4×750 µg) were required to achieve a significant clinical effect [20]. In a related study, Pène et al. [22] demonstrated the protective effect of peptide treatment on airway responses to whole allergen challenge. Similarly, modest efficacy was also reported in preliminary data from a study evaluating the clinical response of allergic individuals to peptides derived from ragweed [23]. More recently, Muller et al. [24] have, in an open study, demonstrated clinical efficacy in a small group of bee venom-sensitized patients treated with three peptides derived from the sequence of phospholipase A$_2$.

In addition to reactions within the first hour of treatment, Norman et al. [20] also observed asthma-like symptoms commencing several hours after administration of IPC1/IPC2. Although these reactions were not documented with objective measurement of lung function, they were manifest by shortness of breath and wheeze. In this sense, they were reminiscent of isolated late asthmatic reactions. We hypothesized that these reactions were the result of direct, MHC-restricted activation of allergen-specific T cells. To determine whether T-cell peptides could induce isolated, IgE-independent LAR, we designed and produced three short Fel d 1 chain 1-derived peptides (FC1P;16/17 residues, fig. 1), based upon our own studies of T-cell proliferative responses of cat-allergic individuals in vitro. Peptides were administered to cat-allergic asthmatic subjects by intradermal injection (80µg of each of the three peptides). Furthermore, by repeated administration of peptides, we tested the hypothesis that specific hyporesponsiveness could be induced. A second injection of the same dose of FC1P was administered after a few weeks of the initial exposure or after a period of greater than 1 year.

```
EICPAVKRDVDLFLTGTPDEYVEQVAQYKALPVVLENARILKNCVDAKMTEEDKENALSLLDKIYTSPLC


LFLTGTPDEYVEQVAQY


EQVAQYKALPVVLENA


KALPVVLENARILKNCV
```

Fig. 1. Sequence of FC1P. Peptides of 16/17 amino acids were synthesized by Fmoc chemistry and purified by HPLC prior to sequencing and endotoxin analysis.

Results and Discussion

Each of the three FC1P peptides was capable of inducing proliferative responses in peripheral blood mononuclear cells (PBMC) from a proportion of cat-allergic individuals. Histamine release assays were used to determine that FC1P peptides were unable to release histamine from basophil-enriched preparations of PBMC [25]. Following intradermal injection of FC1P, 9 out of 40 cat-allergic asthmatic subjects experienced a fall in FEV_1 which started at 3–4 h and reached a plateau by 6 h (fig. 2) [25]. No immediate lung reactions were observed. We hypothesized that these responses represented isolated Th2 cell-dependent LARs. Recognition of antigenic peptides by T cells requires that the peptide be presented to the T cell in the context of an approriate MHC molecule or 'restriction element'. Since not all individuals developed a response, the HLA-DRB1 haplotype of all subjects was determined. Allergen-specific T-cell lines derived from the study subjects prior to peptide injection were used together with fibroblast cell lines (FCL) transfected with appropriate HLA-DR alleles to determine that peptide FC1P3 bound to and could be presented to T cells by both DR1 (HLA-DRB1*0101) and DR13 (HLA-DRB1*1301 and HLA-DRB1*1302) [25] leading to proliferation and secretion of IL-5 (fig. 3). Additionally peptide FC1P2 was presented by DR4 (HLA-DRB1*0405) to T cells derived from both an autologous (HLA-DRB1*0405) subject and to an individual expressing the closely related microvariant HLA-DRB1*0408. Thus, FC1P-mediated induction of LAR could be accounted for by virtue of the 9 individuals who developed reactions expressing a DR1, DR4 or DR13 allele. These findings support the hypothesis that direct, MHC-restricted activation of Th2 lymphocytes by allergen-derived peptides leads to the development of the LAR.

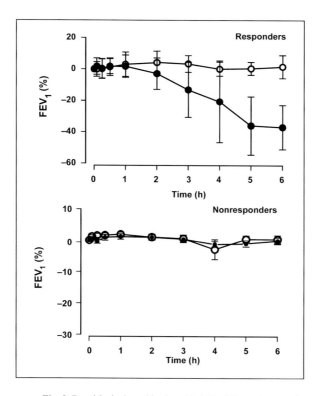

Fig. 2. Peptide-induced isolated LARs. Mean changes in FEV_1 (%) following intradermal injection of FC1P (●) and during a control day (○) of 9 responders and 31 nonresponders. Arrows indicate therapy with inhaled bronchodilator and inhaled corticosteroids. Error bars denote SEM.

Recognition of two peptides in the context of more than one MHC molecule suggests that the peptides described are capable of binding to multiple allelic products (promiscuous binding). The latter observation may be significant as it has been suggested that the use of peptides for disease-modulating immunotherapy in humans may be impractical due to the variability in MHC haplotypes. However, our findings suggest that individual peptides are capable not only of binding to more than one MHC molecule, but that there is a degree of degeneracy in TcR recognition, since a TcR from an HLA-DRB1*0408 individual recognized FC1P2 when presented in the context of HLA-DRB1*0405. Thus, a relatively small number of carefully selected peptides from an allergen may be effective in the treatment of allergic disease.

During the course of these investigations, 3 subjects displaying an isolated LAR were given a further injection of the same dose of peptide and this was

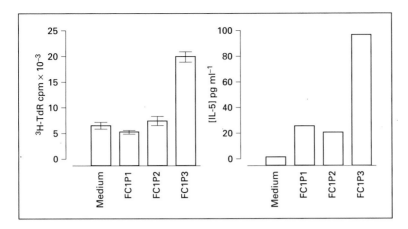

Fig. 3. Restriction of T-cell responses to FC1P3 in the context of DRB1*0101. Proliferation and IL-5 production by a cat allergen extract-specific T-cell line from a cat-allergic asthmatic subject expressing DRB1*0101, cultured with an FCL transfected with DRB1*0101 in the presence of medium alone and peptides FC1P1, 2, 3. Presentation of FC1P3 by DRB1*0101 resulted in proliferation and IL-5 production.

followed by an attenuated or absent response [25]. This observation suggests that T-cell hyporesponsiveness had been induced by the initial injection and that when peptide was re-injected, peptide-specific T cells were already functionally inactive. However, a further peptide injection was administered to three study subjects more than 1 year after the first. In this case, LARs of similar magnitude to the initial response were observed [25]. We concluded that peptide-induced hyporesponsiveness followed the induction of LAR and lasted for more than several weeks, but less than 1 year. More recent studies have suggested that a single peptide injection may confer hyporesponsiveness for a period of several months.

The cellular mechanisms which underlie peptide-induced, MHC-restricted reactions and subsequent hyporesponsiveness described here remain to be elucidated. Several hypothetical mechanisms may be responsible for the observations including the deletion of peptide-specific T cells following activation (activation-induced cell death), the induction of anergy or 'transient tolerance' or a switch in the T-cell cytokine phenotype from Th2 to Th1. Recently, attention has focused on T cells that regulate the immune response. A number of regulatory T-cell populations has been described in animal studies [26–29]. The mechanisms by which these cells modulate Th1 or Th2 responses require further clarification, but cytokines such as IL-10 and TGF-β are likely to be important factors. Future studies will address the mechanisms of both the induction of isolated LAR with allergen-derived peptides and the induction of antigen-specific nonresponsiveness.

Conclusions

Intradermal administration of short overlapping peptides derived from chain 1 of the cat allergen FC1P, which did not cross-link IgE, elicited isolated LARs with no visible early or late response in 9 out of 40 cat-allergic asthmatics. LARs were MHC-restricted. Four of the 9 were HLA-DR13+ as compared with only 1 of 31 nonreactors. The other 5 reactors expressed either DR1 or DR4. To confirm MHC restriction, FCLs transfected with HLA-DR molecules were used to present FC1P peptides to cat allergen-specific T-cell lines derived from subjects prior to peptide injection. FC1P3 was recognized in the context of DRB1*1301/1302 and induced specific T-cell activation. T cells from a DR1+ responder proliferated and produced IL-5 in the presence of FC1P3 and DRB1*0101 FCLs, whereas T cells from a DR4+ subject recognized FC1P2 when presented by DRB1*0405. Thus, short allergen-derived peptides can directly initiate an MHC-restricted, T cell-dependent LAR, without the requirement for an early IgE/mast cell-dependent response, in sensitized asthmatic subjects. Furthermore, re-administration of peptide was accompanied by a markedly reduced or abrogated lung response suggesting that T-cell hyporesponsiveness was induced following the initial LAR.

The ability to directly activate specific T cells using peptides will provide a clinical model in which to investigate the precise role of the T cell in late-phase allergic inflammation. It allows the confounding influence of the early-phase reaction to be removed, and in so doing, allows the identification of the components of the late-phase reaction which are dependent upon a preceding early-phase reaction and those which are not. The ability to dissect the cellular mechanisms of the complex events which give rise to allergic reactions, and lead to chronic allergic inflammation, will lead to a better understanding of how therapeutic approaches may be designed in order to improve clinical outcome measures.

Acknowledgments

The following colleagues and collaborators are sincerely thanked for their contributions to this work: Dr. Brigitte Marie Haselden, Prof. A.B. Kay, Dr. Meinir Jones, Prof. Robert Lechler, Dr. Giovanna Lombardi, Prof. Jonathan Lamb, Dr. Carolyn Katovich-Hurley, Dr. John Richert, Dr. Amanda Bennett and Prof. Martin Church. ALK-Abelló, Copenhagen, Denmark are acknowledged for the generous gift of cat dander extract. This work was supported by the National Asthma Campaign and the Medical Research Council.

References

1   Metzger WJ, Zavala D, Richerson HB, Moseley P, Iwamota P, Monick M, Sjoerdsma K, Hunninghake GW: Local allergen challenge and bronchoalveolar lavage of allergic asthmatic lungs. Description of the model and local airway inflammation. Am Rev Respir Dis 1987;135:433–440.

2   Sedgwick JB, Calhoun WJ, Gleich GJ, Kita H, Abrams JS, Schwartz LB, Volovitz B, Ben-Yaakov M, Busse WW: Immediate and late airway response of allergic rhinitis patients to segmental antigen challenge. Characterization of eosinophil and mast cell mediators. Am Rev Respir Dis 1991;144: 1274–1281.

3   Liu MC, Hubbard WC, Proud D, Stealey BA, Galli SJ, Kagey-Sobotka A, Bleecker ER, Lichtenstein LM: Immediate and late inflammatory responses to ragweed antigen challenge of the peripheral airways in allergic asthmatics. Cellular, mediator, and permeability changes. Am Rev Respir Dis 1991;144:51–58.

4   Bentley AM, Meng Q, Robinson DS, Hamid Q, Kay AB, Durham SR: Increases in activated T lymphocytes, eosinophils, and cytokine mRNA expression for interleukin-5 and granulocyte/macrophage colony-stimulating factor in bronchial biopsies after allergen inhalation challenge in atopic asthmatics. Am J Respir Cell Mol Biol 1993;8:35–42.

5   Ying S, Humbert M, Barkans J, Corrigan CJ, Pfister R, Menz G, Robinson DS, Larché M, Durham SR, Kay AB: Expression of IL-4 and IL-5 mRNA and protein product by CD4 + and CD8 + T cells, eosinophils, and mast cells in bronchial biopsies obtained from atopic and nonatopic (intrinsic) asthmatics. J Immunol 1997;158:3539–3544.

6   Ying S, Robinson DS, Meng Q, Rottman J, Kennedy R, Ringler DJ, Mackay CR, Daugherty BL, Springer MS, Durham SR, Williams TJ, Kay AB: Enhanced expression of eotaxin and CCR3 mRNA and protein in atopic asthma. Association with airway hyperresponsiveness and predominant co-localization of eotaxin mRNA to bronchial epithelial and endothelial cells. Eur J Immunol 1997; 27:3507–3516.

7   Fahy JV, Fleming HE, Wong HH, Liu JT, Su JQ, Reimann J, Fick RB Jr, Boushey HA: The effect of an anti-IgE monoclonal antibody on the early- and late-phase responses to allergen inhalation in asthmatic subjects. Am J Respir Crit Care Med 1997;155:1828–1834.

8   Hendeles L, Davison D, Harman E, Sherman JM: The effect of Cys LT1 receptor blockade on airway responses to allergen. Pharmacotherapy 1999;19:1243–1251.

9   Alexander AG, Barnes NC, Kay AB. Trial of cyclosporin A in corticosteroid-dependent chronic severe asthma. Lancet 1992;339:324–328.

10 Kon OM, Sihra BS, Compton CH, et al: Randomised, dose-ranging, placebo-controlled study of chimeric antibody to CD4 (keliximab) in chronic severe asthma. Lancet 1998;352:1109–1113.

11 Jorgensen JL, Reay PA, Ehrich EW, Davis MM: Molecular components of T-cell recognition. Annu Rev Immunol 1992;10:835–873.

12 Schwartz RH: Costimulation of T lymphocytes: The role of CD28, CTLA-4, and B7/BB1 in interleukin-2 production and immunotherapy. Cell 1992;71:1065–1068.

13 Larché M, Till SJ, Haselden BM, North J, Barkans J, Kay AB, Robinson DS: Co-stimulation through CD86 is involved in airway presenting cell and T cell responses to allergen in atopic asthmatics. J Immunol 1998;161:6375–6382.

14 Schwartz RH: T cell clonal anergy. Curr Opin Immunol 1997;9:351–357.

15 Lamb JR, Skidmore BJ, Green N, Chiller JM, Feldmann M: Induction of tolerance in influenza virus-immune T lymphocyte clones with synthetic peptides of influenza hemagglutinin. J Exp Med 1983;157:1434–1447.

16 Briner TJ, Kuo MC, Keating KM, Rogers BL, Greenstein JL: Peripheral T-cell tolerance induced in naive and primed mice by subcutaneous injection of peptides from the major cat allergen Fel d1. Proc Natl Acad Sci USA 1993;90:7608–7612.

17 Hoyne GF, O'Hehir RE, Wraith DC, Thomas WR, Lamb JR: Inhibition of T cell and antibody responses to house dust mite allergen by inhalation of the dominant T cell epitope in naive and sensitized mice. J Exp Med 1993;178:1783–1788.

18 O'Hehir RE, Garman RD, Greenstein JL, Lamb JR: The specificity and regulation of T-cell responsiveness to allergens. Annu Rev Immunol 1991;9:67–95.

19   Higgins JA, Lamb JR, Marsh SG, Tonks S, Hayball JD, Rosen-Bronson S, Bodmer JG, O'Hehir RE: Peptide-induced nonresponsiveness of HLA-DP restricted human T cells reactive with *Dermatophagoides* spp. (house dust mite). J Allergy Clin Immunol 1992;90:749–756.

20   Norman PS, Ohman JL Jr, Long AA, Creticos PS, Gefter MA, Shaked Z, Wood RA, Eggleston PA, Hafner KB, Rao P, Lichtenstein LM, Jones NH, Nicodemus CF: Treatment of cat allergy with T-cell reactive peptides. Am J Respir Crit Care Med 1996;154:1623–1628.

21   Simons FE, Imada M, Li Y, Watson WT, Hayglass KT. Fel d 1 peptides: Effect on skin tests and cytokine synthesis in cat-allergic human subjects. Int Immunol 1996;8:1937–1945.

22   Pène J, Desroches A, Paradis L, Lebel B, Farce M, Nicodemus CF, Yssel H, Bousquet J: Immunotherapy with Fel d 1 peptides decreases IL-4 release by peripheral blood T cells of patients allergic to cats. J Allergy Clin Immunol 1998;102:571–578.

23   Creticos PS, Hebert J, Phillip G, et al: Efficacy of Allervax ragweed peptides in the treatment of ragweed-induced allergy. J Allergy Clin Immunol 1997;99(abstr 1631).

24   Muller U, Akdis CA, Fricker M, Akdis M, Blesken T, Bettens F, Blaser K: Successful immunotherapy with T-cell epitope peptides of bee venom phospholipase A_2 induces specific T-cell anergy in patients allergic to bee venom. J Allergy Clin Immunol 1998;101:747–754.

25   Haselden BM, Kay AB, Larché M: Immunoglobulin E-independent major histocompatibility complex-restricted T cell peptide epitope-induced late asthmatic reactions. J Exp Med 1999;189:1885–1894.

26   Weiner HL, Inobe J, Kuchroo V, Chen Y: Induction and characterisation of TGFβ secreting Th3 cells. FASEB J 1996;10:A1444.

27   Powrie F, Carlino J, Leach MW, Mauze S, Coffman RL: A critical role for transforming growth factor-β but not IL-4 in the suppression of T helper type 1-mediated colitis by CD45RB(low) CD4+ T cells. J Exp Med 1996;183:2669–2674.

28   Groux H, O'Garra A, Bigler M, Rouleau M, Antonenko S, de Vries JE, Roncarolo MG: A CD4+ T-cell subset inhibits antigen-specific T-cell responses and prevents colitis. Nature 1997;389:737–742.

29   Bridoux F, Badou A, Saoudi A, Bernard I, Druet E, Pasquier R, Druet P, Pelletier L: Transforming growth factor beta (TGF-beta)-dependent inhibition of T helper cell 2 (Th2)-induced autoimmunity by self-major histocompatibility complex (MHC) class II-specific, regulatory CD4(+) T cell lines. J Exp Med 1997;185:1769–1775.

Mark Larché, PhD, Allergy and Clinical Immunology, Imperial College School of Medicine, National Heart and Lung Institute, Dovehouse Street, London SW3 6LY (UK)
Tel. +44 20 7351 8181, Fax +44 20 7376 3138 E-Mail m.larche@ic.ac.uk

Robinson DS (ed): Immunological Mechanisms in Asthma and Allergic Diseases.
Chem Immunol. Basel, Karger, 2000, vol 78, pp 39–49

....

The Role of the T Cell in the Immunopathogenesis of Asthma

C. J. Corrigan

Department of Respiratory Medicine and Allergy, Guy's, King's and
St. Thomas' School of Medicine, Guy's Hospital, London, UK

Introduction

It is salutary to reflect on the fact that, barely a decade ago, the role of
the T cell in the pathogenesis of the bronchial mucosal inflammation which
characterizes asthma was scarcely recognized, and moreover doubted by many
workers in the field. During this decade, scientific opinion has undergone a
complete reversal in this regard. Currently, T cells are thought to play a
fundamental role in orchestrating the eosinophil-rich inflammatory response
which characterizes asthma. An understanding of the role of T cells in asthma
has been refined by the emergence of new techniques which have permitted
the characterization of the activation status and spectrum of cytokine production of T cells actually within the target organ. In recounting my own studies
in this field, which follow in the paragraphs below, I would like to pay tribute
to Professor Barry Kay, in whose laboratory this work was commenced and
through whose vision this revolutionary understanding of the role of T cells
in the disease had its origin. Much of the work described below was performed
in Professor Kay's laboratory in the Department of Allergy and Clinical Immunology at the National Heart and Lung Institute, now part of the Imperial
College School of Medicine. Some of my studies were subsequently performed
with Drs Steve Durham and Steve Till in the Department of Upper Respiratory
Medicine, National Heart and Lung Institute, and at Charing Cross Hospital,
now also a campus of the Imperial College School of Medicine, and most
recently at Guy's Hospital in the Department of Respiratory Medicine and
Allergy. The work of my remaining colleagues, who are too numerous to
mention individually, but without whom none of this work would have been

possible, will be apparent from the lists of authors in the attached references. To these collaborators and friends, in addition to Professor Kay himself, I extend my thanks and respect.

T Cells in Asthmatic Inflammation

In a sense, T cells may be regarded as responsible for initiating all inflammatory processes within the human body, since these cells are the only cells capable of recognizing very low concentrations of foreign antigens and instituting an immune response. Even humoral immune reactions generally require initiation by T cells, which then activate antigen-specific B cells to make specific antibodies. In the case of asthma, T cells are a major source of the cytokines IL-3, IL-5 and GM-CSF. These cytokines have a number of effects on eosinophils, which are thought to be the principal pro-inflammatory effector cells of the asthmatic inflammatory process. In particular, they promote the differentiation of eosinophils in the bone marrow, their local adhesion to vascular endothelial adhesion molecules, their priming and activation within the target organ for release of elevated quantities of their pro-inflammatory products, and their enhanced survival within the tissues. All of these properties may account for the striking and specific bronchial mucosal accumulation of eosinophils which is characteristic of asthma.

One of the first suggestions that T cells may be involved in asthma pathogenesis was the observation that elevated percentages of CD4, but not CD8, T cells expressing surface activation markers could be detected by flow cytometry in the peripheral blood of patients with acute severe asthma [1, 2]. The percentages of CD4 T cells expressing these markers could be correlated with disease severity. Furthermore, amelioration of the disease in association with systemic glucocorticoid therapy was associated with reductions in the percentages of these activated peripheral blood T cells, again to an extent which correlated with the degree of clinical improvement. Molecular analysis of the function of these T cells suggested that, in addition to displaying an activated phenotype, they also secreted elevated quantities of asthma-relevant cytokines in patients with severe asthma. For example, in one study using polymerase chain reaction amplification of reverse transcribed cytokine messenger RNA products [3], peripheral blood T cells from patients with acute severe asthma expressed elevated quantities of the asthma-relevant cytokine IL-5 as compared with controls, and this expression was reduced in association with glucocorticoid therapy of the asthmatics and clinical improvement. Similarly, it was shown [4] that elevated percentages of CD4, but not CD8, peripheral blood T cells from acute severe asthmatics expressed and released cytokines relevant to eosinophil accumulation and survival (broadly the so-called 'Th2-type' cytokines) and that this was associated with elevated release of these cytokines into culture supernatants. This differential production of cytokines by CD4, but not CD8, T cells in asthma was broadly concurrent with the preferential expression of activation markers on CD4 T cells in the work described above.

It was also possible to identify elevated concentrations of asthma-relevant cytokines in the serum of these severe asthmatic patients [5, 6]. Once again, systemic glucocorticoid therapy of these patients was associated with reductions in serum IL-5 concentrations concomitant with clinical improvement.

Along with these studies, the role of T cells in asthma pathogenesis was emerging from the studies of the target organ. Through immunohistochemical techniques at the beginning of the 1980s, it became apparent that infiltration of the bronchial mucosa with activated CD4 T cells and eosinophils was essentially a universal feature of asthma regardless of its clinical context (atopic, nonatopic or occupational). Development of in situ hybridization techniques enabled the demonstration of elevated IL-5 messenger RNA expression in the bronchial mucosa of asthmatics as compared with controls [7]. Similar analysis of bronchoalveolar lavage T cells from milder atopic asthmatics showed that elevated percentages of these cells expressed asthma-relevant cytokines such as IL-5 and IL-4 in the context of a 'Th2-type' pattern [8]. Further development of these techniques, particularly the technique of sequential immunohistochemistry and in situ hybridization, allowed the definition of the phenotype of cells expressing mRNA encoding particular cytokines within the asthmatic bronchial mucosa. In two such studies [9, 10], it was shown that the numbers of cells expressing mRNA encoding IL-4 and IL-5, but not IL-2 and IFN-γ, were elevated in atopic asthmatics as compared with controls. Furthermore, approximately 80% of these cells were identified as T cells. The remainder of the inflammatory cells expressing IL-5 and IL-4 mRNA were eosinophils and mast cells. Finally, it was demonstrated that asthmatics have elevated concentrations of IL-5 in induced sputum [11], suggesting that cytokines such as IL-5 are released from activated T cells in the asthmatic bronchial mucosa and also within the bronchial lumen. Taken together, these studies are all consistent with the hypothesis that asthma is orchestrated, at least in part, by the release of eosinophil-active cytokines from activated CD4 T cells within the bronchial mucosa and lumen. These observations are also consistent with the hypothesis that glucocorticoid therapy ameliorates asthma at least partly through inhibition of activation of these T cells and their elevated production of asthma-relevant cytokines.

Glucocorticoid-Resistant Asthma

While the vast majority of asthmatics respond to topical or systemic glucocorticoid therapy with disease improvement, there remains a small but clinically very significant group of asthmatics who exhibit little or no clinical response to systemic glucocorticoid therapy. Early studies of this phenomenon by myself and others helped to establish a working clinical definition of glucocorticoid resistance. It is currently defined as the failure of an asthmatic patient, with a baseline FEV_1 of less than 75% of the predicted value, to exhibit a 15% or greater improvement in this baseline FEV_1 following a 2-week course of oral prednisolone at a dosage of 40 mg daily, despite an improvement in FEV_1 of 15% or more acutely in response to β_2-agonist therapy. We were able to show that there were no fundamental differences between glucocorticoid-sensitive and -resistant asthmatics in terms of the uptake and elimination of orally administered prednisone from their serum [12]. What was apparent, however, was that peripheral blood T cells from these patients were markedly more resistant to the effects of glucocorticoids in inhibiting lectin-induced proliferation and cytokine production in vitro [13]. This was not an absolute phenomenon, but reflected a shift of the concentration-response curve to glucocorticoid such that significant T-cell inhibition would have been achieved in these patients only with dosages of glucocorticoids considered far in excess of a safe and reasonable dosage for long-term administration. The precise mechanism of this resistance is still in the process of being elucidated. It could not be attributed to increased intracellular metabolism of glucocorticoid by T cells from the resistant asthmatic patients [14]. Although it was noted that the glucocorticoid receptors in the T cells of resistant patients showed on average a slightly reduced ligand affinity as compared with receptors from the T cells of sensitive patients [12], this was not felt to account for the rightward shift of the glucocorticoid concentration-response curve of two decades or more in T cells from resistant, as compared with those from sensitive asthmatics. Other workers in this field have claimed, however, that this reduced binding affinity of the glucocorticoid receptor in T cells from glucocorticoid-resistant asthmatics may have some physiological role and may at least partly explain their relative resistance to glucocorticoid inhibition. In contrast to this differential sensitivity to glucocorticoid, T cells from glucocorticoid-sensitive and -resistant asthmatics were inhibited by other immunosuppressive drugs such as cyclosporin A and rapamycin with equivalent potency, and at concentrations of these drugs within the therapeutic range [13–15]. These observations provided further evidence in support of the hypothesis that T cells play a fundamental role in regulating asthma severity and that glucocorticoids ameliorate asthma through inhibition of T-cell activation (except in that small minority of asthmatics where they are apparently ineffective in this regard at therapeutic concentrations). They also suggested that immunosuppressive drugs which can inhibit T-cell proliferation and cytokine production in vitro might also be useful for the therapy of asthmatics, particularly those patients who are relatively glucocorticoid-resistant.

Immunosuppressive Therapy in Asthma

Data from the experiments described in the preceding paragraph formed the basis of studies by my colleagues in Professor Kay's laboratory investigating the possible therapeutic efficacy of cyclosporin A in chronic, severe, glucocorticoid-dependent asthma [16, 17]. These studies were performed in a blinded fashion and showed that concomitant cyclosporin A therapy of patients who continue to have chronic severe asthma despite systemic glucocorticoid therapy showed a degree of clinical improvement and were also able to reduce the amount of this concomitant glucocorticoid therapy. Although these severe asthmatic patients were not formally classified as glucocorticoid-sensitive or -resistant according to the criteria mentioned above, it seems not unreasonable to hypothesize that such patients would be overrepresented in any group of chronic, severe, glucocorticoid-dependent asthmatic patients. The wider use of cyclosporin A therapy for such patients has been somewhat held back by fears about the unwanted effects of chronic therapy, even at the relatively low dosages used to treat these asthmatic patients, and also the fact that only a proportion of patients show any useful clinical response. In contrast to the situation with glucocorticoid therapy, the clinical response of these asthmatics to cyclosporin A therapy could not be correlated with the sensitivity of their peripheral blood T cells to cyclosporin A inhibition in vitro [18]. With regard to the T-cell hypothesis of asthma, although these data are consistent with the proposition that cyclosporin A ameliorates asthma through T-cell inhibition, it must be borne in mind that cyclosporin is inhibitory to a wide range of other inflammatory cells, such as mast cells and basophils, antigen-presenting cells and eosinophils. For example, we were able to show that cyclosporin A showed some inhibitory effects on IL-5-induced eosinophil degranulation and prolonged survival [19]. Nevertheless, the observation [20] that clinical improvement of these chronic severe asthmatics in association with cyclosporin A therapy was accompanied by reductions in their serum concentrations of soluble CD25, a secreted form of the β-chain of the T-cell IL-2 receptor, suggested a role for T-cell inhibition in disease amelioration, as in the case of glucocorticoids. We were also able to show a selective inhibitory effect of cyclosporin A on CD4, as compared with CD8 T cells in vitro, at least in terms of their re-expression of these surface molecules on the following lectin-induced activation [21].

In summary, the T-cell hypothesis of chronic asthma has led in a logical fashion to a development of other new therapies for the disease, most particularly for those asthmatic patients who retain severe symptoms in the face of systemic glucocorticoid therapy and are thus in desperate need of such new approaches. Although cyclosporin A is not the perfect alternative drug, these observations have reinforced the opinion that one fundamental aspect of any new approach to asthma therapy should involve inhibition of the function of CD4 T cells, or alternatively their asthma-relevant cytokine products.

Paediatric Asthma

Paediatric asthma is treated along much the same lines as adult asthma, implying similarities in the pathogenesis of the disease in both adults and children. Nevertheless, the pathogenesis of asthma in children has been very little studied, principally because of the practical and ethical difficulties of obtaining access to the target organ in children through fibreoptic bronchoscopy. Our observations that peripheral blood T cells appear to share many of the functional properties of bronchial mucosal T cells in patients with asthma prompted us to study the function of peripheral blood T cells in asthmatic children. As in adults, we were able to show elevated percentages of activated CD4 T cells in the peripheral blood of child asthmatics as compared with controls [22]. Interestingly, in contrast to adult asthmatics, there was some additional suggestion of activation of CD8 T cells in the peripheral blood of these paediatric patients. In a further study, we addressed cytokine messenger RNA expression by peripheral blood T cells from child asthmatics before and after a period of treatment with inhaled glucocorticoids which was associated with disease improvement [23]. As with studies in adults, it was quite clear that elevated percentages of peripheral blood T cells in these child asthmatics expressed messenger RNA encoding asthma-relevant cytokines including IL-3, IL-4, IL-5 and GM-CSF ('Th2-type' cytokines) but not 'Th1-type' cytokines such as IFN-γ and IL-2. Again, during the course of inhaled glucocorticoid therapy and disease amelioration, the percentages of peripheral blood T cells expressing these cytokines was markedly reduced. These limited data nevertheless suggest that the pathogenesis of asthma in children and adults is broadly similar, and provides some scientific justification for treating childhood asthma along similar lines to that of adults.

Intrinsic and Extrinsic Asthma

In the United Kingdom and Europe it has long been customary to separate asthmatics clinically according to their atopic status. Nonatopic ('intrinsic') asthmatics typically have disease beginning later in life, and this is typically more difficult to control than the milder asthma associated with atopy ('extrinsic') which is seen in children and younger adults. Since IL-4 and IL-13 are the only cytokines known which are capable of promoting B cells to 'switch' to IgE synthesis during the course of differentiation, and thereby induce the atopic phenotype, the hypothesis had already been put forward, based on some preliminary clinical data, that there was a fundamental difference between the pathogenesis of intrinsic and extrinsic asthma with regard to production of these cytokines within the target organ. In a large study of carefully documented atopic and nonatopic asthmatics, along with control subjects matched for atopic status, we used the techniques of polymerase chain mRNA amplification, in situ hybridization and immunohistochemistry to address this question [24]. We were able to show that, in addition to the similar cellular infiltrate in the bronchial mucosa of atopic and nonatopic asthmatics, both groups were characterized by elevated expression of IL-4, as well as IL-5 within cells in the bronchial mucosa and the bronchoalveolar lavage fluid as compared with controls. This study was extended [25] to demonstrate similar and elevated expression of mRNA encoding IL-3 and GM-CSF, as well as the eosinophil attractant CC chemokines RANTES and MCP-3. Overall, the molecular immunopathology of extrinsic and intrinsic asthma, at least in terms of expression of these particular cytokines and chemokines, appeared to be essentially identical. Thus, although intrinsic asthmatics do not produce any detectable circulating allergen-specific IgE, they still overexpress IL-4 in their bronchial mucosa. These observations raise the question of whether, in addition to playing a fundamental role in the regulation of IgE synthesis, IL-4 could also be implicated, along with IL-5 and other eosinophil-active cytokines, in regulating asthma severity. In fact, when studying the expression of IL-5 and IL-4 mRNA in the bronchial mucosa of the same groups of atopic and nonatopic asthmatics and corresponding controls, we were able to show [26] that bronchial mucosal IL-5 mRNA expression correlated very closely within the asthmatics with a number of measures of disease severity, whereas IL-4 mRNA expression did not. Conversely, IL-4 expression correlated very well with total serum IgE concentrations in these asthmatics, whereas IL-5 expression did not. In summary, these data suggest that, whereas both IL-4 and IL-5 are overexpressed in the bronchial mucosa of both atopic and nonatopic asthmatics, IL-5 can be implicated in regulating disease severity whereas IL-4 can be implicated in regulating circulating IgE concentrations. At first sight this detracts from a role for IL-4 in the pathogenesis of asthma (as opposed to the pathogenesis of atopy). Nevertheless, many more questions remain to be answered. Is it possible, for example, that IL-4 directs the local synthesis of IgE within the bronchial mucosa of nonatopic asthmatics, a process which is not reflected by changes in circulating IgE concentrations?

The Role of Allergen-Specific T-Cell Responses in Asthma

The precise stimuli which activate T cells in the bronchial mucosa and peripheral blood of asthmatic patients have yet to be characterized. It has long been assumed, despite a great paucity of direct evidence, that at least some of these T cells recognize inhaled aeroallergens. This would serve as a putative direct mechanism for asthma exacerbation following allergen exposure, which need not necessarily be dependent on the presence of allergen-specific IgE. We have begun to address the properties of allergen-specific T cells in the peripheral blood and bronchial lumen of sensitized atopic asthmatics. We were able to show that allergen-induced proliferation and IL-5 production by T cells from the peripheral blood of sensitized atopic asthmatics in vitro was related to the severity of expression of atopic disease [27]. This was associated with concomitant elevated expression of IL-13, but not Th1-type cytokines such as IFN-γ [28]. These observations suggest a link between T cells' responses to allergen, the production of asthma-relevant cytokines and the likelihood of development of asthma. With regard to the target organ, following preliminary data from experiments showing that T-cell lines established from the bronchoalveolar lavage fluid of atopic asthmatics produced elevated quantities, on a per cell basis, of IL-5 and GM-CSF as compared with cells from atopic nonasthmatics and normal controls [29], we went on to address the hypothesis that at least some of these T cells recognized inhaled aeroallergens. We were able to demonstrate allergen-induced proliferation and IL-5 production by both bronchoalveolar lavage and peripheral blood T cells obtained contemporaneously from sensitized atopic asthmatics following local segmental bronchial allergen challenge [30]. These data provided the first direct demonstration of allergen-specific T cells within the bronchial lumen of asthmatics, and substantiated the possibility that inhaled allergens may be one direct T-cell stimulus in this disease. It was also noted that, although the overall proliferative responses of equivalent numbers of bronchoalveolar lavage and peripheral blood T cells to allergen were equivalent in these patients, suggesting that there was no preferential accumulation of allergen-specific T cells in the lungs as compared with the peripheral blood, there was nevertheless markedly elevated production of IL-5 by the bronchoalveolar lavage T cells as compared with equivalent numbers of peripheral blood T cells, suggesting that, in the process of migrating from the peripheral blood to the bronchial lumen, these allergen-specific T cells acquire new functional properties which enhances their production of asthma-relevant cytokines in response to an allergen stimulus.

In summary: Taken together, all these observations provide overwhelming evidence in support of the general hypothesis that asthma severity is regulated, at least in part, by cytokine products of activated CD4 T cells. These observations have done much to consolidate the view that inhibition of T-cell function, or alternatively cytokine products of activated T cells, will continue to form one fundamental basis for new approaches to asthma therapy. Nevertheless, the large number of other mediators implicated in asthma pathogenesis, as well as the inherent redundancy in the overlapping functions of individual cytokines, suggest that caution is necessary when trying to identify effective therapeutic targets. In particular, it would appear to be wise to concentrate on those mediators which have clearly been shown to have a role in regulating asthma severity. The last two decades have seen a revolution in our understanding of the role of T cells in asthma pathogenesis, and it is to be hoped that further advances in management based on these fundamental observations will continue to be made.

References

1   Corrigan CJ, Hartnell A, Kay AB: T-lymphocyte activation in acute severe asthma. Lancet 1988; i:1129–1132.
2   Corrigan CJ, Kay AB: CD4 T-lymphocyte activation in acute severe asthma: Relationship to disease severity and atopic status. Am Rev Respir Dis 1990;141:970–977.
3   Doi S, Gemou-Engesaeth V, Kay AB, Corrigan CJ: Polymerase chain reaction quantification of cytokine messenger RNA expression in peripheral blood mononuclear cells of patients with acute exacerbations of asthma: Effect of glucocorticoid therapy. Clin Exp Allergy 1994;24:854–867.
4   Corrigan CJ, Hamid Q, North J, Barkans J, Moqbel R, Durham S, Kay AB: Peripheral blood CD4, but not CD8 T lymphocytes in patients with exacerbation of asthma transcribe and translate messenger RNA encoding cytokines which prolong eosinophil survival in the context of a Th2-type pattern: Effect of glucocorticoid therapy. Am J Respir Cell Mol Biol 1995;12:567–578.
5   Corrigan CJ, Haczku A, Gemou-Engesaeth V, Doi S, Kikuchi Y, Takatsu K, Durham SR, Kay AB: CD4 T-lymphocyte activation in asthma is accompanied by increased serum concentrations of interleukin-5: Effect of glucocorticoid therapy. Am Rev Respir Dis 1993;147:540–547.
6   Alexander AG, Barkans J, Moqbel R, Barnes NC, Kay AB, Corrigan CJ: Serum interleukin-5 concentrations in atopic and non-atopic patients with glucocorticoid-dependent chronic severe asthma. Thorax 1994;49:1231–1233.
7   Hamid Q, Azzawi M, Ying S, Moqbel R, Wardlaw AJ, Corrigan CJ, Bradley B, Durham SR, Collins JV, Jeffery PK, Quint DJ, Kay AB: Expression of mRNA for interleukin-5 in mucosal bronchial biopsies from asthma. J Clin Invest 1991;87:1541–1546.

8   Robinson DS, Hamid Q, Ying S, Tsicopoulos A, Barkans J, Bentley AM, Corrigan CJ, Durham SR, Kay AB: Predominant Th2-type bronchoalveolar lavage T-lymphocyte population in atopic asthma. N Engl J Med 1992;326:298–304.

9   Ying S, Durham SR, Corrigan CJ, Hamid Q, Kay AB: Phenotype of cells expressing mRNA for Th2-type (interleukin-4 and interleukin-5) and Th1-type (interleukin-2 and interferon-γ) cytokines in bronchoalveolar lavage and bronchial biopsies from atopic asthmatics and normal control subjects. Am J Respir Cell Mol Biol 1995;12:477–487.

10   Ying S, Humbert M, Barkans J, Corrigan CJ, Pfister R, Menz G, Larché M, Robinson DS, Durham SR, Kay AB: Expression of IL-4 and IL-5 mRNA and protein product by CD4+ and CD8+ T cells, eosinophils and mast cells in bronchial biopsies obtained from atopic and non-atopic (intrinsic) asthmatics. J Immunol 1997;158:3539–3544.

11   Keatings VM, O'Connor BJ, Wright LG, Huston DP, Corrigan CJ, Barnes PJ: Late phase response to allergen is associated with increased concentrations of TNF- and IL-5 in induced sputum. J Allergy Clin Immunol 1997;99:693–698.

12   Corrigan CJ, Brown PH, Barnes NC, Szefler SJ, Tsai JJ, Frew AJ, Kay AB: Glucocorticoid resistance in chronic asthma: Glucocorticoid pharmacokinetics, glucocorticoid receptor characteristics and inhibition of peripheral blood T cell proliferation by glucocorticoids in vitro. Am Rev Respir Dis 1991;144:1016–1025.

13   Corrigan CJ, Brown PH, Barnes NC, Tsai JJ, Frew AJ, Kay AB: Glucocorticoid resistance in chronic asthma: Peripheral blood T-lymphocyte activation and a comparison of the T-lymphocyte inhibitory effects of glucocorticoids and cyclosporin A. Am Rev Respir Dis 1991;144:1026–1032.

14   Corrigan CJ, Bungre JK, Cooper AE, Seddon H, Kay AB: Glucocorticoid-resistant asthma: T-lymphocyte steroid metabolism and sensitivity to glucocorticoids and immunosuppressive agents. Eur Respir J 1996;9:2077–2086.

15   Haczku A, Alexander A, Brown P, Assoufi B, Li B, Kay AB, Corrigan CJ: The effect of dexamethasone, cyclosporine and rapamycin on T-lymphocyte proliferation in vitro: Comparison of cells from patients with glucocorticoid-sensitive and glucocorticoid-resistant chronic asthma. J Allergy Clin Immunol 1994;93:510–519.

16   Alexander AG, Barnes NC, Kay AB: Trial of cyclosporin in corticosteroid-dependent chronic severe asthma. Lancet 1992;239:324–328.

17   Lock SH, Kay AB, Barnes NC: Double-blind, placebo-controlled study of cyclosporin A as a corticosteroid-sparing agent in corticosteroid-dependent asthma. Am J Respir Crit Care Med 1996;153:509–514.

18   Alexander AG, Barnes NC, Kay AB, Corrigan CJ: Can clinical response to cyclosporin in chronic severe asthma be predicted by an in vitro T-lymphocyte proliferation assay? Eur Respir J 1996;9:1421–1426.

19   Meng Q, Ying S, Corrigan CJ, Wakelin M, Assoufi B, Moqbel R, Kay AB: Effects of rapamycin, cyclosporin A and dexamethasone on interleukin-5-induced eosinophil degranulation and prolonged survival. Allergy 1997;52:1095–1101.

20   Alexander AG, Barnes NC, Kay AB, Corrigan CJ: Clinical response to cyclosporin in chronic severe asthma is associated with a reduction in serum soluble interleukin-2 receptor concentrations. Eur Respir J 1995;8:574–578.

21   Haczku A, Kay AB, Corrigan CJ: Inhibition of re-expression of surface CD4, but not CD8, on activated human T-lymphocytes by the immunosuppressive drugs dexamethasone and cyclosporine A: Correlation with inhibition of proliferation. Int J Immunopharmacol 1996;18:45–52.

22   Gemou-Engesaeth V, Kay AB, Bush A, Corrigan CJ: Activated peripheral blood CD4 and CD8 T lymphocytes in childhood asthma: Correlation with eosinophilia and disease severity. Paediatr Allergy Immunol 1994;5:170–177.

23   Gemou-Engesaeth V, Bush A, Kay AB, Hamid Q, Corrigan CJ: Inhaled glucocorticoid therapy of childhood asthma is associated with reduced peripheral blood T cell activation and 'Th2-type' cytokine mRNA expression. Paediatrics 1997;99:695–703.

24   Humbert M, Durham SR, Ying S, Kimmitt P, Barkans J, Assoufi B, Pfister R, Menz G, Robinson DS, Kay AB, Corrigan CJ: IL-4 and IL-5 messenger RNA and protein in bronchial biopsies from patients with atopic and non-atopic asthma: Evidence against 'intrinsic' asthma being a distinct immunopathologic entity. Am J Respir Crit Care Med 1996;154:1497–1504.

25   Humbert M, Ying S, Corrigan C, Menz G, Barkans J, Pfister R, Meng Q, Van Damme J, Opdenakker G, Durham SR, Kay AB: Bronchial mucosal expression of the genes encoding chemokines RANTES and MCP-3 in symptomatic atopic and non-atopic asthmatics: Relationship to the eosinophil-active cytokines interleukin (IL)-5, granulocyte/macrophage colony-stimulating factor and IL-3. Am J Respir Cell Mol Biol 1997;16:1–8.

26   Humbert M, Durham SR, Kimmitt P, Till SJ, Kay AB, Corrigan CJ: The relationship between IL-4 and IL-5 mRNA expression and disease severity in atopic asthma. Am J Respir Crit Care Med 1997;156:704–708.

27   Till S, Dickason R, Huston D, Humbert M, Robinson D, Larché M, Durham S, Kay AB, Corrigan C: IL-5 secretion by allergen-stimulated CD4+ T cells in primary culture: Relationship to expression of allergic disease. J Allergy Clin Immunol 1997;99:563–569.

28   Till S, Durham S, Dickason R, Huston D, Bungre J, Walker S, Robinson D, Kay AB, Corrigan C: IL-13 production by allergen-stimulated T cells is increased in allergic diseases and associated with IL-5, but not IFN-γ expression. Immunology 1997;91:53–57.

29   Till SJ, Li B, Durham S, Humbert M, Assoufi B, Huston D, Dickason R, Jeannin P, Kay AB, Corrigan CJ: Secretion of the eosinophil-active cytokines interleukin-5, granulocyte/macrophage colony-stimulating factor and interleukin-3 by bronchoalveolar lavage CD4+ and CD8+ T cell lines in atopic asthmatics, and atopic and non-atopic controls. Eur J Immunol 1995;25:2727–2731.

30   Till SJ, Durham SR, Rajakulasingam K, Humbert M, Huston D, Dickason R, Kay AB, Corrigan CJ: Allergen-induced proliferation and IL-5 production by bronchoalveolar lavage and blood T cells following segmental allergen challenge. Am J Respir Crit Care Med 1998;158:404–411.

Dr. C.J. Corrigan, MA, MSc, PhD, FRCP, Department of Respiratory Medicine and Allergy,
Guy's, King's and St. Thomas' School of Medicine, 5th Floor,
Thomas Guy House, Guy's Hospital, London SE1 9RT (UK)
Tel. +44 20 7955 4571, Fax +44 20 7403 8640, E-Mail chris.corrigan@kcl.ac.uk

Robinson DS (ed): Immunological Mechanisms in Asthma and Allergic Diseases.
Chem Immunol. Basel, Karger, 2000, vol 78, pp 50–61

....

The Th1 and Th2 Concept in Atopic Allergic Disease

Douglas S. Robinson

Allergy and Clinical Immunology, Imperial College School of Medicine,
National Heart and Lung Institute, London, UK

Introduction

The Th1/Th2 paradigm

The description of two subtypes of T-helper cells based on cytokine profiles by Mosmann and Coffman [1] in 1986 was a major step forward in thinking on control of immune responses. Building on previous divisions of responses into predominantly humoral or predominantly cell-mediated [2] they described murine T-cell clones that could be divided into either Th1 producing IFN-γ and IL-2 but not IL-4 and IL-5 or Th2 which produces IL-4 and IL-5 but not IFN-γ [1]. The functional consequences of this division follow from the observation that IFN-γ was required for activation of macrophage function and cytotoxic T-cell responses in cell-mediated immunity [3], whereas IL-4 unopposed by IFN-γ was essential in switching B cells to IgE synthesis [4] and IL-5 was involved in eosinophil development and survival [5]. This was seen most elegantly in the response of different mouse strains to Leishmania infection which was shown to be largely determined by the genetic tendency to mount either a healing Th1 response or an inappropriate Th2 response leading to disseminated disease [6–8]. The potential relevance of Th2 responses to atopic disease was rapidly apparent since IL-4 and IL-5 could explain both IgE and eosinophilic inflammation.

Human Th1 and Th2 Cells
Although a variety of cytokine profiles were described from human T-helper clones, the work of the groups of Romagnani [9] and Kapsenberg [10]

firmly established that polarized Th1 and Th2 clones could indeed be derived from humans, and in particular that Th2 responses were prominent in allergen-specific CD4+ T-cell clones. Although the principle of the Th1/Th2 concept applies in both mice and men, there are differences both in the cytokine profiles observed, the factors determining the response and the apparent stability of cytokine profile. Thus the work from study of murine T cells and animal models needs to be confirmed in humans.

The Potential Role of Th2 Cytokines in Allergic Disease

IgE Regulation. The defining hallmark of atopic disease is production of specific IgE to allergens. The molecular regulation of IgE production from B cells has been well defined [11, 12]. In particular, IL-4 or IL-13 are essential for the first step in isotype switching: generation of the I_ε immature mRNA transcript. A second signal, such as that from CD40/CD40L interaction, is required for IgE production. Other cytokines including IL-5 [13], IL-6 [14] and IL-9 [15] can enhance IgE production, whereas IFN-γ and IL-12 inhibit both isotype switch and IgE production. Thus a Th2 cytokine profile favours generation of specific IgE. It is of note that non-T cells can also produce IL-4, and mast cells and basophils are capable of IgE switching [16]. However, without cognate MHC/TCR interaction, such IgE will not be allergen-specific. IL-13 can be produced by human Th1 as well as Th2 T cells, although IFN-γ from Th1 cells would inhibit IgE switching.

IL-5 and Eosinophils. Just before the description of Th1 and Th2 cells, IL-5 had been defined as a cytokine with specific action in the development, priming and survival of eosinophils [5]. Some activity is also seen on basophils and human B cells [17, 18]. Although IL-5 shares a common β-receptor subunit with IL-3 and GM-CSF [19, 20], and initial studies suggested that all three cytokines could act to cause eosinophil development from bone marrow progenitors [21], our recent studies suggest that IL-5 itself, but not IL-3 or GM-CSF, upregulates IL-5Rα expression and that human eosinophil development is largely IL-5-dependent [22].

Evidence for Th2 T-Cell Involvement in Atopic Allergic Disease

Baseline Disease. Assessment of mRNA expression in bronchoalveolar lavage (BAL) cells from atopic asthmatic subjects showed a predominant Th2 pattern [23], and numbers of cells expressing both IL-4 and IL-5 mRNA were correlated with measures of disease severity such as bronchial responsiveness or forced expiratory volume in 1 s [24]. In addition, IL-4 and IL-5 but not IFN-γ protein levels were increased in BAL fluid from atopic asthmatics when compared to control subject [25], and allergen-specific Th2-type clones could be isolated from the respiratory mucosa of atopic subjects [26]. Similarly, allergen-specific Th2 cells were isolated from lesional skin in atopic dermatitis, and a Th2 cytokine mRNA profile was demonstrated in skin biopsies. More recently, allergen-specific T-cell lines from BAL of atopic asthmatics were shown to produce IL-5: this was from both CD4 and CD8 cells [27]. In addition, by combining immunohistochemical staining to identify cell phenotype with in situ hybridization for cytokine mRNA, IL-4 and IL-5 mRNA were predominantly localized to CD4 + cells in the airway mucosa from asthmatic subjects, with lesser contributions from CD8 + cells, mast cells and eosinophils [28]. Other Th1 and Th2 cytokines have been assessed in asthma: some reports find increased expression of IL-10 [29], and increased IL-13 expression is also reported [30].

Nonatopic Asthma

Nonatopic asthma is characterized by asthma, generally occurring later in life than atopic asthma, without clinical or laboratory evidence of IgE sensitization to aeroallergens. Bronchial biopsies from such asthmatics show eosinophil infiltration and activated T cells in the bronchial mucosa, as in atopic asthma [31]. Although one study did not detect IL-4 in concentrated BAL fluid from nonatopic subjects, more recent biopsy studies have reported a Th2 cytokine profile at both mRNA and protein level [32]. In addition, increased numbers of cells bearing high-affinity IgE receptor were detected in bronchial biopsies from nonatopic asthmatics when compared to control subjects [23]. What the role of IgE in this nonatopic variant of asthma is, and whether it is directed against specific antigens, remains to be established. It is of note that Valenta et al. [34] have recently described a human IgE binding 'autoallergen'.

Allergen Challenge

The late-phase response to allergen challenge has been used to model chronic allergic inflammation, and is characterized by T-cell activation and eosinophil and neutrophil infiltration [35, 36]. Studies of cytokine mRNA expression also support activation of a Th2-type response in skin, nose and lung biopsies obtained 24 h after allergen challenge [37–39].

Response to Treatment

Numbers of cells expressing mRNA for IL-4 or IL-5 both fell after corticosteroid treatment of asthma in a double-blind placebo-controlled study [40], and there was a small increase in IFN-γ mRNA expressing cells. That such changes might be relevant to clinical improvement was supported by the work of Leung et al. [41] who showed a similar fall in IL-5 mRNA expressing cells in subjects responding to oral prednisone, but not in a group of subjects whose asthma did not improve with steroid therapy. The role of T cells in asthma was also supported by the demonstration of clinical efficacy and steroid-sparing activity of cyclosporin A in severe asthma, and by the inhibition of the late, but not early, asthmatic response to allergen challenge by this inhibitor of T-cell activation [42–44]. In addition, a nondepleting anti-CD4 monoclonal antibody was also shown to improve lung function in severe steroid-dependent asthmatics [45].

Allergen immunotherapy has been used to control atopic allergic disease for many years, and evidence also suggests that this too may target Th2 T-cell activation, since reduced allergen-induced IL-4 and IL-5 production with increased IFN-γ responses were seen after clinically successful treatment [46–48].

Animal Models of Allergic Disease

Mouse models of allergic asthma yield varying data in different mouse strains and different sensitization and challenge regimens. Most models involve initial sensitization by intraperitoneal route with adjuvant and subsequent inhaled challenge. They are thus models of allergen challenge and some way from human asthma. Nonetheless, such models can elicit airway eosinophilia and hyperresponsiveness, and allow careful molecular dissection of the immunology of such responses. Although some caution must be applied in extrapolating to human disease, data from genetic studies and from gene manipulation in such models has elegantly identified themes for future research in human disease.

Gene knockout studies and use of blocking antibodies established the importance of IL-4 and IL-5 in eosinophilic and IgE responses and AHR in animal models of allergen challenge, although the relative role of these cytokines varies according to the strain studied [49–51]. Targeting T cells with anti-CD4 antibodies and experiments with adoptive transfer of antigen-specific Th2 cells have shown that Th2 cells can certainly induce airway eosinophilia and BHR [52, 53]. Recent experiments suggest that IL-4 and IL-5 are not the only route to T-cell-dependent AHR. Hogan et al. [51] showed that in IL-4 gene-targeted BALB/c mice anti-IL-5 antibody treatment reduced airway eosinophila but did not block AHR, whereas depleting CD4 + T cells in mice lacking both IL-4 and IL-5 did abolish residual AHR. More recently an important role for IL-13 was suggested. Wills-Karp et al. [54] showed that a soluble IL-13Rα-human IgG-Fc fusion protein, which blocks mouse IL-13 but not IL-4, could inhibit AHR in a mouse allergen challenge model, without reducing airway eosinophilia or serum antigen-specific IgE. Grunig et al. [55] showed similar data, although their experiments did suggest some reduction in eosinophilia, and went on to show that IL-4R-deficient mice did not acquire the AHR upon Th2 transfer that was seen in wild-type controls. These data suggest that IL-13, and IL-4, may act to produce AHR by mechanisms that do not involve IgE or eosinophils. Whether this is also so in humans remains to be established.

Transgenic expression of IL-5, IL-9, IL-11 or IL-13 under the control of a promoter directing lung-specific overexpression of these cytokines can induce AHR in mice without allergen challenge [56–59]. The airway pathology in such models varies, but variable mast cell and eosinophil expansion is seen. It is likely that such experiments induce a cascade of cytokines and chemokines in the lung, and definition of the patterns seen may pinpoint important contributers to the AHR seen in these models. Some such transgenic animals, in particular those overexpressing IL-11 and IL-13, also show some evidence of changes reminiscent of the airway remodelling that characterizes chronic asthma, such as subepithelial collagen deposition, and may give information on these processes.

Animal models have also defined the interaction of IL-5 with eotaxin and other chemokines in eosinophil mobilization from the bone marrow. Collins et al. [60, 61] showed synergy between systemically delivered IL-5 with local eotaxin in recruitment of eosinophils, and both were shown to act in release of a bone marrow pool of eosinophils. Wang et al. [56] went on to show that reconstitution of IL-5 knockout mice with gene transfer directing systemic production of IL-5 could restore eosinophil and AHR response to inhaled antigen, whereas pulmonary IL-5 gene delivery did not.

Factors Regulating Th2 Development, Recruitment and Phenotype Expression

Development of Th1 and Th2 Cells

A variety of factors have been shown to act in driving developing naïve T-cell responses in either the Th1 or Th2 direction. The best defined is the cytokine environment, but the antigen dose, antigen-presenting cell, local hormone and prostaglandin milieu can also influence the outcome [62]. As the molecular control of T-cell differentiation is defined, these data can be better understood. An important factor in Th1/Th2 development is the loss or retention of IL-12 responsiveness, determined at the level of expression of IL-12Rβ2. IL-4, unopposed by IFN-γ, or IFN-α in human cells, directs loss of IL-12Rβ2 expression and thus drives to Th2 phenotype [63, 64]. In contrast, IFN-γ (IFN-α in humans) directs retention of IL-12Rβ2, and thus in the presence of IL-12, Th1 development. More recently, the role of IL-1 family members induced in innate immune responses has been shown. In particular IL-18 synergizes with IL-12 in Th1 phenotype expression, whereas Th2 cells are responsive to IL-1α [65]. Indeed IL-18R has been suggested as a phenotypic marker of Th1 cells, whereas another IL-1R family member ST2/T1 appears restricted to Th2 cells [66, 67]. The ligand for ST2/T1 remains to be defined.

Studies of transcriptional regulation of cytokine expression suggest a number of factors important in determining murine IL-4 production, including GATA3, c-maf, NIP-45 and NFAT [68]. Indeed overexpression of GATA3 was suggested to favour Th2 development [69]. However, other investigators suggest that GATA3, together with NFκB, may be more important in control of IL-5 expression [70, 71], and retroviral gene transfer to Th1 cells downregulated IFN-γ production, suggesting that effects on IL-4 may be indirect [72]. It will be important to define whether similar mechanisms apply in regulating Th2 phenotype expression in humans, although increased GATA3 expressing cells were seen in bronchial biopsies from asthmatic subjects [73]. Recent data suggest that IL-4, and IL-2, expression is regulated in a monoallelic fashion [74]. Thus only one of the two IL-4 alleles is expressed in developing Th2 cells. In addition, further experiments are elucidating the epigenetic modification including histone deacetylation and DNA methylation involved in directing gene expression, together with the role of cell cycling and passage of such epigenetic imprinting to determine, for example, IL-4 cells in progeny [75]. Understanding the molecular regulation of human Th2 cytokine expression may help in understanding the complex genetics of asthma and atopy, and provide opportunities for regulating cytokine production in disease.

Although much work has been done on murine Th1 and Th2 development, and some of this has been extended to human T cells, there is still a need for information on the factors driving Th2 responses during initiation of allergic disease and in maintaining the Th2 phenotype in human allergen-specific memory T cells.

Recruitment of Th1 and Th2 Cells
With the explosion of information on chemokines it has become clear that Th1 and Th2 cells can express different chemokine receptors and respond to different chemokines. It is also clear that chemokine receptor expression by T cells varies with activation status and cytokine environment, so that the

picture in vivo may be different from that seen in isolated T-cell clones. Current evidence suggests that human polarized Th1 cells express CXCR3 and are more responsive to its ligand IP-10, whereas Th2 lines express CCR3, CCR4 and CCR8 and respond to eotaxin, TARC and I-309 [76, 77]. Th2 clones were reported to have reduced expression of CCR5. It will be interest to determine the chemokine receptor profile and responsiveness of allergen-specific T cells in vivo, and to determine whether different chemokines are involved in recruitment, retention and activation of Th2 cells at sites of allergic inflammation.

Differential responses of Th1 and Th2 cells to p- and e-selectin have been reported, and whether different adhesion pathways act in selection of Th1 or Th2 responses in humans remains to be established [78].

Genetics of Atopy and Asthma

A number of studies have implicated genetic polymorphism associated with the Th2 gene cluster on chromosome 5q23 in BHR [79]. In particular, linkage studies have implicated IL-9, IL-4 and IL-13. Murine studies also show that IL-9 is linked to BHR. In addition, receptor variants of IL-4 and IL-9 have been described [80, 81]. It is of note that murine studies of BHR and genetic susceptibility to Leishmania infection identify regions that may be syntenic with human atopy and asthma candidate regions [82, 83]. This may be due to common pathways controlling Th2 expression. If such genes are expressed mono-allelically, this may also impact on genetic studies of asthma and atopy.

Conclusion and Potential for Regulating Th2 Responses

There is now considerable evidence that Th2-type T-cell responses play a role in human atopic allergic disease. The factors that drive such a response in initiating the allergic diathesis will be important, and may act even in utero [84]. The relative role of continued 'new' Th2 T cells and memory responses in perpetuating human allergic disease and control of these processes will be important. The role of individual cytokines of the Th2 'family' will become clearer with the use of blocking antibodies in human studies. Although initial understanding of the reciprocal regulation of Th1 and Th2 cells and data from immunotherapy studies were interpreted to suggest that inducing a Th1 response might be benefical in control of allergic inflammation, recent mouse studies suggest otherwise, and an allergen-specific Th1 respose might also induce pathology [85, 86]. Of more interest is the possibility of inducing T-cell unresponsiveness, as had been described for both conventional allergen immunotherapy [87] and peptide therapy [88, 89]. In particular, the description of regulatory T cells, such as the murine Th3, or murine and human Tr1, that inhibit through cytokines such as IL-10 and TGF-β is of interest [90, 91]. Further understanding of normal immunological regulation of Th1 and Th2 responses may hold the key to targeted manipulation of pathological Th2 responses in atopic allergic disease.

References

1   Mosmann TR, Cherwinski H, Bond MW, Gieldin MA, Coffman RL: Two types of murine helper T cell clone. I. Definition according to profiles of lymphokine activities and secreted proteins. J Immunol 1986;136:2348–2357.
2   Parish CR, Liew FY: Immune response to chemically modified flagellin. 3. Enhanced cell-mediated immunity during high and low zone antibody tolerance to flagellin. J Exp Med 1972;135:298–311.
3   Fong TA, Mosmann TR: The role of IFN-γ in delayed-type hypersensitivity mediated by Th1 clones. J Immunol 1989;143:2887–2893.
4   Del Prete GF, Maggi E, Parronchi P, Chretien I, Tiri A, Macchia D, Ricci M, Banchereau J, de Vries J, Romagnani S: IL-4 is an essential factor for the IgE synthesis induced in vitro by human T cell clones and their supernatants. J Immunol 1988;140:4193–4198.
5   Sanderson CJ: Interleukin-5, eosinophils and disease. Blood 1992;79:3101–3109.
6   Heinzel FP, Sadick MD, Holaday BJ, Coffman RL, Locksley RM: Reciprocal expression of interferon-γ or interleukin-4 during the resolution or progression of murine leishmaniasis. Evidence for expansion of distinct helper T cell subsets. J Exp Med 1989;169:59–72.
7   Scott P, Natovitz P, Coffman RL, Pearce E, Sher A: Immunoregulation of cutaneous leishmaniasis. T cell lines that transfer protective immunity or exacerbation belong to different T helper subsets and respond to distinct parasite antigens. J Exp Med 1988;168:1675–1684.
8   Guler ML, Gorham J, Hsieh CS, Mackey AJ, Steen RG, Dietrich WF, Murphy KM: Genetic susceptibility to Leishmania: IL-12 responsiveness in TH1 cell development. Science 1996;271: 984–987.
9   Parronchi P, Macchia D, Piccinni MP, Biswas P, Simonelli C, Maggi E, Ricci M, Ansari AA, Romagnani S: Allergen- and bacterial antigen-specific T-cell clones established from atopic donors show a different profile of cytokine production. Proc Natl Acad Sci USA 1991;88:4538–4542.
10 Wierenga EA, Snoek M, de Groot C, Chretien I, de Bos J, Jansen HM, Kapsenberg ML: Evidence for compartmentalization of functional subsets of CD4+ T lymphocytes in atopic patients. J Immunol 1990;144:4651–4656.
11 Geha RS: Regulation of IgE synthesis in humans. J Allergy Clin Immunol 1992;90:143–150.
12 Sutton BJ, Gould HJ: The human IgE network. Nature 1993;366:421–428.
13 Pene J, Rousset F, Briere F, Chretien I, Wideman J, Bonnefoy JY, de Vries JE: Interleukin-5 enhances interleukin-4-induced IgE production by normal human B cells. The role of soluble CD23 antigen. Eur J Immunol 1988;18:929–935.
14 Vercelli D, Jabara HH, Arai K, Yokota T, Geha RS: Endogenous IL-6 plays an oligatory role in IL-4-induced human IgE synthesis. Eur J Immunol 1989;19:1419–1422.
15 Dugas B, Renauld JC, Pene J, Bonnefoy JY, Peti-Frere C, Braquet P, Bousquet J, Van-Snick J, Mencia Huerta JM: Interleukin-9 potentiates the interleukin-4-induced immunoglobulin (IgG, IgM and IgE) production by normal human B lymphocytes. Eur J Immunol 1993;23:1687–1692.
16 Gauchat JF, Henchoz S, Mazzei G, Aubry JP, Brunner T, Blasey H, Life P, Talabot D, Flores-Romo L, Thompson J, Kishi K, Butterfield J, Dahinden C, Bonnefoy JY: Induction of human IgE synthesis in B cells by mast cells and basophils. Nature 1993;365:340–343.
17 Denburg JA, Silver JE, Abrams JS: Interleukin-5 is a human basophilopoietin: Induction of histamine content and basophilic differentiation of HL-60 cells and of peripheral blood basophil-eosinophil progenitors. Blood 1991;77:1462–1468.

18   Huston MM, Moore JP, Mettes HJ, Tavana G, Huston DP: Human B cells express IL-5 receptor messenger ribonucleic acid and respond to IL-5 with enhanced IgM production after mitogenic stimulation with *Moraxella catarrhalis*. J Immunol 1996;156:1392–1401.

19   Tavernier J, Devos R, Cornelis S, Tuypens T, Van der Heyden J, Fiers W, Plaetinck G: A human high affinity interleukin-5 receptor is composed of an IL-5-specific α chain and a β chain shared with the receptor for GM-CSF. Cell 1991;66:1175–1184.

20   Kitamura T, Sato N, Arai K, Miyajima A: Expression cloning of the human interleukin-3 receptor cDNA reveals a shared β subunit for the human IL-3 and GM-CSF receptors. Cell 1991;66:1165–1174.

21   Clutterbuck EJ, Hirst EM, Sanderson CJ: Human interleukin-5 regulates the production of eosinophils in human bone marrow cultures: Comparison and interaction with IL-1, IL-3, IL-6, and GM-CSF. Blood 1989;73:1504–1512.

22   Tavernier J, Van der Heyden J, Verhee A, Brusselle G, Van Ostade X, Vandekerckhove J, North J, Rankin SM, Kay AB, Robinson DS: Interleukin-5 regulates the isoform expression of its own receptor α-subunit. Blood 2000;95:1600–1607.

23   Robinson DS, Hamid Q, Sun Ying, Tsicopoulos A, Brakans J, Bentley AM, Corrigan CJ, Durham SR, Kay AB: Predominant Th2-like bronchoalveolar T-lymphocyte population in atopic asthma. N Engl J Med 1992;326:298–304.

24   Robinson DS, Ying S, Bentley AM, Meng Q, North J, Durham SR, Kay AB, Hamid Q: Relationships among numbers of bronchoalveolar lavage cells expressing messenger ribonucleic acid for cytokines, asthma symptoms, and airway methacholine responsiveness in atopic asthma. J Allergy Clin Immunol 1993;92:397–403.

25   Walker C, Bode E, Boer L, Hansel TT, Blaser K, Virchow JC Jr: Allergic and non-allergic asthmatics have distinct patterns of T-cell activation and cytokine production in peripheral blood and bronchoalveolar lavage. Am Rev Respir Dis 1992;146:109–115.

26   Del Prete GF, De Carli M, D'Elios MM, Maestrelli P, Ricci M, Fabbri L, Romagnani S: Allergen exposure induces the activation of allergen-specific Th2 cells in the airway mucosa of patients with allergic respiratory disorders. Eur J Immunol 1993;23:1445–1449.

27   Till S, Li B, Durham S, Humbert M, Assoufi B, Huston D, Dickason R, Jeannin P, Kay AB, Corrigan CJ: Secretion of the eosinophil-active cytokines interleukin-5, granulocyte/macrophage colony-stimulating factor and interleukin-3 by bronchoalveolar lavage CD4+ and CD8+ T cell lines in atopic asthmatics, and atopic and non-atopic controls. Eur J Immunol 1995;25:2727–2731.

28   Ying S, Humbert M, Barkans J, Corrigan CJ, Pfister R, Menz G, Larche M, Robinson DS, Durham SR, Kay AB: Expression of IL-4 and IL-5 mRNA and protein product by CD4+ and CD8+ T cells, eosinophils, and mast cells in bronchial biopsies obtained from atopic and nonatopic (intrinsic) asthmatics. J Immunol 1997;158:3539–3544.

29   Robinson DS, Tsicopoulos A, Meng Q, Durham S, Kay AB, Hamid Q: Increased interleukin-10 messenger RNA expression in atopic allergy and asthma. Am J Respir Cell Mol Biol 1996;14:113–117.

30   Humbert M, Durham SR, Kimmitt P, Powell N, Assoufi B, Pfister R, Menz G, Kay AB, Corrigan CJ: Elevated expression of messenger ribonucleic acid encoding IL-13 in the bronchial mucosa of atopic and nonatopic subjects with asthma. J Allergy Clin Immunol 1997;99:657–665.

31   Bentley AM, Menz G, Storz C, Robinson DS, Bradley B, Jeffery PK, Durham SR, Kay AB: Identification of T-lymphocytes, macrophages and activated eosinophils in the bronchial mucosa in intrinsic asthma: Relationship to symptoms and bronchial responsiveness. Am Rev Respir Dis 1992;146:500–506.

32   Humbert M, Durham SR, Ying S, Kimmitt P, Barkans J, Assoufi B, Pfister R, Menz G, Robinson DS, Kay AB, Corrigan CJ: IL-4 and IL-5 mRNA and protein in bronchial biopsies from patients with atopic and nonatopic asthma: Evidence against 'intrinsic' asthma being a distinct immunopathologic entity. Am J Respir Crit Care Med 1996;154:1497–1504.

33   Humbert M, Grant JA, Taborda-Barata L, Durham SR, Pfister R, Menz G, Barkans J, Ying S, Kay AB: High affinity IgE receptor (FcεRI)-bearing cells in bronchial biopsies from atopic and nonatopic asthma. Am J Respir Crit Care Med 1996;153:1931–1937.

34   Valenta R, Natter S, Seiberler S, Wichlas S, Maurer D, Hess M, Pavelka M, Grote M, Ferreira F, Szepfalusi Z, Valent P, Stingl G: Molecular characterization of an autoallergen, Hom s 1, identified by serum IgE from atopic dermatitis patients. J Invest Dermatol 1998;111:1178–1183.

35 Frew AJ, Kay AB: The relationship between infiltrating CD4 + lymphocytes, activated eosinophils, and the magnitude of the allergen-induced late phase cutaneous reaction in man. J Immunol 1988; 141:4158–4164.

36 Robinson DS, Hamid Q, Bentley AM, Ying S, Kay AB, Durham SR: CD4 + T cell activation, eosinophil recruitment and interleukin(IL)-4, IL-5 and GM-CSF messenger RNA expression in bronchoalveolar lavage after allergen inhalation challenge of atopic asthmatics. J Allergy Clin Immunol 1993;92:313–324.

37 Kay AB, Ying S, Varney V, Gaga M, Durham SR, Moqbel R, Wardlaw AJ, Hamid Q: Messenger RNA expression of the cytokine gene cluster, interleukin(IL)-3, IL-4, IL-5, and granulocyte/macrophage colony-stimulating factor, in allergen-induced late-phase cutaneous reactions in atopic subjects. J Exp Med 1991;173:775–778.

38 Durham SR, Ying S, Varney VA, Jacobson MR, Sudderick RM, Mackay IS, Kay AB, Hamid QA: Cytokine messenger RNA expression for IL-3, IL-4, IL-5 and granulocyte macrophage colony-stimulating factor in the nasal mucosa after allergen provocation: Relationship to tissue eosinophilia. J Immunol 1992;148:2390–2394.

39 Bentley AM, Meng Q, Robinson DS, Hamid Q, Kay AB, Durham SR: Increases in activated T lymphocytes, eosinophils, and cytokine messenger RNA expression or IL-5 and GM-CSF in bronchial biopsies after allergen inhalation challenge in atopic asthmatics. Am J Respir Cell Mol Biol 1993;8:35–42.

40 Robinson DS, Hamid Q, Ying S, Bentley AM, Assoufi B, North J, Meng Q, Durham SR, Kay AB: Prednisolone treatment in asthma is associated with modulation of bronchoalveolar lavage cell interleukin-4, interleukin-5 and interferon-γ cytokine gene expression. Am Rev Respir Dis 1993; 148:401–406.

41 Leung DYM, Martin RJ, Szefler SJ, Sher ER, Ying S, Kay AB, Hamid Q: Dysregulation of interleukin-4, interleukin-5, and interferon-γ expression in steroid-resistant asthma. J Exp Med 1995;181:33–40.

42 Alexander AG, Barnes NC, Kay AB: Trial of cyclosporin A in corticosteroid-dependent chronic severe asthma. Lancet 1992;339:324–328.

43 Lock SH, Kay AB, Barnes NC: Double-blind, placebo-controlled study of cyclosporin A as a corticosteroid-sparing agent in corticosteroid-dependent asthma. Am J Respir Crit Care Med 1996; 153:509–514.

44 Sihra BS, Durham SR, Walker S, Kon OM, Barnes NC, Kay AB: Inhibition of the allergen-induced late asthmatic response by cyclosporin A. Effect of cyclosporin A on the allergen-induced late asthmatic reaction. Thorax 1997;52:447–452.

45 Kon OM, Sihra BS, Compton CH, Leonard TB, Kay AB, Barnes NC: Randomised, dose-ranging, placebo-controlled study of chimeric antibody to CD4 (keliximab) in chronic severe asthma. Lancet 1998;352:1109–1113.

46 Jutel M, Pichler WJ, Skrbic D, Urwyler A, Dahinden C, Muller UR: Bee venom immunotherapy results in decrease of IL-4 and IL-5 and increase of IFN-γ secretion in specific allergen-stimulated T cell cultures. J Immunol 1995;154:4187–4194.

47 Secrist H, Chelen CJ, Wen Y, Marshall JD, Umetsu DT: Allergen immunotherapy decreases interleukin-4 production in CD4 + T cells from allergic individuals. J Exp Med 1993;178:2123–2130.

48 Durham SR, Ying S, Varney VA, Jacobson MR, Sudderick RM, Mackay IS, Kay AB, Hamid QA: Grass pollen immunotherapy inhibits allergen-induced infiltration of CD4 + T lymphocytes and eosinophils in the nasal mucosa and increases the number of cells expressing messenger RNA for interferon-γ. J Allergy Clin Immunol 1996;97:1356–1365.

49 Corry DB, Folkesson HG, Warnock ML, Erle DJ, Matthay MA, Wiener-Kronish JP, Locksley RC: Interleukin-4, but not interleukin-5 or eosinophils, is required in a murine model of acute airway hyperreactivity. J Exp Med 1996;183:109–117.

50 Foster PS, Hogan SP, Ramsay AJ, Matthaei KI, Young IG: IL-5 deficiency abolishes eosinophilia, airways hyperreactivity, and lung damage in a mouse asthma model. J Exp Med 1995;183:195–201.

51 Hogan SP, Matthaei KI, Young JM, Koskinen A, Young IG, Foster PS: A novel T cell-regulated mechanism modulating allergen-induced airways hyperreactivity in BALB/c mice independently of IL-4 and IL-5. J Immunol 1998;161:1501–1509.

52   Gavett SH, Chen X, Finkelman F, Wills-Karp M: Depletion of murine CD4+ T lymphocytes prevents antigen-induced airway hyperreactivity and pulmonary eosinophilia. Am J Respir Cell Mol Biol 1994;10:587–593.

53   Li XM, Schofield BH, Wang QF, Kim KH, Huang SK: Induction of pulmonary allergic responses by antigen-specific Th2 cells. J Immunol 1998;160:1378–1384.

54   Wills-Karp M, Luyimbazi J, Xu X, Schofield B, Neben TY, Karp CL, Donaldson DD: Interleukin-13: Central mediator of allergic asthma. Science 1998;282:2258–2261.

55   Grunig G, Warnock M, Wakil AE, Venkayya R, Brombacher F, Rennick DM, Sheppard D, Mohrs M, Donaldson DD, Locksley RM, Corry DB: Requirement for IL-13 independently of IL-4 in experimental asthma. Science 1998;282:2261–2263.

56   Wang J, Palmer K, Lotval J, Milan S, Feng X, Matthaei KI, Gauldie J, Inman MD, Jordana M, Xing Z: Circulating, but not local lung IL-5 is required for the development of antigen-induced airways eosinophilia. J Clin Invest 1998;102:1132–1141.

57   Temann UA, Geba GP, Rankin JA, Flavell RA: Expression of interleukin-9 in the lungs of transgenic mice causes airway inflammation, mast cell hyperplasia and bronchial hyperresponsiveness. J Exp Med 1998;188:1307–1320.

58   Tang W, Geba GP, Zheng T, Ray P, Homer RJ, Kuhn C, Flavell RA, Elias JA: Targeted expression of IL-11 in the murine airway causes lymphocytic inflammation, bronchial remodeling, and airways obstruction. J Clin Invest 1996;98:2845–2853.

59   Zhu Z, Homer RJ, Wang Z, Chen Q, Geba GP, Wang J, Zhang Y, Elias JA: Pulmonary expression of interleukin-13 causes inflammation, mucus hypersecretion, subepithelial fibrosis, physiologic abnormalities and eotaxin production. J Clin Invest 1999;103:779–788.

60   Collins PD, Marleau S, Griffiths-Johnson DA, Jose PJ, Williams TJ: Cooperation between interleukin-5 and the chemokine eotaxin to induce eosinophil accumulation in vivo. J Exp Med 1995;182:1169–1174.

61   Palframan RT, Collins PD, Williams TJ, Rankin SM: Eotaxin induces a rapid release of eosinophils and their progenitors from the bone marrow. Blood 1998;91:2240–2248.

62   O'Garra A: Cytokines induce the development of functionally heterogeneous T helper cell subsets. Immunity 1998;8:275–283.

63   Szabo SJ, Dighe AS, Gubler U, Murphy KM: Regulation of the interleukin-12R β2 subunit expression in developing T helper (Th)1 and Th2 cells. J Exp Med 1997;185:817–824.

64   Rogge L, Barberis-Maino L, Biffi M, Passini N, Presky DH, Gubler U, Sinigaglia F: Selective expression of an interleukin-12 receptor component by human T helper 1 cells. J Exp Med 1997;185:825–831.

65   Robinson D, Shibuya K, Mui A, Zonin F, Murphy E, Sana T, Hartley SB, Menon S, Kastelein R, Bazan F, O'Garra A: IGIF does not drive Th1 development but synergizes with IL-12 for interferon-γ production and activates IRAK and NFκB. Immunity 1997;7:571–581.

66   Xu D, Chan WL, Leung BP, Huang FP, Wheeler R, Piedrafita D, Robinson JH, Liew FY: Selective expression of a stable cell surface molecule on type 2 but not type 1 helper T cells. J Exp Med 1998;187:787–794.

67   Xu D, Chan WL, Leung BP, Hunter D, Schulz K, Carter RW, McInnes IB, Robinson JH, Liew FY: Selective expression and functions of interleukin-18 receptor on T helper (Th) type 1 but not Th2 cells. J Exp Med 1998;188:1485–1492.

68   Szabo SJ, Glimcher LH, Ho IC: Genes that regulate interleukin-4 expression in T cells. Curr Opin Immunol 1997;9:776–781.

69   Zheng W, Flavell RA: The transcription factor GATA-3 is necessary and sufficient for Th2 cytokine gene expression in CD4 T cells. Cell 1997;89:587–596.

70   Zhang DH, Yang L, Ray A: Differential responsiveness of the IL-5 and IL-4 genes to transcription factor GATA-3. J Immunol 1998;161:3817–3821.

71   Yang L, Cohn L, Zhang DH, Homer R, Ray A, Ray P: Essential role of nuclear factor κB in the induction of eosinophilia in allergic airway inflammation. J Exp Med 1998;188:1739–1750.

72   Ouyang W, Ranganath SH, Weindel K, Bhattacharya D, Murphy TL, Sha WC, Murphy KM: Inhibition of Th1 development mediated by GATA-3 through an IL-4-independent mechanism. Immunity 1998;9:745–755.

73 Nakamura Y, Ghaffar O, Olivenstein R, Taha RA, Soussi-Gounni A, Zhang DH, Ray A, Hamid Q: Gene expression of the GATA3 transcription factor is increased in atopic asthma. J Allergy Clin Immunol 1999;103:215–222.

74 Riviere I, Sunshine MJ, Littman DR: Regulation of IL-4 expression by activation of individual alleles. Immunity 1998;9:217–228.

75 Bird J, Brown DR, Mullen AC, Moskowitz NH, Mahowald MA, Sider JR, Gajewski TF, Wang CR, Reiner SL: Helper T cell differentiation is controlled by the cell cycle. Immunity 1998;9:229–237.

76 Sallusto F, Lenig D, Mackay CR, Lanzavecchia A: Flexible programs of chemokine receptor expression on human polarised T helper 1 and 2 lymphocytes. J Exp Med 1998;187:875–883.

77 Zingoni A, Soto H, Hedrick JA, Stoppaccio A, Storlazzi CT, Sinigaglia F, D'Amrosio D, O'Garra A, Robinson DS, Rocchi M, Santoni A, Zlotnick A, Napolitano M: The chemokine receptor CCR8 is preferentially expressed in Th2 but not Th1 cells. J Immunol 1998;161:547–551.

78 Austrup F, Vestweber D, Borges E, Lohning M, Brauer R, Herz U, Renz H, Hallmann R, Scheffold A, Radbruch A, Hamann A: P- and E-selectin mediate recruitment of T-helper-1 but not T-helper-2 cells into inflamed tissues. Nature 1997;385:81–83.

79 Wilkinson J, Holgate ST: Evidence for and against chromosome 5q as a region of interest in asthma and atopy. Clin Exp Allergy 1996;26:861–864.

80 Mitsuyasu H, Izuhara K, Mao XQ, Gao PS, Arinobu Y, Enomoto T, Kawai M, Sasaki S, Dake Y, Hamasaki N, Shirakawa T, Hopkin JM: Ile50Val variant of IL4R α upregulates IgE synthesis and associates with atopic asthma. Nat Genet 1998;19:119–120.

81 Grasso L, Huang M, Sullivan CD, Messler CJ, Kiser MB, Dragwa CR, Holroyd KJ, Renauld JC, Levitt RC, Nicolaides NC: Molecular analysis of human interleukin-9 receptor transcripts in peripheral blood mononuclear cells. J Biol Chem 1998;273:24016–24024.

82 Wills-Karp M, Ewart SL: The genetics of allergen-induced airway hyperresponsiveness in mice. Am J Respir Crit Care Med 1997;156:S89–S96.

83 Beebe AM, Mauze S, Schork NJ, Coffman RL: Serial backcross mapping of multiple loci associated with resistance to Leishmania major in mice. Immunity 1997;6:551–557.

84 Prescott SL, Macaubas C, Smallacombe T, Holt BJ, Sly PD, Holt PG: Development of allergen-specific T-cell memory in atopic and normal children. Lancet 1999;353:196–200.

85 Randolph DA, Carruthers CJ, Szabo SJ, Murphy KM, Chaplin DD: Modulation of airway inflammation by passive transfer of allergen-specific Th1 and Th2 cells in a mouse model of asthma. J Immunol 1999;162:2375–2383.

86 Hansen G, Berry G, DeKruyff RH, Umetsu DT: Allergen-specific Th1 cells fail to counterbalance Th2 cell-induced hyperreactivity but cause severe airway inflammation. J Clin Invest 1999;103:175–183.

87 Akdis CA, Akdis M, Blesken T, Wymann D, Alkan SS, Muller U, Blaser K: Epitope-specific T cell tolerance to phospholipase A$_2$ in bee venom immunotherapy and recovery by IL-2 and IL-15 in vitro. J Clin Invest 1996;98:1676–1683.

88 Norman PS, Ohman JL Jr, Long AA, Creticos PS, Gefter MA, Shaked Z, Wood RA, Eggleston PA, Hafner KB, Rao P, Lichtenstein LM, Jones NH, Nicodemus CF: Treatment of cat allergy with T-cell reactive peptides. Am J Respir Crit Care Med 1996;154:1623–1628.

89 Haselden BM, Kay AB, Larche M: IgE-independent MHC-restricted T cell peptide epitope-induced late asthmatics reactions. J Exp Med 1999;189:1885–1894.

90 Fukaura H, Kent SC, Pietrusewicz MJ, Khoury SJ, Weiner HL, Hafler DA: Induction of circulating myelin basic protein and proteolipid protein-specific transforming growth factor-β1-secreting Th3 T cells by oral administration of myelin in multiple sclerosis patients. J Clin Invest 1996;98:70–77.

91 Groux H, O'Garra A, Bigler M, Rouleau M, Antonenko S, de Vries JE, Roncarolo MG: A CD4+ T-cell subset inhibits antigen-specific T-cell responses and prevents colitis. Nature 1997;389:737–742.

Douglas S. Robinson, MA, MD, FRCP, Senior Lecturer, Allergy and Clinical Immunology,
Imperial College School of Medicine, National Heart and Lung Institute,
Dovehouse Street, London SW3 6LY (UK)
Tel. +44 171 351 8116, Fax +44 171 376 3138, E-Mail d.s.robinson@ic.ac.uk

Robinson DS (ed): Immunological Mechanisms in Asthma and Allergic Diseases.
Chem Immunol. Basel, Karger, 2000, vol 78, pp 62–71

....

The Bronchial Epithelial Origins of Asthma

Stephen T. Holgate

Respiratory Cell and Molecular Biology Research Division,
School of Medicine, University of Southampton, UK

The bronchial epithelium provides an important physical barrier between the external environment and internal tissue milieux. The suprabasal cells are attached to each other and to basal cells, but they may make contact with the basement membrane that is not attached to this structure [1]. Thus, the bronchial epithelium covering the intermediate and large airways may best be described as stratified rather than pseudostratified as often stated. In asthma there is evidence that the epithelium is abnormal. This review makes a case that the epithelium is not only structurally abnormal, but also functionally abnormal to orchestrate many of the airway changes that are characteristic of chronic disease.

Structural Changes in Asthmatic Epithelium

While it has long been recognized that the epithelium is disrupted in severe asthma, there has been debate over whether or not this occurs in milder forms of the disease, the argument being that the biopsy procedure itself leads to artefactual damage to the epithelium. Based on a series of independent studies, there is consensus that, while the epithelium may not appear physically detached in asthma, it exists in a fragile form. This means that with minimal trauma, e.g. bronchoscopy, lavage, columnar cells separate from their basal attachments [2]. Further evidence to support the view that the epithelium is abnormal in asthma is provided by overexpression of the epidermal growth factor receptor (EGFR; *c-erb B1*) [3] and the epithelial isoform of the adhesion molecule CD44 in up to 80% of the airway epithelium [4], events which occur in tissue culture when epithelial cells are stressed or injured and lose contact with their neighbouring cells [5, 6]. The stratified normal epithelium in medium and large airways consists of basal cells that are attached to the basement membrane via hemidesmosomes containing the integrin $\alpha_6\beta_4$ which provides tight binding to laminin [1]. The columnar, goblet and Clara cells are attached to the basal cells by desmosomes, complex adhesion structures that, in addition to providing 'spot welds' to hold the epithelium together, also have important signalling properties. Tight junctions and intermediate junctions are further complex adhesion structures that provide control mechanisms over paracellular transport of small- and large-molecular-weight solutes. Intercellular communication is provided by numerous gap junctions between adjacent epithelial cells. These structures are susceptible to proteolytic cleavage and intracellular control [7].

It has been suggested that the arginine-rich granule proteins of the eosinophil, specifically major basic protein (MBP), are responsible for the epithelial disruption in asthma [8]. While MBP is cytotoxic at high concentration and can activate and detach epithelial cells at lower concentrations, the eosinophil is equipped with additional mechanisms for attacking this structure. The eosinophil is a rich source of the metalloproteinase MMP-9 (gelatinase B) and also contains the naturally occurring tissue inhibitor, TIMP-1 [9]. Bronchoalveolar lavage fluid from patients with active asthma contains high concentrations of MMP-9 assessed by gelatin zymography. MMP-9 is secreted at the leading edge of migrating leukocytes to facilitate their passage through tissues enriched with collagen and other matrix proteins. The epithelium is also able to generate MMP-9 following injury, as well as MMP-2. Following segmental allergen provocation, MMP-9 and TIMP-1 levels increase in airway lining fluid between 2 and 24 h in parallel with eosinophil recruitment. Immunostaining of bronchial biopsies for MMP-9 in patients with mild and severe asthma demonstrates marked extracellular deposition of MMP-9 in the epithelium and matrix [10]. Analysis of MMP-9 and TIMP-1 levels in bronchial biopsies has revealed a close positive relationship in mild asthma, whereas in severe disease the TIMP-1/MMP-9 ratio is markedly reduced. TIMP-1 is also immunolocalized to the epithelium and endothelium, with incomplete immunostaining of the endothelium being observed in severe asthma when compared to mild disease, suggesting either a defect in TIMP-1 production or its increased destruction [10].

The bronchial epithelium contains a rich network of professional antigen-presenting cells – dendritic cells. These are derived from CD34+ precursors that originate in the bone marrow. In the circulation they resemble monocytes, but on recruitment into the airways they lose their CD14 monocyte-like cell surface marker and acquire high levels of expression of MHC class II molecules and CD1. For effective antigen signalling to T cells in local lymphoid collection, dendritic cells need to uptake the antigen efficiently, process this by cathepsin degradation and then select a peptide to present in the cleft of the MHC class II heterodimer to the T-cell receptor (TCR) [11]. Commitment of naïve T cells to a memory phenotype and proliferation of polarized Th-1- or Th-2-like cytokine production requires two additional signals – an interaction between co-stimulatory molecules expressed on dendritic cells and T cells and secretion of selective cytokines from dendritic cells. Of key importance in producing Th-2 cytokines in asthma is an interaction between B7 (CD80 or CD86) on dendritic cells and CD28 on T cells. In the presence of high concentrations of IL-12, antigen presentation by dendritic cells along with co-stimulation polarizes the T-cell response to a Th-1-like phenotype whereas reduced ambient IL-12 (e.g. via PGE_2) and IL-10 polarizes the responses to Th-2 cells. In the asthmatic mucosa the obligatory requirement for these cell-cell interactions has been shown using bronchial explants incubated with allergen for 24 h. Allergen exposure released substantial amounts of IL-5 and IL-13 that was accompanied by increased cytokine gene transcription in the explants [12]. Almost complete abrogation of the Th-2 cytokine response to allergen was achieved by co-incubation with a CTLA-4 immunoglobulin fusion protein [12] or blocking antibodies [13] which intervenes between CD80/86/CD28 signalling to provide a negative signal to the T cell.

The factors that direct the maturation and migration of dendritic cells into the mucosa in asthma are largely unknown. They are known to differentiate from precursors in the presence of GM-CSF and migrate to the lymphatics when exposed to TNF-α [14] and MMP-9 [15]. Dendritic cells in the asthmatic airways also overexpress FcεR1 which greatly increases allergen uptake [16]. Recent studies suggest that the β chain of FcεR1 improves the efficiency of receptor FCεR1 signalling and is under the control of the Th-2 cytokine, IL-4.

Epidemiological studies have provided convincing evidence that atopy (the predisposition to generate IgE to common environmental allergens) is one of the strongest risk factors in asthma, with exposure to allergens in the domestic environment being particularly important. However, while up to 50% of the population may be atopic, only 7–10% of the adult population have diagnosed asthma [17]. Since allergen sensitization most likely occurs throughout the inhaled route, the discrepancy between atopy and clinical asthma deserves explanation. Bronchial biopsy studies in atopic nonasthmatic subjects have revealed low levels of mast cell activation and eosinophil infiltration, suggesting that the lower airway Th-2 response is 'capped' in these subjects. This phenomenon is relevant to why established asthma in childhood may remit during adolescence despite continued allergen exposure. Equally, the ability of low levels of allergen exposure presented repeatedly to the airways in sensitized subjects to enhance rather than diminish airway responsiveness and indices of eosinophil engagement deserves further study since this is opposite to the 'capping' effect observed in animal models with repeated inhaled antigen exposure.

We have used the DO11.10 TCR transgenic mouse to investigate mechanisms of lung-specific downregulation of the pulmonary response to repeated ovalbumin (OA) exposure [18]. These mice express a transgene that expresses a TCR of 16 amino acids of OA. When the transgene is back-crossed onto Balb-c mice, the T cells expressing the clonotypic TCR can be identified in tissues or by flow cytometry using a clonotypic monoclonal antibody. Repeated exposure of the original TCR transgenic mice to aerosolized OA results in a lung eosinophilia over the first 5 days but, on continuing this exposure up to 8–12 days, the T-cell proliferative, IL-2-producing capacity and the inflammatory lung response is lost. Examination of the T-cell contents in the lung of these OA nonresponsive animals showed no changes in total OA-TCR cell numbers but, in contrast to clonotypic T cells isolated from the spleen on draining mediastinal lymph nodes of these animals, the proliferation response to OA or OA peptide was absent. Of considerable interest, the removal of adherent macrophages/monocytes from dispersed lung cells of OA refractory mice restored the OA proliferative response to OA on the OA peptide, suggesting a strong negative signal being provided by the macrophages. Further characterization of these cells indicates that they express many of the markers of dendritic cells but in addition express high concentrations of E-cadherin on adhesion molecules that implicates an interaction between these cells and the epithelium. Whether or not suppressor macrophage/dendritic cells exist in human lungs needs to be determined.

In a further development of this model [18], OA-specific transgenic T cells were polarized in vitro to either a Th-1 phenotype (using IFN-γ and anti-IL-4 Mab) on a Th-2 phenotype (using IL-4 and anti-IFN-γ). Either Th-1 or Th-2 cells were infused into naïve Balb-c mice and the animals were then exposed to consecutive inhalation of OA daily for 8 days and the lung inflammatory and T-cell response followed. Initial OA inhalation cause an eosinophilia in those mice receiving Th-2 cells and a neutrophilia in those receiving Th-1 cells. In both cases, repeated inhalation caused a reduction in T-cell proliferative response and IL-2 production associated with a reduced inflammatory response that again could be restored in vitro by removing the adherent macrophages. In addition, inhibition of cyclooxygenase also enhanced and helped maintain the local immune and inflammatory responses suggesting a key role for cyclooxygenase products. Since a cyclooxygenase-2 inhibitor was equally effective as indomethacin in restoring the responses, it seems likely that it is the inducible enzyme that is important in mediating the actions of these drugs [19].

We suggest that the local downregulation or capping of the T-cell response in both wild-type and TCR transgenic mice is a protective response to prevent the lung becoming overwhelmed with antigen-driven proliferating T cells. The recent observation by Jordana and co-workers [20] that adenoviral gene transfer of GM-CSF to the airway epithelium of mice is able to restore the proliferative and cytokine responses to inhalation challenge suggests that epithelial-derived GM-CSF plays a key role in maintaining an ongoing airway inflammatory response in diseases such as asthma. In this regard, GM-CSF production by the asthmatic epithelium is increased in asthma, an abnormality that we have recently shown persists when asthmatic epithelial cells are grown in tissue culture.

The Epithelium as a Source of Inflammatory Mediators in Asthma

The epithelium in asthma becomes an important source of pro-inflammatory mediators. The altered epithelial phenotype expresses inducible enzymes for mediators (iNOS, cPLA$_2$, COX2, 15-LO and endothelin-1), cytokines (IL-1β, TNF-α, IL-6, oncostatin M, IL-11 and chemokines) and growth factors (EGF, PDGF, GM-CSF, bFGF, TGF-α, TGF-β_1-β_2 and IGF-1) [21]. While these may be induced by cytokines released by inflammatory cells infiltrating the airways such as IFN-γ and TNF-α, an alternative explanation is that these epithelial pro-inflammatory genes are induced by growth factors generated as an integral component of an epithelial repair response. For example, epidermal growth factor (EGF) generated by perturbed epithelial cells can itself active c-erb B receptors on these cells by autocrine mechanisms which, through activation of the transcription factors STAT-1 and STAT-3 leads to the expression of inducible genes such as iNOS and COX-2 [3, 5]. Nuclear factor κ B (NFκB) is another transcription factor linked to epithelial cell stress which is overexpressed at baseline in the asthmatic bronchial epithelium [22] and is further activated by a wide range of epithelial stimuli (e.g. viruses, pollutants, cytokines) and partially suppressed by inhaled corticosteroids [23]. These inflammatory manifestations of tissue stress involving NFκB and TNF-α are not dissimilar to those reported in other chronic inflammatory disorders such as rheumatoid arthritis. Taken together, there are strong indications that stimulated and repairing epithelium plays a key role in augmenting and sustaining airway inflammation.

The Epithelium in Airway Wall Remodelling

In addition to the release of rapidly acting autacoid mediators in asthma, the architecture of the airway wall changes. The most widely recognized change is the deposition of interstitial collagens (type I, V and VI) in the subepithelial lamina reticularis beneath the true basement membrane [24]. This collagen is accompanied by fibronectin developmental forms of laminin and tenascin. The thickness of this collagen band has variously been reported to be dependent of the severity or duration of asthma [25, 26], may occur within the first year or two of life prior to the onset of asthma [27] and may be partially reversed by inhaled corticosteroids or by removal from a causative sensitizing agent (e.g. occupational reactive small-molecular-weight chemicals). The cells responsible for secreting this new collagen are myofibroblasts with the capacity to generate matrix proteins, pro-inflammatory cytokines and whose number correlates with the thickness of the sub-basement membrane layer [28]. These cells also contract with certain spasmogens (e.g. endothelin-1) and maybe precursors of the increased smooth muscle in the asthmatic airway.

In tissue culture, airway myofibroblasts proliferate in the presence of a range of fibroblast growth factors. Many of these, such as TGF-β, EGFs, bFGF, IGF-1, PDGF and endothelin-1, are synthesized by the epithelium and are upregulated in asthma [21]. As with other epithelial-derived mediators, upregulation of secretion appears to be linked to epithelial injury and repair processes [29]. Following segmental allergen provocation of sensitized asthmatic airways, both bFGF and TGF-β are released onto the airway surface but with differing time courses, bFGF being detected within 15 min whereas TGF-β reaches maximum at 24 h. The factors controlling the generation and release of these growth factors have yet to be determined although, in a composite human bronchial epithelial/myofibroblast model, in vitro damage to the overlying epithelium results in proliferation of myofibroblasts that can be inhibited with a cocktail of blocking monoclonal antibodies against bFGF, PDGF, TGF-β, IGF-1 and endothelin-1 antagonist [30]. These and other growth factors may also contribute to the increase in microvasculature and smooth muscle associated with chronic asthma [11, 29]. Little is known about how the airway smooth muscle is regulated in asthma but, along with subepithelial myofibroblasts, they are capable of undergoing a phenotypic change to adopt secretory as well as contractile properties when exposed to PDGF or TGF-β or deprived of serum [31]. Whether or not changes in airway smooth muscle account for the BHR characteristic of asthma is still debated, although many now feel that thickening of the submucosa and adventitial regions of the airway is sufficient to account for the loss of the plateau observed in normal subjects with increasing stimulation. There is also evidence that airway smooth muscle may behave abnormally in chronic asthma by more readily entering a 'latch' phase with loss of actin-myosin cross-link cycling [32].

The Epithelium in Exacerbations of Asthma

Exposure of the airways in asthma to respiratory viruses and ambient air pollutants, such as ozone, oxides of nitrogen and suspended particulates, results in disease exacerbations and progression. We suggest that the epithelium which is abnormal in asthma integrates these environmental signals to create enhanced airway inflammation and remodelling [29].

Respiratory viruses are the most frequent cause of severe exacerbations of asthma both in children and adults. In the case of human rhinoviruses (RV), infection of the epithelium occurs by utilizing the adhesion molecule ICAM-1 which binds to the cavern region of the major class of RV [33]. Once inside the cell, the virus is able to replicate and through an NFκB-dependent pathway upregulate chemokine and other mediator secretion [34]. Of particular interest is the capacity of RV to upregulate its own receptor involving NFκB transcription. A recent finding is the capacity of RV to initiate increased expression of VCAM-1, an adhesion molecule of major importance in eosinophil recruitment and signalling. Epithelial VCAM-1 expression is under the influence of NFκB and GATA-3 transcriptional control. Through the release of cytokines, such as TNF-α and IFN-γ, the presence of ongoing mucosal inflammation characteristic of asthma would render the lower epithelium more susceptible to RV infection by inducing ICAM-1 expression which is under the transcriptional regulation of NFκB. Although >50% of exacerbations of asthma are associated with RV infection [35], it is conceivable that similar mechanisms may operate to increase the susceptibility of the lower airways to other respiratory viruses and microorganisms. Using PCR-based virus detection, exacerbations of asthma have been linked to coronaviruses, adenoviruses, respiratory syncytial viruses, influenza and parainfluenza as well as *Chlamydia pneumonae* and *Myocoplasma pneumonae*, all of which gain access to the lower airway via the respiratory epithelium. Application of PCR to lavage cells and in situ hybridization to lower airway biopsies, RV has been shown to invade the lower airway and colonize the epithelium [36]. Although in asthma this is associated with enhanced allergen sensitivity and prolonged eosinophil recruitment, the mechanisms responsible for these events require clarification.

Ambient air pollutants including ozone, NO_2 and suspended particulates (PM_{10} and $PM_{2.5}$) which accompany summer and winter air pollution episodes also activate the bronchial epithelium via NFκB-dependent pathways leading to enhanced epithelial mediator release and adhesion molecule expression.

The antioxidant status of the airway mucosa and lining fluid is of critical importance in protecting the airway from oxidant-induced air pollutant injury [37]. Our present work would suggest that the air pollutant injury and respiratory virus infection may interact in causing asthma to deteriorate and strengthen the view that, in addition to allergen exposure, these environmental factors are important in directing the airway inflammatory response and clinical expression of asthma. The recent association between asthma and dietary antioxidant status might also be explained on this basis.

Concluding Comments

The bronchial epithelium would seem to be ideally placed for orchestrating the initiation, maintenance and progression of asthma [38, 39]. Taking advantage of the CC-10 Clara cell promoter gene to express cytokine transgenes in mice, restricted to the epithelium, the Th-2 cytokine, IL-13, when expressed solely through this structure, leads to an eosinophil and T-cell-mediated inflammatory response accompanied by subepithelial fibrosis, goblet cell metaplasia and bronchial hyperresponsiveness throughout the airway wall similar to that seen in chronic asthma [40]. Expression of IL-11 results in sub-basement membrane collagen deposition, myofibroblast proliferation, increased airway smooth muscle and BHR similar to the remodelled airway in asthma but in the absence of eosinophilia [41]. These findings provide strong evidence that the epithelium alone is capable of orchestrating much of observed immunopathology of asthma. If true, this view provides a strong rationale for delivering antiasthma drugs that control asthma by the inhaled route so that their pharmacological benefit, such as inhibition of NFκB expression, can be manifest in the epithelium itself in addition to the submucosal cells [42] and raises the interesting question over whether asthma itself starts as a primary abnormality of this structure.

References

1   Montefort SL, Baker J, Roche WR, Holgate ST: The distribution of adhesive mechanisms in the normal bronchial epithelium. Eur Resp J 1993;6:1257–1263.
2   Montefort S, Roberts JA, Beasley CR, Holgate ST, Roche WR: The site of disruption of the bronchial epithelium in asthmatics and non-asthmatics. Thorax 1992;47:499–503.
3   Puddicombe SM, Polosa R, Richter A, Krishna MT, Howarth PH, Holgate ST, et al: The involvement of the epidermal growth factor receptor in epithelial repair in asthma. FASEB J 2000;14:1362–1374.
4   Lackie PM, Baker JE, Günthert U, Holgate ST: Expression of CD44 isoforms is increased in the airway epithelium of asthmatic subjects. Am J Respir Cell Mol Biol 1997;16:14–22.
5   Davies DE, Polosa R, Puddicombe SM, Richter A, Holgate ST: The epidermal growth factor receptor and its ligand family: Their potential role in repair and remodelling in asthma. Allergy 1999;54:771–783.

6   Leir SH, Baker JE, Holgate ST, Lackie PM: Increased CD44 expression in bronchial epithelial repair following mechanical damage or plating at low cell densities. Am J Physiol 2000, in press.

7   Wan H, Winton HL, Soeller C, Tovey ER, Gruenert DC, Thompson PJ, Stewart GA, Taylor GW, Garrod DR, Cannell MB, Robinson C: Der p 1 facilitates transepithelial allergen delivery by disruption of tight junctions. J Clin Invest 1999;104:123–133.

8   Seminario MC, Adeolphson CR, Gleich GJ: Eosinophils: Granule proteins; in Holgate ST, Busse WW (eds): Inflammatory Mechanisms in Asthma. Lung Biology in Health and Disease. New York, Dekker, 1998, vol 117, pp 157–177.

9   Mantino G, Capony F, Bousquet J: Balance in asthma between matrix metalloproteases and their inhibitors. J Allergy Clin Immunol 1999;104:530–533.

10 Dahlén B, Shute JK, Howarth PH: Immunohistochemical localisation of the matrix metalloproteases MMP-3 and MMP-9 within the airways in asthma. Thorax 1999;54:590–596.

11 Holt PH, Macaubus C, Stumbles PA, Sly PD: The role of allergy in the development of asthma. Nature 1999;403(suppl):B12–B17.

12 Jaffar ZH, Roberts K, Pandit A, Linsley P, Djukanovic R, Holgate ST: B7 costimulation is required for IL-5 and IL-13 secretion by bronchial biopsy tissue of atopic asthmatic subjects in response to allergen stimulation. Am J Respir Cell Mol Biol 1999;20:153–162.

13 Jaffar ZH, Stanciu L, Pandit A, Lordan J, Holgate ST, Roberts K: Essential role for both CD80 and CD86 costimulation, but not CD40 interactions, in allergen-induced Th2 cytokine production from asthmatic bronchial tissue: Role for $\alpha\beta$, bot not $\gamma\delta$, T cells. J Immunol 1999;163:6283–6291.

14 Holt PG, McWilliam AS: Macrophage and dendritic cell populations in airway tissues; in Holgate ST, Busse WW (eds). Inflammatory Mechanisms in Asthma. Lung Biology in Health and Disease. New York, Dekker, 1998, vol 117, pp 401–441.

15 Kobayashi Y, Matsumoto M, Kotani M, Makino T: Possible involvement of matrix metalloproteinase-9 in Langerhans cell migration and maturation. J Immunol 1999;163:5989–5993.

16 Turner H, Kinet JP: Signalling through the high affinity IgE receptor, FcεR1. Nature 1999;402(suppl): B24–B30.

17 Pearce N, Pekkanen J, Beasley R: How much asthma is really attributable to atopy? Thorax 1999; 54:268–272.

18 Lee SC, Jaffar Z, Wan KS, Bodey K, Holgate ST, Roberts K: Regulation of pulmonary T cell responses to inhaled antigen: Role of Th1- and Th2-mediated inflammation. J Immunol 1999;162: 6867–6879.

19 Wan KS, Jaffar ZH, Holgate ST, Roberts K: The role of prostaglandins in regulating Th-1 and Th-2 responses. Immunology 1999;98(suppl 1):38.

20 Stämpli MR, Wiley RE, Neigh GS, Gajewsk BU, Lei XF, Snider DP, Xing Z, Jordana M: GM-CSF transgene expression in the airways allows aerosolised ovalbumin to induce allergic sensitisation in mice. J Clin Invest 1998;102:1704–1714.

21 Chung KF, Barnes PF: Cytokines in asthma. Thorax 1999;54:825–857.

22 Wilson SJ, Leon BA, Anderson D, Manning A, Holgate ST: Immunohistochemical analysis of the activation of NFκB and expression of associated cytokines and adhesion molecules in models of allergic inflammation. J Pathol 1999;189:265–272.

23 Wilson SJ, Wallin A, Della-Cioppa G, Sandström T, Holgate ST: Effects of budesonide and formoterol on NFκB, adhesion molecules and cytokines in asthma. Submitted for Publication.

24 Roche WR, Beasley R, Williams J, Holgate ST: Subepithelial fibrosis in the bronchi of asthmatics. Lancet 1989;i:520–524.

25 Minshall EM, Leung DYM, Martin RJ, Song YL, Cameron L, Ernst P, Hamid Q: Eosinophil-associated TGF-β_1 mRNA expression and airways fibrosis in asthma. Am J Respir Cell Mol Biol 1997;17:326–333.

26 Chetta A, Foresi A, Del Donno M, Bertorelli G, Pesci A, Olivieri D: Airways remodelling is a distinctive feature of asthma and is related to severity of disease. Chest 1997;III:852–857.

27 Warner JO, Marguet C, Rao R, Roche WR, Pohunek P: Inflammatory mechanisms in childhood asthma. Clin Exp Allergy 1998;28(suppl 5):71–75.

28 Brewster CED, Howarth PH, Djukanovic R, Wilson J, Holgate ST, Roche WR: Myofibroblasts and subepithelial fibrosis in asthma. Am J Respir Cell Mol Biol 1990;3:507–511.

29   Holgate ST, Lackie PM, Davies DE, Roche WR, Walls AF: The bronchial epithelium as a key regulator of airway inflammation and remodelling in asthma. Clin Exp Allergy 1999;29(suppl 2): 90–95.

30   Zhang S, Smartt H, Holgate ST, Roche WR: Growth factors secreted by bronchial epithelial cells control myofibroblasts proliferation: An in vitro co-culture model of airway remodelling in asthma. Lab Invest 1999;79:395–405.

31   Solway JJ, Fredberg JJ: Perhaps airway smooth muscle dysfunction contributes to asthmatic bronchial hyperresponsiveness after all. Am J Respir Cell 1997;17:144–146.

32   Fredberg J, Inouye DS, Mijailovich SM, Butler JP: Perturbed equilibrium of myosin-binding in airway smooth muscle and its implications in bronchospasm. Am J Respir Crit Care Med 1999; 159:959–967.

33   Ohlin A, Hoover-Litty H, Sanderson G, Paessens A, Johnston SL, Holgate ST, Huguenel E, Greve JM: Spectrum of activity of soluble intercellular adhesion molecule 1 against rhinovirus reference strains and field isolates. Antimicrob Agents Chemother 1994;38:1413–1415.

34   Gern JE, Lemanske RF, Busse WW: The role of rhinoviruses in virus-induced asthma; in Marone G, Austen K, Holgate ST, Kay AB, Lichtenstein LM (eds): Asthma and Allergic Diseases: Physiology, Immunopharmacology and Treatment. London, Academic Press, 1998, pp 293–320.

35   Johnston SL, Pattemore PK, Sanderson G, Smith S, Lampe F, Josephs L, Symington P, O'Toole S, Myint SH, Tyrrell DAJ, Holgate ST: Community study of role of viral infections in exacerbations of asthma in school children in the community. Br Med J 1995;310:1225–1229.

36   Papadopoulos NG, Bates PJ, Bardin PG, Papi A, Leir SH, Fraenhel DJ, Holgate ST, Johnston SB: Rhinovirus infect the lower airways. J Infect Dis 2000, in press.

37   Krishna MT, Madden J, Teran LT, Biscione GL, Lau LCK, Withers NJ, Sandström T, Mudway I, Kelly FJ, Walls A, Frew AJ, Holgate ST: Effects of 0.2 ppm ozone on biomarkers of inflammation in bronchoalveolar lavage fluid and bronchial mucosa of healthy human subjects. Eur Resp J 1998; 11:1294–1300.

38   Elias JA, Zhu Z, Chupp G, Homer RJ: Airway remodelling in asthma. J Clin Invest 1999;104: 1001–1006.

39   Busse W, Elias J, Sheppard D, Banks-Schlegel S: NHLBI Workshop. Airway remodelling and repair. Am J Respir Crit Care Med 1999;160:1035–1042.

40   Zhu Z, Homer RJ, Wang Z, Chen Q, Geba GP, Wang J, Zhang Y, Elias JA: Pulmonary expression of interleukin-13 causes inflammation, mucus hypersecretion, subepithelial fibrosis, physiologic abnormalities and eotaxin production. J Clin Invest 1999;103:779–788.

41   Tang W, Geba GP, Zheng T, Ray P, Homer RJ, Kuhn C III, Flavell RA: Targeted expression of IL-11 in the murine airway causes airway obstruction, bronchial remodelling and lymphocytic inflammation. J Clin Invest 1996;98:2845–2853.

42   Barnes PJ: Therapeutic strategies for allergic diseases. Nature 1999;402(suppl):B31–B38.

Stephen T. Holgate, MRC Clinical Professor of Immunopharmacology,
Director, Respiratory Cell and Molecular Biology Research Division, School of Medicine,
University of Southampton, Level D, Centre Block, Southampton General Hospital,
Southampton SO16 6YD (UK)
Tel. +44 23 80 796960/794730, Fax +44 23 80 701771, E-Mail sth@soton.ac.uk

Robinson DS (ed): Immunological Mechanisms in Asthma and Allergic Diseases.
Chem Immunol. Basel, Karger, 2000, vol 78, pp 72–80

....

Molecular Basis for Corticosteroid Action in Asthma

Peter J. Barnes

Department of Thoracic Medicine, National Heart and Lung Institute,
Imperial College, London, UK

Introduction

Corticosteroids are by far the most effective treatment currently available for asthma. The widespread use of glucocorticoids is in asthma and inhaled glucocorticoids have revolutionized treatment and have now become the mainstay of therapy for patients with chronic disease [1]. There have been important advances in our understanding of how glucocorticoids suppress inflammation [2].

I am pleased to contribute to this Special Supplement celebrating Barry Kay's 60th birthday. Barry and I have worked closely and productively together for over 10 years since I joined the National Heart and Lung Institute and have had many long and fruitful discussions about asthma mechanisms. His research has identified key cellular targets for the anti-inflammatory actions of corticosteroid in asthma and he has had a long-standing interest in the mechanisms of action of corticosteroids in asthma. He was one of the first to recognize the existence of corticosteroid resistance in asthma and has contributed enormously to our understanding of the mechanisms involved. Elucidating the molecular action of corticosteroid in asthma may help understand the mechanisms involved in the complex chronic inflammatory process in asthma and may point the way to the development of improved glucocorticoids and more specific anti-inflammatory therapies in the future.

Glucocorticoid Receptors

Glucocorticoid receptors (GR) are members of the nuclear receptor superfamily that includes other steroids (oestrogen, progesterone) and receptors for vitamins (vitamins A and D) and thyroid hormone. GR are transcription factors, proteins that bind to DNA to regulate the transcription of several steroid-responsive target genes [3]. GR are expressed in most types of cell and in human lung there is a high level of expression in airway epithelium and the endothelium of bronchial vessels [4]. GR mRNA and protein expression in bronchial biopsies and epithelial cell brushings is unchanged in asthmatic and COPD patients compared with normal subjects [4, 5].

The inactive GR is bound to a protein complex which includes two molecules of 90 kDa heat-shock protein (hsp90) and an immunophilin, which act as molecular chaperones, protecting the nuclear localization site. Glucocorticoids bind to GR in the cytoplasm, resulting in dissociation of these molecules and rapid nuclear localization and DNA binding. GR form homodimers to interact with glucocorticoid response elements (GRE) with the sequence 5'-GGTACAnnnTGTTCT-3', resulting in histone acetylation on lysines 5 and 16 of histone H4 [6] and increased gene transcription. GR utilizes the co-activator molecule CREB-binding protein (CBP) to enhance transcription, an effect that is blocked by the adenovirus protein E1A [7]. GR interacts with CBP either directly [8] or through binding of GR to an accessory coactivator, such as steroid receptor coactivator-1 (SRC-1) [9].

Relatively few genes have GRE sequences. One well-studied example is the human β_2-adrenergic receptor gene which has at least three GREs [10]. Corticosteroids increase transcription of β_2-receptors in animal and human lung and this may prevent tolerance to the effects of β_2-agonists by compensating for their down-regulation [11, 12]. Corticosteroids also increase the transcription of several anti-inflammatory proteins, including lipocortin-1, secretory leukoprotease inhibitor, CC-10 and IL-1 receptor antagonist and these effects are presumably also mediated via GREs in the promoter regions of these genes [2]. Corticosteroids have also been reported to increase the expression of IκB-α in lymphocytes and thus to inhibit nuclear factor-κB (NF-κB), a transcription factor that regulates the expression many inflammatory genes that are expressed in asthmatic airways [13, 14], but this has not been seen in other cell types, including airway epithelial cells [15–17]. The IκB-α gene does not appear to have any GRE consensus sequence so any effect of corticosteroids is probably mediated via other transcription factors.

The major effect of corticosteroids in inflammation is to repress the expression of multiple inflammatory genes. Although this was once believed to be due to an interaction with negative GRE sequences, very few true negative GREs have been identified. One example is the osteocalcin gene which is involved in bone formation. Osteocalcin is repressed by GR acting through a positive GRE overlapping the TATA box at the start site of transcription, thus blocking binding of the basal transcription complex and blocking mRNA expression [18].

Interaction with Other Transcription Factors

Few, if any, of the inflammatory and immune genes that are switched off by steroids in asthma appear to have negative GREs in their promoter sequences, suggesting that there must be some less direct inhibitory mechanism. The inhibitory effect of corticosteroids appears to be due largely to an inhibitory effect on the action of proinflammatory transcription factors, such as AP-1, NF-κB and C/EBPβ, that mediate the expression of multiple inflammatory genes [2]. This may be mediated via a direct protein-protein interaction between ligand-activated GR and the activated transcription factors. Direct protein-protein interactions have been demonstrated between GR and AP-1 [19], between the p65 component of NF-κB [20–22] and some STAT (signal transduction-activated transcription) proteins, such as STAT3 [23], STAT5 [24] and STAT6 [25], suggesting that glucocorticoids modulate either the binding or activation of these transcription factors and thus modify the expression of inflammatory genes. However, there is increasing evidence that these direct protein interactions may be an artefact of the expression systems with transfected cells that have been used to study these interactions. While high concentrations of corticosteroids have an inhibitory effect on NF-κB activation in vitro, this is only partial and yet corticosteroids markedly inhibit the expression of genes that are regulated via this transcription factor [16]. Furthermore, we have found that at therapeutic doses of an inhaled corticosteroid that are effective in suppressing inflammation in patients with asthma there is no inhibition of NF-κB activation in bronchial biopsies [26]. This suggests that some other mechanism must account for the potent inhibitory action of corticosteroids on inflammatory genes in asthma.

Effects on Histone Acetylation

There is increasing evidence that glucocorticoids have effects on the chromatin structure of DNA. The repressive action of steroids may be because of competition between GR and the binding sites on CBP for other transcription factors, including AP-1, NF-κB and STATs [27–30]. Activated GR may bind to several transcription corepressor molecules, such as NCoR1 and GRIP1, that associate with proteins that have histone deacetylase activity [31]. This results in deacetylation of histones, increased tightening of DNA round histone residues and thus reduced access of transcription factors such as AP-1 and NF-κB to their binding sites and repression of inflammatory genes [32] (fig. 1). Corticosteroids, at low concentrations, may activate histone deacetylation by recruitment of histone deacetylases to the transcriptional complex, thus revers-

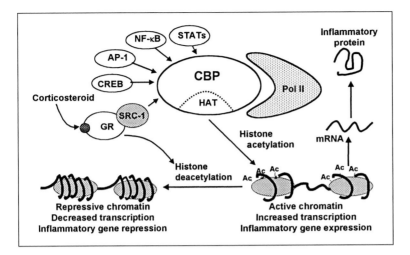

Fig. 1. The effect of corticosteroids on gene transcription is mediated via effects on histone acetylation and deacetylation. Transcription factors, such as STATs, AP-1 and NF-κB, bind to the coactivator molecule CREB-binding protein (CBP), which has intrinsic histone acetyltransferase (HAT) activity, resulting in acetylation (Ac) of histone proteins around which DNA is wound in the chromosome. This leads to unwinding of DNA (active chromatin structure) and this allows increased binding of transcription factors resulting in increased gene transcription through the activation of RNA polymerase II (Pol II). Glucocorticoid receptors (GR) after activation by high concentrations of corticosteroids bind to a steroid receptor coactivator molecule (SRC-1) which interacts with CBP, resulting in acetylation of histone, with increased transcription of genes, such as anti-inflammatory genes. Low concentrations of corticosteroids interact with GR to result in deacetylation of histone and this reverses the acetylation induced by transcription factors, such as NF-κB and AP-1, thus silencing the transcription of inflammatory genes.

ing the increased transcription of inflammatory genes induced by inflammatory stimuli such as IL-1β and TNF-α [33].

Recently, corticosteroids have also been shown to prevent c-Jun phosphorylation by Jun-N-terminal kinase (JNK), and thus the activation of AP-1 and other JNK-activated transcription factors, such as Elk-1 and ATF-2 [34, 35]. Interference with the JNK signalling pathway represents an alternative mechanism by which corticosteroids may antagonize AP-1 activation.

Anti-Inflammatory Actions in Asthma

Corticosteroids are very effective in suppressing inflammation in asthmatic airways, but have little effect in COPD. In asthmatic airways many different inflammatory genes are repressed, including cytokines, inflammatory enzymes, adhesion molecules and receptors and this is likely to involve the interaction of GR with several transcription factors through the molecular mechanisms described above [36].

Corticosteroids may suppress airway inflammation by increasing the transcription for anti-inflammatory genes. For example, inhaled corticosteroids increase the expression of IL-1 receptor antagonist in airway epithelial cells in asthmatic patients [37]. Inhaled corticosteroids also increase the release of IL-10, a potent anti-inflammatory cytokine, from alveolar macrophages of asthmatic patients [38]. At one time it was proposed that lipocortin-1 (annexin-1), which has phospholipase A_2 inhibitory activity, might account for the anti-inflammatory effects of corticosteroids through inhibition of prostaglandin and leukotriene synthesis. However, inhaled corticosteroids appear to have no effect on the release of lipocortin-1 in asthmatic patients [39].

It is more likely that the major anti-inflammatory effect of corticosteroids is mediated by an inhibitory effect on the transcription factors, such as AP-1 and NF-κB, that are responsible for the increased expression of inflammatory genes and proteins in asthma. These proteins include inflammatory cytokines (such as IL-1, TNF-α, IL-6), chemokines involved in eosinophil recruitment (such as eotaxin and RANTES), adhesion molecules (ICAM-1, VCAM-1), inflammatory enzymes (inducible nitric oxide synthase, inducible cyclooxygenase, cytosolic phospholipase A_2) and inflammatory receptors (neurokinin-1, neurokinin-2, bradykinin-1 and IL-2 receptors). Corticosteroids potently inhibit the expression of IL-5 in T-lymphocytes and this is likely to be mediated via an inhibitory effect on AP-1, which is a critical component of the transcription factor nuclear factor of activated T cells (NF-AT) [40].

Corticosteroid-Resistant Asthma

A small proportion of asthmatic patients are corticosteroid-resistant and fail to respond to even high doses of oral steroids [41, 42]. Similar resistance is reported in other chronic inflammatory diseases, such as inflammatory bowel disease and rheumatoid arthritis, but the phenomenon has been studied most carefully in patients with asthma. Monocytes and T lymphocytes isolated from these patients have an impaired response to corticosteroids in vitro [43, 44]. In some patients there is a reduction in the number or affinity of GR and this can be mimicked by incubation of T cells with IL-2 and IL-4 1 [45]. These changes are reversed by the p38 MAPK inhibitor SB203580, suggesting that this pathway may be contributory to corticosteroid resistance [46]. The relatively small changes in GR affinity cannot fully account for the lack of effect of corticosteroids in these patients, however. There is also a marked impairment of GRE binding after exposure of mononuclear cells to corticosteroids in vitro compared to cells from normal individuals and corticosteroid-sensitive asthmatics [47]. This is associated with a marked reduction in the number of activated GR within the nucleus that are available for binding. In the same patients there is a reduced inhibitory effect of corticosteroids on AP-1 activation, but not on NF-κB or CREB activation [48]. Furthermore, there is an increase in the baseline activity of AP-1 and activation of AP-1 with phorbol esters shows a greatly exaggerated expression of c-Fos due to increased gene transcription [49]. This appears to be due to excessive activation of JNK at baseline and in response to TNF-α [50]. The increased activation of AP-1 may result in sequestration of GR so that no receptors are available for inhibiting NF-κB, C/EBP etc., thus resulting in steroid resistance. This resistance will be seen at the site of inflammation where cytokines are produced – i.e. in the airways of asthmatic patients, but not at noninflamed sites. This may explain why patients with steroid-resistant asthma are not resistant to the endocrine and metabolic effects of steroids, and thus develop steroid side effects [51]. Whether this abnormality is inherited is not yet certain, although there is often a positive family history of asthma in patients with steroid-resistant asthma, indicating that genetic factors may be important.

Therapeutic Implications

The two actions of the GR, transactivation and transrepression, can be distinguished in cell lines by mutations of the DNA-binding site or the dimerization domain [52]. In addition, several novel steroid ligands, such as RU24858, RU486 and ZK98299, distinguish between corticosteroid-induced transactivation and inhibition of NF-κB and AP-1 in reporter gene assays [15, 52, 53]. In a T-cell line transfected with a mutant form of GR it has been possible to differentiate interactions with AP-1 and NF-κB [54]. The clinical relevance of these effects of GR mutants is indicated by the construction of a GR dimerization-deficient mutant mouse model in which GR is unable to dimerize and therefore bind to DNA, thus separating the transactivation and transrepression activities of corticosteroids [55]. These animals, in contrast to GR knockout animals, survive to adulthood and allow dexamethasone to suppress AP-1-driven collagenase gene expression but not several GRE-mediated functions, such as cortisol suppression. Interestingly, T-cell apoptosis was not affected. Studies on the anti-inflammatory effects of corticosteroids in these animals are waiting to be determined. These studies raise the possibility that corticosteroids may be developed that can suppress inflammation, but may have less side effects which are largely mediated by transactivation effects and DNA binding.

The recognition that transactivation of genes by corticosteroids is mediated by increased histone acetylation and that transrepression is linked to deacetylation may allow a clearer separation of these actions and the development of novel drugs that might retain most of the anti-inflammatory effects, while avoiding side effects of corticosteroids, such as effects on bone metabolism, connective tissue and adrenal suppression.

References

1   Barnes PJ: Inhaled glucocorticoids for asthma. N Engl J Med 1995;332: 868–875.
2   Barnes PJ: Anti-inflammatory actions of glucocorticoids: Molecular mechanisms. Clin Sci 1998;94: 557–572.
3   Beato M, Herrlich P, Schutz G: Steroid hormone receptors: Many actors in search of a plot. Cell 1995;83:851–857.
4   Adcock IM, Gilbey T, Gelder CM, Chung KF, Barnes PJ: Glucocorticoid receptor localization in normal human lung and asthmatic lung. Am J Respir Crit Care Med 1996;154:771–782.
5   Vachier I, Chiappara G, Vignola AM, et al: Glucocorticoid receptors in bronchial epithelial cells in asthma. Am J Respir Crit Care Med 1998;158:963–970.
6   Ito K, Adcock IM, Barnes PJ: Different histone acetylation induced by glucocorticoids and by IL-1β in human epithelial cells (A549). Am J Respir Crit Care Med 1999;159:A442.
7   Smith CL, Onate SA, Tsai MJ, O'Malley BW: CREB binding protein acts synergistically with steroid receptor coactivator-1 to enhance steroid receptor-dependent transcription. Proc Natl Acad Sci USA 1996;93:8884–8888.
8   Torchia J, Rose DW, Inostroza J, Kamei Y, Westin S, Glass CK, Rosenfeld MG: The trancriptional coactivator p/CIP binds CBP and mediates nuclear receptor function. Nature 1997;387:677–684.
9   Spencer TE, Jenster G, Burcin MM, et al: Steroid receptor coactivator-1 is a histone acetyltransferase. Nature 1997;389:194–198.
10 Collins S, Altschmied J, Herbsman O, Caron MG, Mellon PL, Lefkowitz RJ: A cAMP element in the β₂-adrenergic receptor gene confers autoregulation by cAMP. J Biol Chem 1990;265:19930–19935.
11 Mak JCW, Nishikawa M, Barnes PJ: Glucocorticosteroids increase β2-adrenergic receptor transcription in human lung. Am J Physiol 1995;12:L41–L46.
12 Mak JCW, Nishikawa M, Shirasaki H, Miyayasu K, Barnes PJ: Protective effects of a glucocorticoid on down-regulation of pulmonary β₂-adrenergic receptors in vivo. J Clin Invest 1995;96:99–106.
13 Auphan N, DiDonato JA, Rosette C, Helmberg A, Karin M: Immunosuppression by glucocorticoids: Inhibition of NF-κB activity through induction of IκB synthesis. Science 1995;270:286–290.
14 Barnes PJ, Karin M: Nuclear factor-κB: A pivotal transcription factor in chronic inflammatory diseases. N Engl J Med 1997;336:1066–1071.
15 Heck S, Bender K, Kullmann M, Gottlicher M, Herrlich P, Cato AC: I κBα-independent down-regulation of NF-κB activity by glucocorticoid receptor. EMBO J 1997;16:4698–4707.
16 Newton R, Hart LA, Stevens DA, Bergmann M, Donnelly LE, Adcock IM, Barnes PJ: Effect of dexamethasone on interleukin-1β-induced nuclear factor-κB and κB-dependent transcription in epithelial cells. Eur J Biochem 1998;254:81–89.
17 Adcock IM, Nasuhara Y, Stevens DA, Barnes PJ: Ligand-induced differentiation of glucocorticoid receptor trans-repression and transactivation: Preferential targeting of NF-κB and lack of I-κB involvement. Br J Pharmacol 1999;127:1003–1011.
18 Meyer T, Carlstedt-Duke J, Starr DB: A weak TATA box is a prerequisite for glucocorticoid-dependent repression of the osteocalcin gene. J Biol Chem 1997;272:30709–30714.

19   Pfahl M: Nuclear receptor/AP-1 interaction. Endocr Rev 1993;14:651–658.

20   Ray A, Prefontaine KE: Physical association and functional antagonism between the p65 subunit of transcription factor NF-κB and the glucocorticoid receptor. Proc Natl Acad Sci USA 1994;91: 752–756.

21   Caldenhoven E, Liden J, Wissink S, et al: Negative cross-talk between RelA and the glucocorticoid receptor: A possible mechanism for the anti-inflammatory action of glucocorticoids. Mol Endocrinol 1995;9:401–412.

22   Adcock IM, Brown CR, Gelder CM, Shirasaki H, Peters MJ, Barnes PJ: The effects of glucocorticoids on transcription factor activation in human peripheral blood mononuclear cells. Am J Physiol 1995; 37:C331–C338.

23   Zhang Z, Jones S, Hagood JS, Fuentes NL, Fuller GM: STAT3 acts as a co-activator of glucocorticoid receptor signaling. J Biol Chem 1997;272:30607–30610.

24   Stocklin E, Wissler M, Gouilleux F, Groner B: Functional interactions between Stat5 and the glucocorticoid receptor. Nature 1996;383:726–728.

25   Moriggl R, Berchtold S, Friedrich K, et al: Comparison of the transactivation domains of Stat5 and Stat6 in lymphoid cells and mammary epithelial cells. Mol Cell Biol 1997;17:3663–3678.

26   Hart L, Lim S, Adcock I, Barnes PJ, Chung KF: Effects of inhaled corticosteroid therapy on expression and DNA-binding activity of nuclear factor-κB in asthma. Am J Respir Crit Care Med 2000;161:224–231.

27   Arias J, Alberts AS, Brindle P, et al: Activation of cAMP and mitogen responsive genes relies on a common nuclear factor. Nature 1994;370:226–229.

28   Kamei Y, Xu L, Heinzel T, et al: A CBP integrator complex mediates transcriptional activation and AP-1 inhibition by nuclear receptors. Cell 1996;85:403–414.

29   Zhang JJ, Vinkemeier U, Gu W, Chakravarti D, Horvath CM, Darnell JE: Two contact regions between STAT1 and CBP/p300 in interferon-γ signalling. Proc Natl Acad Sci USA 1996;93:15092–15096.

30   Perkins ND, Felzien LK, Betts JC, Leung K, Beach DH, Nabel GJ: Regulation of NF-κB by cyclin-dependent kinases associated with the p300 coactivator. Science 1997;275:523–526.

31   Ding XF, Anderson CM, Ma H, Hong H, Uht RM, Kushner PJ, Stallcup MR: Nuclear receptor-binding sites of coactivators glucocorticoid receptor interacting protein 1 (GRIP1) and steroid receptor coactivator 1 (SRC-1): Multiple motifs with different binding specificities. Mol Endocrinol 1998;12:302–313.

32   Wolffe AP: Sinful repression. Nature 1997;387:16–17.

33   Ito K, Adcock IM, Barnes PJ: Different histone acetylation induced by glucocorticoids and IL-1β in human epithelial cells (A549). Am J Respir Crit Care Med 1999;159:A442.

34   Caelles C, Gonzalez-Sancho JM, Munoz A: Nuclear hormone receptor antagonism with AP-1 by inhibition of the JNK pathway. Genes Dev 1997;11:3351–3364.

35   Swantek JL, Cobb MH, Geppert TD: Jun N-terminal kinase/stress-activated protein kinase (JNK/SAPK) is required for lipopolysaccharide stimulation of tumor necrosis factor α (TNF-α) translation: Glucocorticoids inhibit TNF-α translation by blocking JNK/SAPK. Mol Cell Biol 1997;17:6274–6282.

36   Barnes PJ: Mechanism of action of glucocorticoids in asthma. Am J Respir Crit Care Med 1996; 154:S21–S27.

37   Sousa AR, Trigg CJ, Lane SJ, Hawksworth R, Nakhosteen JA, Poston RN, Lee TH: Effect of inhaled glucocorticoids on IL-1β and IL-1 receptor antagonist (IL-1 ra) expression in asthmatic bronchial epithelium. Thorax 1997;52:407–410.

38   John M, Lim S, Seybold J, Robichaud A, O'Connor B, Barnes PJ, Chung KF: Inhaled corticosteroids increase IL-10 but reduce MIP-1α, GM-CSF and IFN-γ release from alveolar macrophages in asthma. Am J Respir Crit Care Med 1998;157:256–262.

39   Hall SE, Lim S, Witherden IR, Tetley TD, Barnes PJ, Kamal AM, Smith SF: Lung type II cell and macrophage annexin I release: Differential effects of two glucocorticoids. Am J Physiol 1999; 276:L114–L121.

40   Mori A, Kaminuma O, Suko M, et al: Two distinct pathways of interleukin-5 synthesis in allergen-specific human T-cell clones are suppressed by glucocorticoids. Blood 1997;89:2891–2900.

41 Barnes PJ, Greening AP, Crompton GK: Glucocorticoid resistance in asthma. Am J Respir Crit Care Med 1995;152:125S–140S.

42 Szefler SJ, Leung DY: Glucocorticoid-resistant asthma: Pathogenesis and clinical implications for management. Eur Respir J 1997;10:1640–1647.

43 Corrigan C, Brown PH, Barnes NC, Szefler SJ, Tsai J, Frew AJ, Kay AB: Glucocorticoid resistance in chronic asthma: Glucocorticoid pharmacokinetics, glucocorticoid receptor characteristics and inhibition of peripheral blood T cell proliferation by glucocorticoids in vitro. Am Rev Respir Dis 1991;144:1016–1025.

44 Corrigan CJ, Brown PH, Barnes NC, Tsai J, Frew AJ, Kay AB: Peripheral blood T lymphocyte activation and comparison of the T lymphocyte inhibitory effects of glucocorticoids and cyclosporin A. Am Rev Respir Dis 1991;144:1026–1032.

45 Kam JC, Szefler SJ, Surs W, Sher FR, Leung DYM: Combination IL-2 and IL-4 reduces glucocorticoid-receptor binding affinity and T cell response to glucocorticoids. J Immunol 1993;151: 3460–3466.

46 Matthews JG, Irusen E, Chung KF, Barnes PJ, Adcock IM: p38 mitogen-activated protein kinase mediates IL-2 and IL-4 mediated changes in glucocorticoid receptor affinity. Am J Respir Crit Care Med 1999;157:A336.

47 Adcock IM, Lane SJ, Brown CA, Peters MJ, Lee TH, Barnes PJ: Differences in binding of glucocorticoid receptor to DNA in steroid-resistant asthma. J Immunol 1995;154:3000–3005.

48 Adcock IM, Lane SJ, Brown CA, Lee TH, Barnes PJ: Abnormal glucocorticoid receptor/AP-1 interaction in steroid resistant asthma. J Exp Med 1995;182:1951–1958.

49 Lane SJ, Adcock IM, Richards D, Hawrylowicz C, Barnes PJ, Lee TH: Corticosteroid-resistant bronchial asthma is associated with increased c-Fos expression in monocytes and T-lymphocytes. J Clin Invest 1998;102:2156–2164.

50 Adcock IM, Brady H, Lim S, Karin M, Barnes PJ: Increased JUN kinase activity in peripheral blood monocytes from steroid-resistant asthmatic subjects. Am J Respir Crit Care Med 1997;155: A288.

51 Lane SJ, Atkinson BA, Swimanathan R, Lee TH: Hypothalamic-pituitary axis in corticosteroid-resistant asthma. Am J Respir Crit Care Med 1996;153:1510–1514.

52 Heck S, Kullmann M, Grast A, Ponta H, Rahmsdorf HJ, Herrlich P, Cato ACB: A distinct modulating domain in glucocorticoid receptor monomers in the repression of activity of the transcription factor AP-1. EMBO J 1994;13:4087–4095.

53 Vayssiere BM, Dupont S, Choquart A, et al: Synthetic glucocorticoids that dissociate transactivation and AP-1 transrepression exhibit anti-inflammatory activity in vivo. Mol Endocrinol 1997;11: 1245–1255.

54 Ramdas J, Harmon JM: Glucocorticoid-induced apoptosis and regulation of NF-κB activity in human leukemic T cells. Endocrinology 1998;139:3813–3821.

55 Reichardt HM, Kaestner KH, Tuckermann J, et al: DNA binding of the glucocorticoid receptor is not essential for survival. Cell 1998;93:531–541.

Prof. P.J. Barnes, National Heart and Lung Institute, Imperial College,
Dovehouse Street, London SW3 6LY (UK)
Tel. +44 171 351 8174, Fax +44 171 351 5675, E-Mail p.j.barnes@ic.ac.uk

Robinson DS (ed): Immunological Mechanisms in Asthma and Allergic Diseases.
Chem Immunol. Basel, Karger, 2000, vol 78, pp 81–92

....

Mast Cell-Eosinophil-Fibroblast Crosstalk in Allergic Inflammation

S.J. Smith[a, b]*, F. Levi-Schaffer*[b]

[a] Department of Allergy and Clinical Immunology, Imperial College School of
Medicine, National Heart and Lung Institute, London, UK and
[b] Department of Pharmacology, School of Pharmacy, The Hebrew University-
Hadassah Medical School, Jerusalem, Israel

It is well established that triggering of mast cells, by an IgE-dependent
mechanism, causes the early stage of an allergic reaction through the release
of preformed mediators, the production and release of cytokines and the
de novo synthesis of arachidonic acid metabolites. Together these mediators
not only orchestrate the early phase, but also influence the development of
the late phase reaction. The late phase, which occurs several hours after the
degranulation of mast cells, is characterized by an influx of inflammatory cells
to the site of activation, notably the eosinophils.

It is evident that during the late phase of an allergic reaction both mast
cells and eosinophils are in an environment which promotes continued and
repeated activation. Prolonged or repeated activation of these cells can lead
to their extended survival, recruitment of other inflammatory cells and to
further secretion of inflammatory mediators resulting in tissue damage. Usually
when such damage occurs, there follows a process of repair in which fibroblasts
are the predominant cell type. Biopsies of asthmatic subjects demonstrate an
increased number of fibroblasts, which may be due to both the growth and
chemotaxis of fibroblasts to the site of allergic inflammation. In particular,
there are increased numbers of myofibroblasts in the bronchial mucosa of
asthmatic subjects compared to normal controls [1].

In some circumstances an exaggerated and unbalanced repair process
takes place, which eventually leads to fibrosis and tissue remodelling. One can
speculate that the mast cell-eosinophil interaction is one of the ways that
promotes the activation of these cells during the later stages of allergic inflam-

mation and that this interaction can also affect fibroblast function, thereby influencing the repair process. It is the crosstalk of mast cells, eosinophils and fibroblasts that is the focus of our research and the present review.

Mast Cell Influences on Eosinophils

Mast cells are typically found adjacent to blood vessels and in asthmatics they are closely associated with bronchial smooth muscle. Recruitment of eosinophils from blood vessels into the tissue during the late asthmatic response thus brings them into close proximity to resident mast cells. Furthermore, tissue eosinophils, for example those analysed in bronchoalveolar lavage (BAL) fluid of asthmatics, are found to have a different phenotype compared to peripheral blood eosinophils and this may reflect a more activated state [2, 3].

The activation of mast cells, by the cross-linking of receptor-bound IgE molecules, causes the secretion of preformed and de novo synthesis of an array of arachidonic acid metabolites and an array of cytokines which can have effects on eosinophil recruitment, activation and survival.

Degranulation of mast cells is clearly evident in asthma, given the increased levels of tryptase, histamine and PGD_2 in BAL fluid from asthmatics [4]. Human mast cells of the respiratory tract and nasal mucosa have been shown to produce a plethora of cytokines that include IL-4, IL-6 and TNF-α and also the eosinophil 'survival/activation' cytokines, namely IL-3, IL-5 and GM-CSF [5, 6]. In particular, the release of IL-5 from lung mast cells following IgE-dependent triggering has recently been shown to have pronounced effects on eosinophils, including enhancing their survival, degranulation and adhesion to the vascular endothelium [7].

Following the identification of cytokines and chemokines as soluble mediators, it was thought that these glycoproteins would form the basis for crosstalk between cells. However, it has been demonstrated that although cytokines and chemokines are involved in influencing cells, other mediators are also important. For example, mast cell mediators such as histamine have been demonstrated to have functional effects on eosinophils. Histamine is chemotactic for eosinophils and promotes eosinophil activation by increasing metabolic activity and upregulation of certain membrane receptors [8–10].

The majority of in vitro studies determine the effects of isolated or purified mediators, or those generated by recombinant technology. However, in order to determine the role of specific mediators produced by one cell type in the presence of other substances generated by the same cell type, cell sonicates, cell lysates, supernatants of activated cells or coculture of cells are used. It is then possible to identify the responsible mediator(s) using neutralizing antibodies or receptor antagonists. Using these preparations it is possible to evaluate the synergistic or antagonistic action of mediators that cannot be fully determined using isolated ones.

Using such methodology we have recently demonstrated that purified human peripheral blood eosinophils exhibit enhanced survival when incubated with a rat peritoneal mast cell sonicate or the supernatant from mast cells activated in vitro by compound 48/80 [11]. The sonicate of mast cells caused increased viability of eosinophils thereby suggesting that the factor(s) responsible is both preformed and soluble. Using neutralizing antibodies to identify which factor(s) caused this effect, TNF-α was found to be predominantly responsible for this activity, through an autocrine induction of GM-CSF. In addition to enhancing viability, mast cell sonicates also caused eosinophils to release preformed granule proteins as evident by EPO release [11].

In another experimental system, culture supernatant from mast cells, which had been activated by cross-linking of receptor-bound IgE, was found to contain GM-CSF at levels that enhance eosinophil viability and cause release of ECP [12].

There is considerable new interest in the significance of the presence of nerve growth factor (NGF) in allergic reactions [13]. NGF can be produced by mast cells [14], fibroblasts [15] and eosinophils [16] during such reactions. Although we have shown that NGF can induce EPO, but not IL-6, release from eosinophils [16], in another study it was shown that it inhibited LTC_4 release [17] and therefore, NGF may have divergent effects on eosinophils.

Other mast cell-derived mediators have also been shown to cause eosinophil activation. For example, histamine and prostaglandin D_2 (PGD_2) have been shown to induce cytosolic calcium mobilization in eosinophils [18] and LTB_4 and PAF caused ECP release [19]. In addition, we have recently detected IL-8 production by eosinophils which is attributable to tryptase [unpubl. data].

Mast cells have been shown to produce stem cell factor (SCF) [20]. Eosinophils express the c-kit receptor and binding of SCF to this receptor on eosinophils has been shown to stimulate VLA-4-mediated adhesion to fibronectin and VCAM-1 [21].

TNF-α which is produced by mast cells, has a multitude of effects on eosinophils, alone and in synergy with other mediators. TNF-α has been shown to be released following anti-IgE triggering of dispersed lung tissue and is produced in sufficient quantities to have effects on eosinophils. It causes eosinophil chemotaxis in vitro and is thought to contribute to eosinophil recruitment in the airways [22]. TNF-α has been shown to increase eosinophil oxidative metabolism, trigger ECP release and IL-8 production and increase eosinophil survival [23–25].

TNF-α and IL-5, both of which can be generated by mast cells, have been demonstrated to act synergistically to induce eosinophil degranulation [25]. Furthermore, TNF-α has recently been shown to act in conjunction with IL-4 and IL-13 to upregulate eosinophil activation and survival [26].

TNF-α appears to be a major mediator of the mast cell-eosinophil crosstalk, since it is both preformed and synthesized de novo by stimulated mast cells. Although it is produced by several other inflammatory cells in the allergic response, such as eosinophils and macrophages, mast cells have been identified in skin biopsies as the predominant cell type expressing both mRNA and protein for TNF-α [27].

Eosinophil Influences on Mast Cells

Considerably less is known about the effects of eosinophils and their mediators on mast cells. Historically, mast cells have been considered to be the primary cells of allergic responses, influencing, but not being influenced by other cells. In addition, even though histamine has been detected during the late phase of allergic reaction it was postulated to be released only from infiltrating basophils. However, we have recently shown that the number of basophils in bronchial biopsies taken from allergic asthmatics are very low, being approximately only 10% of the number of mast cells [28], although in the skin, basophils are more prevalent in late phase reaction [28].

Eosinophil-derived cytokines can act on mast cells. For example, IL-6 and IL-5 which are prestored in the eosinophil granules, have been shown in vitro to promote the survival of mast cells and enhance IgE-mediated histamine release [29].

Recently, we found that eosinophils can produce and secrete SCF [30]. Several studies have highlighted the importance of SCF as being the major cytokine responsible for the maturation of mast cells [31, 32]. However, the effects of SCF are not only related to growth and differentiation of mast cells as it has also been shown to have chemotactic activity [33] and regulates their adhesion to matrix proteins [34]. Furthermore, SCF enhances IgE-dependent mediator release and cytokine release from human mast cells [35, 36].

NGF has potent effects on the differentiation of mast cells and also enhances mast cell survival [37], it has also been shown to cause mast cell degranulation in vitro, inducing PGD_2 and IL-6 production, although inhibiting TNF-α release from mast cells [38].

It has been demonstrated that the eosinophil granule proteins ECP and MBP, although not EDN or EPO, purified from human eosinophils cause histamine and tryptase release and the production of PGD_2 from human cardiac mast cells [39]. The release of mast cell mediators was shown to be both energy and calcium dependent and is, therefore, not attributable to a toxic effect of these proteins. This finding is in accordance with an earlier report of histamine release from rat mast cells stimulated by either MBP or ECP [40]. Interestingly, it was also found that none of these four eosinophil cationic proteins caused mediator release from human skin mast cells, on the other hand they decreased substance P mast cell activation, which may be related to mast cell heterogeneity [41].

All of the previous studies have determined the effects of eosinophil granule proteins using unchallenged naive rat mast cells. However, in terms of assessing the role of mast cells in the late phase reaction it is important to evaluate the effects of eosinophil proteins on mast cells that have already been activated, as happens in the early phase of an allergic response. We have recently shown that rat peritoneal mast cells that have previously been challenged, using an IgE-dependent stimulus and subsequently desensitized to the same stimulus, can be reactivated to release histamine following incubation with an eosinophil sonicate or purified MBP [42]. Furthermore, this activation of mast cells by MBP appears to be a Gi pertussis-sensitive mechanism and therefore is a metabolically active process that cannot be attributed to toxicity of this cationic protein [42].

It is important to point out that the release of histamine and tryptase from mast cells induced by the eosinophil granule proteins can act as a positive feedback loop. Histamine, as mentioned earlier, is chemotactic for eosinophils and also causes their activation. Tryptase can activate complement, the products of which, C3a and C5a, can then further activate mast cells and induce mediator release which potentiates the allergic reaction [43].

Mast Cell and Eosinophil Influences on Fibroblasts (fig. 1)

Historically, Paul Erlich was the first to notice the presence of mast cells in early fibrosis and since then considerable evidence has been brought about to support their participation in this process in several fibrotic diseases with different etiopathology [44, 45]. For example, dynamic changes in the ultrastructure and number of mast cells during fibrosis has been shown. In addition, eosinophils together with mast cells have been associated with many fibrotic diseases, although few studies have been performed to dissect their role in this context [46].

The mast cells and eosinophils by release of a wide range of mediators could be responsible for the modulation of fibroblast functions thereby contributing to tissue repair. Mast cell and eosinophil mediators could potentially

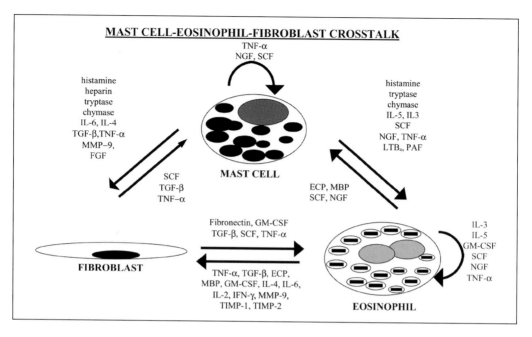

Fig. 1. Mast cell-eosinophil-fibroblast crosstalk. This scheme does not include all the possible mediators released by mast cells/eosinophils/fibroblasts, but highlights those that have already been shown to have a possible effect on these cells.

act antagonistically or synergistically and the actual effector function may also depend on the origin of the fibroblasts themselves.

Several in vitro studies have tried to analyse the effect of mast cells and mast cell products on fibroblast functions, some of the findings are contradictory and this can be attributed to both the type of mast cells and fibroblasts used, or the local milieu.

Histamine, one of the predominant mediators released by mast cells, has been found to stimulate the proliferation of human skin fibroblasts [47] and increase collagen synthesis by guinea pig fibroblasts [48]. The mast cell specific proteases tryptase and chymase have both been shown to be able to degrade collagen type IV and V, laminin and fibronectin and recently human mast cell lines have been demonstrated to produce matrix metalloproteinase-9 (MMP-9) and thus potentially contributing directly to ECM deposition [49]. Furthermore, mast cell tryptase enhances the proliferation of, and also stimulates type I collagen production by, normal lung and skin fibroblasts [50–52].

Another uniquely associated mast cell mediator, heparin, has been shown to inhibit a protein kinase C-dependent induction of the proto-oncogenes c-fos and c-myc, which are necessary for cell proliferation [53]. Heparin can also affect fibroblast growth by binding to extracellular matrix thereby disrupting fibroblast attachment, which is important for fibroblast proliferation [54]. In addition, heparin has also been reported to inhibit gel contraction by fibroblasts in a collagen gel [55].

Mast cells can contribute to fibrosis by the release of cytokines, for example TGF-β, IL-4 and TNF-α, which are found in high concentrations in the airways and are potent stimulators of both collagen and fibronectin synthesis by fibroblasts. TNF-α in particular has also been shown to stimulate fibroblast proliferation and chemotaxis and secretion of matrix proteins, collagenase and cytokines, including IL-6 [56–58]. Furthermore, mast cells have also been shown to produce fibroblast growth factor [59].

Coculture of rat peritoneal mast cells with 3T3 fibroblasts causes the proliferation of fibroblasts. This effect was increased when the mast cells were stimulated and an increase collagen production by fibroblasts was also observed [60].

In order to evaluate the direct effects of mast cell degranulation on fibroblasts, extracts of rat mast cells were added to fibroblasts cultivated in three-dimensional collagen lattices that mimic the in vivo situation in which mast cells and fibroblasts are organized in a three-dimensional tissue structure. In this system we found significant decrease in the speed and intensity of the contraction of the lattices, together with an increase in fibroblast proliferation and collagen and other protein deposition, even at very low mast cell concentrations [61]. The inhibition of the lattice contraction was partially attributed to heparin.

There are limited reports on the effects of eosinophils on fibroblast properties. However, isolated eosinophil mediators have also been shown to cause effects on fibroblasts. For example, ECP was shown to inhibit proteoglycan degradation [62], whereas MBP acts in a synergistic fashion with IL-1 and TGF-β to increase IL-6 production by fibroblasts [63]. Eosinophil-derived cytokines, such as IL-6, IL-4, TGF-β and GM-CSF, can also modulate fibroblast properties. The preformed stores of cytokines by eosinophils facilitates rapid effects. However, the cytokines can act in several different ways. For example, is has been shown that IL-6 and TNF-α are fibrogenic factors and that IL-4 stimulates collagen synthesis of dermal fibroblasts. However, IL-2 and IFN-γ decrease fibroblast proliferation and collagen synthesis [64, 65].

To assess the possible roles of eosinophil mediators we have added either a human peripheral blood sonicate or eosinophil culture supernatant to both human lung and dermal fibroblasts. We found that proliferation and lattice contraction of the three-dimensional collagen lattices were significantly enhanced in a dose-dependent manner. We also found that eosinophils affected collagen production, although the effect was dependent on the source of fibroblasts; collagen production was increased by skin fibroblasts but decreased in lung fibroblasts [66]. Eosinophils can also directly modulate collagen deposition since they were found to contain preformed MMP-9 and tissue inhibitors of metalloproteinases (TIMP-1 and -2). TGF-β is the most potent fibrogenic cytokine, it stimulates the chemotaxis of fibroblasts and extracellular matrix formation. Eosinophils contain preformed TGF-β and in order to evaluate the contribution of this cytokine in these systems we used anti-TGF-β neutralizing antibodies and found that these effects were partially blocked. This demonstrates that TGF-β is involved, although it also suggests that other eosinophil-derived mediators may influence this process [66].

Other earlier reports have shown that human eosinophils can stimulate the DNA synthesis and matrix production of dermal fibroblasts [67] and that guinea pig peritoneal eosinophils enhance the replication of human fetal lung fibroblasts [68].

Therefore, both mast cells and eosinophils through the release of pluripotent mediators can influence fibroblast properties in the same direction and therefore, they are collaborating in tissue repair and possibly in fibrosis. Finally it has to be appreciated that fibroblasts are not just the passive target for inflammatory cells in tissue responses, but they are active players. In fact, fibroblasts have been demonstrated to provide the microenvironment for the differentiation, functional activity and survival of both mast cells and of eosinophils [69–71].

Conclusions

Even though some studies prove that a cross-talk exists between mast cells, eosinophils and fibroblasts, there is still scant evidence for this in vivo. Therefore, more studies are needed in this area. This is particularly important since we believe that the mast cell-eosinophil-fibroblast interactions can be a major cause of worsening and perpetuation of allergic inflammatory reactions. The ultimate aim of elucidating pathways involved in allergic reactions is to define new and specific targets for immunopharmacological modulation.

References

1   Brewster CEP, Howarth PH, Djukanovic R, Wilson JW, Holgate ST, Roche WR: Myofibroblasts and subepithelial fibrosis in bronchial asthma. Am J Respir Cell Mol Biol 1990;3:507–511.
2   Hartnell A, Robinson DS, Kay AB, Wardlaw AJ: CD69 is expressed by human eosinophils activated in vivo in asthma and in vitro by cytokines. Immunology 1993;80:281–286.

3   Mengelers HJ, Maikoe T, Brinkman L, Hooibrink B, Lammers JJ, Koenderman L: Immunophenotyping of eosinophils recovered from blood and BAL of allergic asthmatics. Am J Respir Crit Care Med 1994;149:345–351.

4   Jarjour NN, Calhoun WJ, Schwartz LB, Busse WW: Elevated bronchoalveolar lavage fluid histamine levels in allergic asthmatics are associated with increased airway obstruction. Am Rev Respir Dis 1991;144:83–87.

5   Bradding P, Feather IH, Wilson S: Immunolocalisation of cytokines in the nasal mucosa of normal and perennial rhinitic subjects: The mast cell as a source of IL-4, IL-5 and IL-6 in human allergic mucosal inflammation. J Immunol 1993;151:3853–3865.

6   Bradding P, Roberts JA, Britten KM, Montefort S, Djukanvoic P, Mueller R, Heusser CH, Howarth PH, Holgate ST: Interleukins-4, -5 and -6 and TNF-α in normal and asthmatic airways: Evidence for the human mast cell as an important source of these cytokines. Am J Respir Cell Mol Biol 1994;10:471–480.

7   Okayama Y, Kobayashi H, Ashman LK, Holgate ST, Church MK, Masatomo M: Activation of eosinophils with cytokines produced by lung mast cells. Int Arch Allergy Appl Immunol 1997;114:75–77.

8   Dugas B, Arrock W, Czarlewski W, Bousquet J: Activation of membrane markers from purified human eosinophils by histamine. J Allergy Clin Immunol 1994;93:167.

9   Pincus SH, DiNapoli AM, Schooley WR: Superoxide production by eosinophils: Activation by histamine. J Invest Dermatol 1982;79:53–57.

10   Anwar ARE, Kay AB: Enhancement of human eosinophil complement receptors by pharmacologic mediators. J Immunol 1978;121:1245.

11   Levi-Schaffer F, Temkin V, Malamud V, Feld S, Zilberman Y: Mast cells enhance eosinophil survival in vitro: Role of TNF-α and granulocyte-macrophage colony-stimulating factor. J Immunol 1998;160:5554–5562.

12   Okayama Y, Kobayashi H, Ashman LK, Dobashi K, Nakazawa T, Holgate ST, Church MK, Mori M: Human lung mast cells are enriched in the capacity to produce granulocyte-macrophage colony-stimulating factor in response to IgE-dependent stimulation. Eur J Immunol 1998;28:708–715.

13   Bonini S, Lambiase A, Bonini S, Levi-Schaffer F, Aloe L: Nerve growth factor: An important molecule in allergic inflammation and tissue remodelling. Int Arch Allergy Appl Immunol 1999;118:159–162.

14   Nilsson G, Forsberg-Nilsson K, Xiang L, Hallbrook F, Nillson K, Metcalfe DD: Human mast cells express functional TrK A and are a source of NGF. Eur J Immunol 1997;27:2295–2301.

15   Hattori A, Iwasaki S, Murase K, Tsujimoto M, Sato M, Hayashi K, Kohno M: Tumor necrosis factor is markedly synergistic with interleukin-1 and interferon-γ in stimulating the production of nerve growth factor in fibroblasts. FEBS Lett 1994;340:177–180.

16   Solomon A, Aloe L, Peer J, Frucht-Pery J, Bonini S, Levi-Schaffer F: Nerve growth factor is preformed in and activates human peripheral blood eosinophils. J Allergy Clin Immunol 1998;102:454–460.

17   Takafuji S, Bischoff SC, De Weck AL, Dahinden CA: Opposing effects of tumor necrosis factor-α and nerve growth factor upon leukotriene C_4 production by human eosinophils triggered with N-formyl-methionyl-leucyl-phenylalanine. Eur J Immunol 1992;22:969–974.

18   Raible DG, Schulman ES, Dimuzio J, Cardillo R, Post TJ: Mast cell mediators prostaglandin-D_2 and histamine activate human eosinophils. J Immunol 1992;148:3536–3542.

19   Takafugi S, Tadokoro K, Nakagawa T: Release of granule proteins from human eosinophils stimulated with mast-cell mediators. Allergy 1998;53:951–956.

20   Zhang S, Anderson DF, Bradding P, Coward WR, Baddeley SM, MacLeod JDA, McGill JI, Church MK, Holgate ST, Roche WR: Human mast cells express stem cell factor. J Pathol 1998;186:59–66.

21   Yuan Q, Austen KF, Friend DS, Heidman M, Boyce JA: Human peripheral blood eosinophils express a functional c-kit receptor for stem cell factor that stimulates very late antigen 4 (VLA-4) mediated cell adhesion to fibronectin and vascular cell adhesion molecule 1 (VCAM-1). J Exp Med 1997;186:313–323.

22   Lukacs NW, Strieter RM, Chensue SW, Widmer M, Kunkel SL: TNF-alpha mediates recruitment of neutrophils and eosinophils during airway inflammation. J Immunol 1995;154:5411–5417.

23 Egesten A, Blom M, Calafat J, Janssen H, Knol EF: Eosinophil granulocyte interaction with serum opsonised particles: Binding and degranulation are enhanced by tumor necrosis factor alpha. Int Arch Allergy Appl Immunol 1998;115:121–128.

24 Tsukahara K, Nakao A, Hiraguri M, Miike S, Mamura M, Saito Y, Iwamoto I: Tumor necrosis factor alpha mediates antiapoptotic signals partially via p38 MAP kinase activation in human eosinophils. Int Arch Allergy Appl Immunol 1999;120:54–59.

25 Horie S, Gleich GJ, Kita H: Cytokines directly induce degranulation and superoxide production from human eosinophils. J Allergy Clin Immunol 1996;98:371–381.

26 Luttmann W, Matthiesen T, Matthys H, Virchow JC: Synergistic effects of IL-4 or IL-13 and tumor necrosis factor-α on eosinophil activation in vitro. Am J Respir Cell Mol Biol 1999;20:474–480.

27 Walsh LJ, Trinchieri G, Waldorf HA, Whitaker D, Murphy GF: Human dermal mast cells contain and release tumor necrosis factor alpha, which induces endothelial leukocyte adhesion molecule. Proc Natl Acad Sci USA 1991;88:4220–4224.

28 Macfarlane AJ, Kon OM, Smith SJ, Zeibecoglou K, Khan N, Barata LT, McEuen AE, Buckley MG, Walls AF, Meng Q, Humbert M, Barnes NC, Robinson DS, Ying S, Kay AB: Basophils, eosinophils and mast cells in atopic and non-atopic asthma and in late-phase allergic reactions in the lung and skin. J Allergy Clin Immunol 2000;105:99–107.

29 Yanagida M, Fukamachi H, Ohgami K, Kuwaki T, Ishii H, Uzumaki H, Amano K, Tokiwa T, Mitsui H, Saito H, Iikura Y, Ishizaka T, Nakahata T: Effects of T-helper cytokines, interleukin (IL)-3, IL-4, IL-5 and IL-6 on the survival of cultured human mast cells. Blood 1995;86:3705–3715.

30 Hartman M, Piliponsky A, Temkin V, Levi-Schaffer F: Human peripheral blood eosinophils as a novel source of stem cell factor. J Allergy Clin Immunol 1999;103:700.

31 Tsai M, Takeishi T, Thompson H, Langley KE, Zsebo KM, Metcalfe DD, Geissler EN, Galli SJ: Induction of mast cell proliferation, maturation and heparin synthesis by the rat c-kit ligand, stem cell factor. Proc Natl Acad Sci USA 1991;88:6382–6386.

32 Mitsui H, Furitsu T, Dvorak AM: Development of human mast cells from umbilical cord blood cells by recombinant human and murine c-kit ligand. Proc Natl Acad Sci USA 1993;90:735–739.

33 Meininger CJ, Yano H, Rottadel R, Bernstein A, Zsebo KM, Zetter BR: The c-kit receptor ligand functions as a mast cell chemoattractant. Blood 1992;79:958–963.

34 Dastych J, Metcalfe DD: Stem cell factor induces mast cell adhesion to fibronectin. J Immunol 1994;152:213–219.

35 Bischoff SC, Dahinden CA: c-kit ligand: A unique potentiator of mediator release by human lung mast cells. J Exp Med 1992;175:237–244.

36 Columbo M, Horowitz EM, Botana LM, MacGlashan DW, Bochner BS: The human recombinant c-kit receptor ligand rhSCF, induces mediator release from human cutaneous mast cells and enhances IgE dependent mediator release from both skin mast cells and peripheral blood basophils. J Immunol 1992;149:599–608.

37 Matsuda H, Coyghlin ME, Bienenstock J, Denburg JA: Nerve growth factor promotes haemopoietic colony growth and differentation. Proc Natl Acad Sci USA 1988;85:6508–6512.

38 Marshall JS, Gomi K, Blennerhassett MG, Bienenstock J: Nerve growth factor modifies the expression of inflammatory cytokines by mast cells via a prostanoid-dependent mechanism. J Immunol 1999;162:4271–4276.

39 Patella V, Crescenzo G, Marino I, Genovese A, Adt M, Gleich GJ, Marone G: Eosinophil granule proteins activate human heart mast cells. J Immunol 1996;157:1219–1225.

40 Zheutin LM, Ackerman SJ, Gleich GJ, Thomas LL: Stimulation of basophil and rat mast cell histamine release by eosinophil granule derived cationic proteins. J Immunol 1984;133:2180–2185.

41 Okayama Y, El-Lati SG, Leiferman KM, Church MK: Eosinophil granule proteins inhibit substance P-induced histamine release from human skin mast cells. J Allergy Clin Immunol 1994;93:900–909.

42 Piliponsky A, Pickholtz D, Gleich GJ, Levi-Schaffer F: Eosinophils activate mast cells to release histamine. Int Arch Allergy Appl Immunol 1999;118:202–203.

43 Ellati SG, Dahinden CA, Church MK: Complement peptides C3a-induced and C5a-induced mediator release from dissociated human skin mast cells. J Invest Dermatol 1994;102:803–806.

44 Hawkins RA, Claman HN, Clark RA, Steigerwald JC: Increased dermal mast cell populations in progressive systemic sclerosis: A link in chronic fibrosis? Ann Intern Med 1985;102:182–186.

45   Wichman BE: The mast cell count during the process of wound healing: An experimental investigation on rats. Acta Pathol Microbiol Scand 1955;108:1–35

46   Noguchi H, Kephart GM, Colby TV, Gleich GJ: Tissue eosinophilia and eosinophil degranulation in syndromes associated with fibrosis. Am J Pathol 1992;140:521–528.

47   Jordana M, Befus AD, Newhouse MT, Bienenstock J, Gauldie J: Effect of histamine on proliferation of normal human adult lung fibroblasts. Thorax 1988;43:552–558.

48   Hatamochi A, Kujiwra K, Ueki H: Effects of histamine on collagen synthesis by cultured fibroblasts derived from guinea pig skin. Arch Dermatol Res 1985;277:60–64.

49   Kanbe N, Tanaka A, Kanbe M, Itakura A, Kurosawa M, Matsuda H: Human mast cells produce matrix metalloproteinase 9. Eur J Immunol 1999;29:2645–2649.

50   Gruber BL, Kew RR, Jelaska A, Marchese MJ, Garlick J, Ren S, Schwartz LB, Korn JH: Human mast cells activate fibroblasts: Tryptase is a fibrogenic factor stimulating collagen messenger ribonucleic acid synthesis and fibroblast chemotaxis. J Immunol 1997;158:2310–2317.

51   Abe M, Kurosawa M, Ishikawa O, Miyachi Y, Kido H: Mast cell tryptase stimulates both dermal fibroblast proliferation and type I collagen production. Clin Exp Allergy 1998;28:1509–1517.

52   Cairns JA, Walls AF: Mast cell tryptase stimulates the synthesis of type I collagen in human lung fibroblasts. J Clin Invest 1997;99:1313–1321.

53   Wright TC, Pukac LA, Castellot JJ, Karnovsky MJ, Levine RA, Kimpark HY, Campisi J: Heparin suppresses the induction of c-fos and c-myc messenger RNA in murine fibroblasts by selective inhibition of a protein kinase C dependent pathway. Proc Natl Acad Sci USA 1989;86:3199–3203.

54   Del Vecchio PJ, Bizios R, Holleran LA, Judge TK, Pinto GL: Inhibition of human scleral fibroblast proliferation with heparin. Invest Ophthalmol Vis Sci 1988;29:1272–1276.

55   Guidry C, Grinell F: Heparin modulates the organisation of hydrated collagen gels and inhibits gel contraction by fibroblasts. J Cell Biol 1987;104:1097–1103.

56   Dayer JM, Beutler B, Cerami A: Cachectin/tumor necrosis factor stimulates collagenase and prostaglandin E_2 production by human synovial cells and dermal fibroblasts. J Exp Med 1985;162:2163–2168.

57   Kendall JC, Li XH, Galli SJ, Gordon JR: Promotion of mouse fibroblast proliferation by IgE-dependent activation of mouse mast cells: Role for mast cell TNF-α and TGF-β. J Allergy Clin Immunol 1997;99:113–123.

58   Postlethwaite AE, Seyer JM: Stimulation of fibroblast chemotaxis of human recombinant tumor necrosis factor alpha (TNF-α) and a synthetic TNF-α 31–68 peptide. J Exp Med 1990;172:1749–1756.

59   Qu Z, Lieber JM, Powers MR: Mast cells are a major source of fibroblast growth factor in chronic inflammation and cutaneous hemangioma. Am J Pathol 1995;147:564–573.

60   Levi-Schaffer F, Rubinchik E: Activated mast cells are fibrogenic for 3T3 fibroblasts. J Invest Dermatol 1995;104:999–1003.

61   Levi-Schaffer F, Garbuzenko E, Rubin A, Reich R, Pickholz D, Gillery P, Emonard H, Nagler A, Maquart FX: Human eosinophils regulate human lung and skin derived fibroblast properties in vitro: A role for transforming growth factor β. Proc Natl Acad Sci USA 1999;96:9660–9665.

62   Hernnas J, Sarnstrand B, Lindroth P, Peterson CGP, Venge P, Malstrom A: Eosinophil cationic protein alters proteoglycan metabolism in human lung fibroblast cultures. Eur J Cell Biol 1992;59:352–363.

63   Rochester CL, Ackerman SJ, Zheng T, Elias JA: Eosinophil-fibroblast interactions: Granule major basic protein interacts with IL-1 and transforming growth factor-β in the stimulation of lung fibroblast IL-6-type cytokine production. J Immunol 1996;156:4449–4456.

64   Rubinchik E, Levi-Schaffer F: Interleukin-2 inhibits 3T3 fibroblast proliferation. Life Sci 1996;58:1509–1517.

65   Duncan MR, Berman B: Gamma interferon is the lymphokine and beta-interferon the monokine responsible for inhibition of fibroblast collagen production and late but not early fibroblast proliferation. J Exp Med 1985;162:516–527.

66   Berton A, Levi-Schaffer F, Emonard H, Garbuzenko E, Gillery P, Maquart FX: Activation of fibroblasts in collagen lattices by mast cells extract: A model of fibrosis. Clin Exp Allergy 2000;30:485–492.

67   Birkland TP, Cheavens MD, Pincus SH: Human eosinophils stimulate DNA synthesis and matrix production in dermal fibroblasts. Arch Dermatol Res 1994;286:312–318.
68   Shock A, Rabe KF, Dent G, Chambers RC, Gray RC, Gray AJ, Chung KF, Barnes PJ, Laurent CJ: Eosinophils adhere to and stimulate replication of lung fibroblasts in vitro. Clin Exp Immunol 1991;86:185–190.
69   Levi-Schaffer F, Austen KF, Caulfield JP, Hein A, Bloes WF, Stevens RL: Fibroblasts maintain the phenotype and viability of the rat heparin-containing mast cells in vitro. J Immunol 1985;135: 3454–3462.
70   Levi-Schaffer F, Rubinchik E: Mast cell/fibroblast interactions. Clin Exp Allergy 1994;24:1016–1021.
71   Levi-Schaffer F, Weg VB: Mast cells, eosinophils and fibrosis. Clin Exp Allergy 1997;27:64–70.

Prof. F. Levi-Schaffer, Department of Pharmacology, School of Pharmacy,
The Hebrew University-Hadassah Medical School, POB 12065, Jerusalem 91120 (Israel)
Tel. +972 2 6757512, Fax +972 2 6758741, E-Mail fls@cc.huji.ac.il

Robinson DS (ed): Immunological Mechanisms in Asthma and Allergic Diseases.
Chem Immunol. Basel, Karger, 2000, vol 78, pp 93–111

·····················

The Role of Adhesion in Eosinophil Function

A.J. Wardlaw

Division of Respiratory Medicine, University of Leicester Medical School,
Glenfield Hospital, Leicester, UK

Introduction

Eosinophils are thought to be important in host defence against helminthic parasites and in causing the pathological changes involved in allergic inflammatory disease. Each stage of the life of the eosinophil, from haematopoiesis to engulfment of apoptotic eosinophils by macrophages, involves adhesion-related events, some of which are common to other leucocytes, and some of which, particularly those related to eosinophil adhesion to endothelium, are more eosinophil specific. Leucocyte adhesion is mediated through members of several gene families of membrane glycoproteins which are also involved in biological processes as diverse as wound healing, thrombogenesis, atherogenesis, embryogenesis and maintenance of tissue architecture. I will briefly summarize the major adhesion receptors involved in leucocyte adhesion and their expression in allergic disease before proceeding to a more detailed examination of their role in eosinophil effector function.

Leucocyte Adhesion Receptors

The major gene families of adhesion receptors involved in leucocyte adhesion are the *Selectins* and their counter-receptors, members of the *Integrin* family and members of the Immunoglobulin family.

Selectins and Their Counter-Receptors
There are three selectins. E-selectin expressed on endothelium, P-selectin expressed by platelets and endothelium and L-selectin expressed on most leuco-

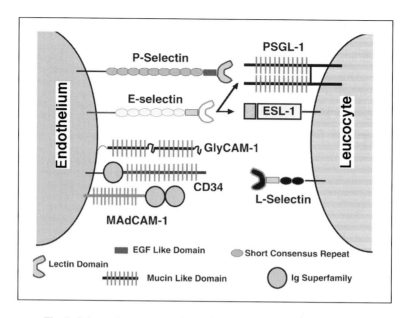

Fig. 1. Schematic representation of the selectin family of adhesion receptors and their ligands. P- and E-selectin are expressed on endothelial cells and bind PSGL-1 and on mouse neutrophils ESL-1 (E-selectin binding protein 1). L-selectin is expressed on mostly leucocytes and binds a number of mucin-like receptors on high endothelial vessels in lymph nodes. There is evidence for another as yet uncharacterized receptor on venular endothelium in other organs.

cytes [1]. All three selectins have a common structure with an N-terminal lectin domain, an EGF-like domain and a variable number of consensus repeats (CR) related to complement binding proteins (fig. 1). E-selectin expression is induced on human umbilical vein endothelial cells (HUVEC) in vitro by stimulation with cytokines including IL-1 and TNF-α with optimal expression at 4 h. In vivo expression is weak or absent on uninflamed tissue but induced during inflammatory processes. E-selectin is particularly well expressed in the skin where it is thought to act as an addressin for skin homing lymphocytes through its ability to bind the carbohydrate antigen CLA expressed on a minority of blood T cells but a majority of T cells in inflamed skin [2]. Like the other selectins, E-selectin binds sialylated fucosylated sugar moieties such as sialyl Lewis x. Expression of these carbohydrate structures is controlled by cell-specific fucosyltransferases such as FucTV11 [3]. The backbone structure which presents these carbohydrates to E-selectin include, on mouse neutrophils a receptor very closely related to a chicken fibroblast growth factor receptor (ESL-1) and in humans P-selectin glycoprotein 1 (PSGL-1), which E-selectin binds with a lower affinity than

P-selectin. Interestingly the carbohydrate antigen CLA which defines skin homing T cells is expressed on a glycoform of PSGL-1 [4]. P-selectin is stored in intracellular granules and expression can be rapidly upregulated on HUVEC by several mediators such as histamine, thrombin and LTC$_4$. Although in the mouse surface expression of P-selectin can be induced by TNF-α and LPS, this is not the case in humans. However, both mRNA and surface expression can be induced for up to 48 h by IL-4, IL-3 and IL-13 [5, and see later]. P-selectin binds PSGL-1 which is expressed on most leucocytes although expression and function are often dissociated, especially on peripheral blood T cells which all express PSGL-1 but only about 20% bind P-selectin [6]. L-selectin is constitutively expressed but shed on cellular activation as a result of the actions of a membrane-bound metalloproteinase. It is the peripheral lymph node homing receptor and several receptors for L-selectin that have been identified on lymph node HEVs. These include GlyCAM-1, CD34 and in the mouse MadCAM-1. Like PSGL-1, these all contain mucin-like regions rich in O-linked sugars such as sialyl Lewis x. The ligand for L-selectin on inflamed venular endothelium has not been identified. Selectins mediate capture of leucocytes under flow conditions. Selectin/carbohydrate bonds mediate a rolling type of interaction. There is considerable overlap in selectin function and single gene deletion mice are relatively healthy. However, type 11 LAD, in which all three selectins are dysfunctional, and a combined E- and P-selectin 'knock out' mouse, both show profound immunodeficiency [7].

Integrins and Their Counter-Structures

Integrins are a large superfamily of heterodimeric glycoproteins involved in a wide range of biological functions including maintenance of tissue homeostasis through binding to matrix proteins [8]. Only a limited number of integrins have been shown to be involved in leucocyte migration. The β2 (CD18) leucocyte integrins comprise four members CD11a-d/CD18. CD11a/CD18 (LFA-1) is expressed on all leucocytes and is involved in a range of functions including transmigration through endothelium and T-cell activation. It has three receptors, ICAM-1 and -2 expressed on endothelium and ICAM-3 expressed on most leucocytes. CD11b/CD18 (Mac-1) is expressed on myelocytes and CD11c/CD18 (p,150.95) is well expressed on tissue macrophages. CD11d/CD18 has as yet been little studied. Mac-1 binds ICAM-1 and has a diverse number of other ligands. It also mediates ICAM-1 independent, granulocyte binding to endothelium through an as yet undefined receptor. Impaired expression of the CD18 integrins as in LAD type 1 leads to profound immunodeficiency, largely as a result of impaired neutrophil migration. ICAM-1 expression is induced on a large number of cell types including epithelium, endothelium and haematopoietic cells by cytokine stimulation.

α4β1 (VLA-4) is expressed on all leucocytes except neutrophils and binds VCAM-1 whose expression on endothelium is selectively upregulated by IL-4 as well as IL-13 [9]. It also binds fibronectin through a C-terminal non-RGD domain. Both VLA-4 and VCAM-1 gene deletion mice are embryonic lethals because of effects on haematopoiesis and cardiac development. α4β7 also binds VCAM-1 and fibronectin as well as MadCAM-1, a receptor largely expressed by gut endothelium consistent with the role of α4β7 as a gut lymphocyte homing receptor [10]. αEβ7 is expressed on a subset of T lymphocytes and binds E-cadherin so mediating localization of intraepithelial lymphocytes [11]. αvβ3 is expressed on endothelium and macrophages and mediates phagocytosis of apoptotic granulocytes [12]. It also binds the widely expressed immunoglobulin-like receptor PECAM which is involved in leucocyte penetration of endothelial basement membrane [13]. The CD18 integrins are unable to capture leucocytes under flow conditions only mediating binding after the cell has become attached to the endothelium and activated. In contrast, the α4β1 and α4β7 integrins can bind ligand under flow conditions [14].

Expression of Adhesion Receptors in Allergic Disease

Endothelial Adhesion Receptors
Adhesion molecule function is regulated in a number of ways including increased expression as with E- and P-selectin, ICAM-1 and VCAM-1, shedding as with L-selectin and conformational changes in the binding affinity of the receptor as seen with many integrins. A number of groups have studied expression of E-selectin, ICAM-1, and VCAM-1 in asthma and other allergic inflammatory conditions. P-selectin expression has been less widely studied, partly because of the difficulty in distinguishing between intracellular and lumenal staining. In general terms, studies in vivo using allergen challenge have been generally consistent with observations in cytokine-stimulated HUVECs. In the skin, low background expression of ICAM-1 is seen with absent expression of E-selectin and VCAM-1. After allergen challenge, increased endothelial expression of all three receptors has been reported [15, 16]. In the airway, Montefort et al. [17] found increased expression of ICAM-1 and E-selectin 6 h after local allergen challenge with no increase in VCAM-1 expression. Bentley et al. [18] reported a trend towards increased VCAM-1 expression (significance was lost through one outlier) with a good correlation between VCAM-1 expression and eosinophil infiltration 24 h after aerosol allergen challenge. In sensitized lung explants, allergen challenge increased ICAM-1, E-selectin and VCAM-1 expression in a manner similar to that seen in HUVEC. Upregulation was mediated by a combination IL-4 and TNF-α [19].

In clinical asthma, findings have been more variable probably reflecting the inherent problems in accurately quantifying small changes in expression using immunohistochemistry. Montefort et al. [20] were unable to detect changes in adhesion receptor expression in atopic asthma and in a study of atopic and nonatopic asthma. Bentley et al. [18] could only detect a modest increase in ICAM-1 and E-selectin expression in their nonatopic asthmatics with relatively high background expression. The E-selectin antibody cross-reacted with P-selectin. In contrast, Gosset et al. [21] found low background expression in normal subjects and could detect increases in adhesion molecule expression in atopic but not nonatopic asthmatics. Ohkawara et al. [22] agreed with these findings in 6 atopic asthmatics, but Fukuda et al. [23] detected no increase in ICAM-1 or E-selectin staining over controls. However, the E-selectin antibody they used also cross-reacted with P-selectin. This group did however find an increase in VCAM-1 expression which correlated with eosinophil counts but only in those subjects with detectable IL-4 in the bronchoalveolar lavage (BAL) fluid. In nasal endothelium, generally weak expression of VCAM-1 has been observed, although increased over normal controls, in both perennial rhinitis and nasal polyps [24]. We have found E-selectin expression to be weak in nasal polyps, lung resection tissue and perennial rhinitis. We have found that P-selectin is widely expressed in both nasal and lung tissue. Strong expression was seen in nasal biopsies from both normal controls and patients with perennial rhinitis with little difference between the two groups either after fixation with acetone or paraformaldehyde which favours surface as opposed to intracellular staining. Similarly, in endobronchial biopsies good expression was observed in sections from both asthmatic and control subjects. Consistent with this observation, P-selectin was well expressed in lung resection tissue from patients with lung cancer. Expression was seen on both bronchial and pulmonary venules but not the pulmonary capillaries. As mentioned above, it is difficult to conclusively distinguish between intracellular and lumenal staining using standard immunohistochemistry. However, the strong expression in the airway does suggest P-selectin rather than E-selectin is the major selectin involved in leucocyte migration into the lung in humans.

ICAM-1 expression on epithelial cells is consistently increased on bronchial epithelium in asthma [18, 25, 26]. Ciprandi et al. [27, 28] demonstrated induction of ICAM-1 within 30 min of allergen challenge on both nasal and conjunctival epithelium. This is considerably faster than the rate at which expression is induced in HUVEC. The role of ICAM-1 as a receptor for the major group of rhinoviruses means that the epithelium in asthmatics may be more vulnerable to viral infection. Expression of CD44, a receptor for the matrix protein hyaluronate, is increased on the bronchial epithelium in asthma although it is also found on normal epithelium [29].

Soluble Adhesion Molecules

Several adhesion molecules can be detected in soluble form circulating in the plasma. Montefort et al. [30] found that concentrations of E-selectin, ICAM-1 and VCAM-1 were not elevated in stable asthma, but there was a significant increase compared with normal controls in concentrations of sE-selectin and sICAM-1 in patients with acute severe asthma. However, concentrations of these molecules did not correlate with disease severity and were therefore not thought useful in clinical management. In another study of 45 atopic and nonatopic asthmatics, serum concentrations of sICAM-1, sE-selectin and sVCAM-1 were increased during 'asthma attacks' when compared with stable periods [31, 32]. Modest increases in concentrations of sICAM-1 and sE-selectin have also been detected in BAL fluid after segmental allergen challenge [33, 34]. Zangrilli et al. [35] measured sVCAM-1 concentrations in BAL fluid 24 h after segmental allergen challenge in 27 ragweed allergic asthmatics and 18 atopic nonasthmatics. A marked increase in sVCAM-1 concentrations were observed in BAL fluid which correlated with increased numbers of eosinophils and concentrations of IL-4 and IL-5. Most of the increase occurred in the late responders. As yet there have been no clear-cut correlations between disease severity and concentration of soluble adhesion receptors, so the significance of these findings in terms of disease pathogenesis or usefulness in monitoring inflammatory activity is still uncertain

Role of Adhesion Receptors in Eosinophil Function

Molecular Basis for Eosinophil Tissue Accumulation

The factors controlling eosinophil traffic and in particular the relatively selective accumulation of eosinophils in allergic disease has been the subject of intensive study for over three decades. In the normal individual, eosinophils make up only 1–5% of the white cell count and in the normal lung there are 50 neutrophils for every 1 eosinophil. In asthma there are 4 eosinophils for every 1 neutrophil in the bronchial submucosa representing an up to 200-fold enrichment of eosinophils over neutrophils [36]. Historically this was thought to be due to a selective chemoattractant. A factor, termed eosinophil chemotactic factor of anaphylaxis (ECF-A), was detected in supernatants from anaphylactically challenged guinea-pig lung which appeared to be selectively chemotactic for eosinophils [37]. This was subsequently found to consist of LTB_4, which is active on guinea-pig eosinophils but less so on human eosinophils, and 15-HETE [38]. ECF-A from human lung was later identified and characterized as two tetrapeptides – Val-Gly-Ser-Glu and Ala-Gly-Ser-Glu

[39]. However, in comparison to PAF these peptides were found to have negligible activity [40]. More recently there has been intense interest in the role of chemokines as selective chemoattractants. It is becoming increasingly clear that selective tissue accumulation of eosinophils is not the result of any single event but occurs because of selective pressure at every stage in the life cycle of the eosinophil, including eosinophilopoiesis and egress from the bone marrow, adhesion mechanisms, chemotaxis and prolonged survival under the influence of locally generated growth factors [41]. The adhesion events involved in selective migration will be discussed here.

Eosinophilopoiesis and Egress from the Bone Marrow

Eosinophils differentiate from bone marrow precursors under the influence of growth factors, especially IL-5. It is likely that eosinophilopoiesis requires adhesion to stromal elements within the bone marrow as has been shown for other leucocytes, but this has not been reported. Increased amounts of IL-5 generated at sites of allergic inflammation act hormonally to increase eosinophil production. The increase in peripheral blood eosinophils in asthma is the consequence of both increased production and egress from the bone marrow. The way in which cells emigrate from the sinuses in the marrow into the peripheral blood is only just becoming understood, but recent work in guinea pigs has shown that IL-5 selectively promotes the egress of eosinophils from the marrow [42]. This is enhanced by eotaxin, an eosinophil-selective chemokine [43] and controlled by the adhesion molecules VLA-4, inhibition of which accelerates egress and Mac-1 whose inhibition prevents egress [44].

Eosinophil Adhesion to Endothelium

Whatever the percentage of circulating eosinophils, unless there are local signals on bronchial post-capillary endothelium leading to adhesion and trans-migration, tissue accumulation of eosinophils will not occur. The pattern of expression of eosinophil adhesion receptors is in general similar to other leucocytes although eosinophils, unlike human neutrophils, express functional forms of VLA-4, VLA-6 and $\alpha 4\beta 7$ [45]. MadCAM-1, the ligand for $\alpha 4\beta 7$ and almost exclusively expressed on gut endothelium, may be important in directing eosinophils to the intestinal wall where they normally reside. Eosinophils also express the newly described member of the $\beta 2$ integrin family $\alpha d\beta 2$, which like VLA-4 binds VCAM-1, although this receptor may be more important in modulating the function of tissue rather than peripheral blood eosinophils [46]. I will discuss selective signals for eosinophil endothelial adhesion in terms of each step of the established paradigm for leucocyte adhesion to endothelium; tethering, activation and firm arrest (fig. 2).

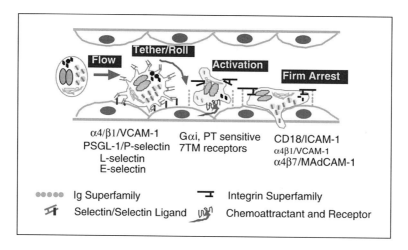

Fig. 2. Schematic representation of the multistage adhesion cascade involved in leucocyte adhesion to endothelium. Cells enter the blood vessel under flow conditions and need to first be captured by the endothelium using selectins and α4 integrin receptors binding to PSGl-1 and VCAM-1 respectively. The close proximity of the leucocytes to endothelial cell surface allows them to become activated which results in engagement of the CD18 integrins with ICAM-1 and 2 leading to firm arrest which is a prerequisite of transmigration. Each step in the cascade is obligatory for successful transmigration to occur.

Tethering

Because of its lack of expression on human neutrophils, VLA-4 has attracted considerable interest as a possible receptor mediating selective eosinophil adhesion. VLA-4 can promote both tethering and firm arrest. IL-4 and IL-13 upregulate expression of VCAM-1, the ligand for VLA-4, on HUVECs and transmigration through IL-4/13-stimulated HUVECs was shown to be dependent on VLA-4 [8]. IL-4/13-induced endothelial expression of VCAM-1 in the absence of a co-stimulus such as TNF-α is however weak, especially on cultured lung microvascular endothelium [47, 48]. Consistent with this, we and others have found variable and often weak expression of VCAM-1 on airway endothelium in clinical asthma with no increase over control subjects [25]. Some investigators have reported increased VCAM-1 expression, although the difference from controls has been modest [49, 50]. A more consistent increase in VCAM-1 has been observed after antigen challenge with a correlation with eosinophil influx [8, 25]. Peripheral blood eosinophils can constitutively bind VCAM-1 via VLA-4, although binding to VCAM-1 and fibronectin can be further enhanced by manganese and activating mAbs such as TS2/16 and 8A2, but not by physiological stimulus such as IL-5 and RANTES which however do upregulate β2 function [51]. VLA-4 can tether eosinophils under flow. Thus the number of eosinophils rolling on IL-1-stimulated rabbit mesenteric vascular endothelium was partially decreased by anti-VLA-4 mAb [52] and eosinophils became tethered to purified VCAM-1 under flow conditions, although at a lower sheer stress than P-selectin [53]. VLA-4 was also important in mediating tethering of eosinophils to TNF-α-stimulated HUVECs [54]. A number of studies, using a variety of animal models, have demonstrated that blocking VLA-4 or VCAM-1 inhibited eosinophil migration into the lung and skin and prevented the development of bronchial hyperresponsiveness (BHR) [8, 25, 55] although these two effects have not always correlated [56].

There is increasing evidence for a role for P-selectin in mediating eosinophil adhesion. Eosinophils bound with greater avidity to purified P-selectin than neutrophils under shear conditions, especially at suboptimal concentrations of P-selectin [33, 57]. The P-selectin gene promoter contains two STAT-6 binding sites [58] and chronic surface expression of P-selectin on HUVECs was induced by IL-4 and IL-13 although, unlike in the mouse, not by IL-1 or TNF-α [5, 59]. Eosinophils, but not neutrophils, were able to adhere to IL-4- or IL-13-stimulated HUVECs under sheer stress and binding was mediated both by antibodies against P-selectin/PSGL-1 and VLA-4/VCAM-1, demonstrating a cooperative effect between these two pairs of receptors [40, 60]. P-selectin was the only selectin involved in eosinophil adhesion to nasal polyp endothelium [61]. The reduced eosinophil infiltration seen in nasal polyps after treatment with fluticasone was associated with a reduction in expression of P-selectin but not VCAM-1 [62]. The importance of P-selectin in eosinophil accumulation in allergic disease has been further underlined by studies in animal models. In a ragweed peritonitis model, eosinophil accumulation was reduced by 75% in P-selectin-deficient mice with an additional contribution from VCAM-1 and ICAM-1 [63]. Eosinophil accumulation was reduced in the airways of P-selectin-deficient mice after antigen challenge [64, 65] and anti-P-selectin, but not E-selectin, reduced eosinophil influx into the pleural cavity in a mouse pleuritis model [66]. In contrast to P-selectin, neutrophils bind with greater avidity to E-selectin than eosinophils [8, 33, 67], although E-selectin did make a minor contribution towards eosinophil adherence to TNF-α-stimulated endothelium [34] and eosinophil influx into the skin in mice, consistent with the preferential expression of E-selectin in this organ [68]. There are no very clear-cut differences in L-selectin function between eosinophils and neutrophils, although anti-L-selectin did partially inhibit eosinophil binding to rabbit mesenteric endothelium [32].

The reasons for the differences in the avidity of eosinophils and neutrophils for E- and P-selectin are not clear. PSGL-1 is a mucin-like homodimeric receptor although expression does not always correlate with function. For example, all lymphocytes express PSGL-1 but only about 15% can bind

P-selectin. The majority of the P-selectin binding function is found in the N-terminal 19 amino acids of PSGL-1 and is crucially dependent on sulphation of at least one of three tyrosine residues as well as the appropriate glyocosylation of a single O-linked sugar residue in this region. In contrast, E-selectin, which can also bind PSGL-1 although with lower affinity than P-selectin, binds to the central, mucin-like, O-linked carbohydrate-rich region of the receptor. E-selectin binding correlates with expression of sialyl Lewis x-like carbohydrate moieties, expression of which is regulated by the glycosyltransferase, fucosyltransferase V11 (FucTVII). Although P-selectin binding function is also dependent on FucTV11, as well as appropriate sulphyltransferases, binding appears to be through sugars other than sialyl Lewis x [69]. Eosinophils, unlike neutrophils, express only low levels of sialyl Lewis x and this probably explains their weak E-selectin binding. Eosinophils express a little more PSGL-l than neutrophils [37] which may explain increased binding affinity. Alternatively there may be as yet to be defined, functionally important differences in glycosylation of PSGL-1 between the two cell types which influence binding.

In summary, the tethering step, which is an essential requirement of leucocyte transmigration into tissue, can play a major part in selective eosinophil migration through the combined effects of VLA-4/VCAM-1 and PSGL-1/P-selectin. Certainly, under conditions in which only IL-4 and IL-13 are expressed, as may be seen in mild to moderate asthma, only eosinophils would be expected to bind to endothelium, with P-selectin playing a major role in eosinophil capture. However, in more florid disease, for example after allergen challenge or in exacerbations of asthma, in which larger amounts of TNF-α and IL-1 are likely to be generated, neutrophils would also be expected to be recruited via E-selectin and VLA-4/VCAM-1 would be the dominant receptor mediating eosinophil capture.

Activation and Firm Arrest

After leucocytes become tethered to the endothelium, activation results in functional up-regulation of integrins which bind to ICAMs and VCAM expressed by the endothelium, resulting in the firm arrest which is a prerequisite of transmigration. The activation step is thought to be mediated by chemoattractants on the endothelium acting through G protein-linked pertussis toxin (PT)-sensitive serpentine receptors [70]. This process can be modeled in vitro by observing the behaviour of leucocytes in flow chambers binding to purified adhesion proteins. Thus when neutrophils flow across slides coated with P- or E-selectin and ICAM-1, they roll but do not stop unless an activating stimulus is exogenously added. Similarly, on HUVECs stimulated with optimal concentrations of TNF-α or IL-1, the majority of tethered neutrophils rapidly arrest. The activating stimulus expressed by the endothelium which stimulates neutrophil β2 integrin-mediated binding in these circumstances include PAF and IL-8 [71]. Some chemoattractants such as PAF and eotaxin, but not RANTES, induced β2- and VLA-4-mediated eosinophil adhesion to HUVECs in static assays [25, 72]. Eosinophil binding to purified adhesion proteins was upregulated by RANTES, MCP-3 and C5a in a VLA-4- and Mac-1-dependent fashion via PT-inhibitable receptors [73]. VLA-4-, unlike Mac-1-, dependent increases in adhesion were transient and relied on actin polymerization. C3a and C5a were able to mediate firm arrest of eosinophils to rabbit mesenteric endothelium under flow conditions [74]. However, despite apparent eosinophil-active chemokine production, eosinophil adhesion to TNF-α- and IFN-γ-stimulated HUVEC under flow was only slightly inhibited by either anti-CCR3, the major chemokine receptor on eosinophils, or PT. When HUVECs were stimulated with IL-4 alone, no eosinophil-active chemokine release was detected, suggesting that under conditions more relevant to allergic disease, CC chemokines may not be playing a major role in the activation step [75]. Consistent with this, we observed only rolling behaviour when eosinophils bound to IL-4- and IL-13-stimulated HUVECs, although this was not the experience of Patel's group [40, 41] who found that all the eosinophils arrested. A confounding factor is VCAM-1 which may be able to promote eosinophil arrest in the absence of an activating stimulus. In our studies of binding to nasal polyp endothelium, whereas neutrophil adhesion was inhibited by PT, an anti-IL-8R antibody and a PAF antagonist, eosinophil adhesion, although activation dependent, was not inhibited by PT or anti-CCR3 [76]. This suggests that alternative endothelial associated pathways may exist for activation of eosinophil β2 integrins.

A number of studies of eosinophil adhesion and transmigration through HUVECs have shown that these events are mediated by a combination of VLA-4/VCAM-1 and the β2 (CD18) integrins binding to ICAM-1, the relative importance of either pathway depending on the cytokines involved in stimulating the endothelium. LFA-1 and Mac-1 are both involved in CD18-mediated binding [8, 25, 27, 28]. Eosinophil accumulation was reduced in ICAM-1 gene-deleted mice and by the use of anti-ICAM-1 mAbs [44, 45, 77]. The contribution from the CD18 integrins remains substantial even in the presence of good VCAM-1 expression, suggesting that this is not a site at which selection of eosinophils versus neutrophils occurs to any great extent. Consistent with this, in the FSA, we found that most of the integrin contribution for both eosinophil and neutrophil migration was via β2 rather than VLA-4/VCAM-1 [57]. Interestingly, in the ICAM-2 gene-deleted mouse, eosinophil accumulation was increased in the lung after antigen challenge through an unknown mechanism [78].

In summary therefore, the major contribution at the adhesion stage for selective eosinophil migration appears to be at the capture step, with P-selectin and VCAM-1 cooperating to tether eosinophils, but not neutrophils, to IL-4- and IL-13-stimulated endothelium. There are however potentially important differences in the activation step between the two cell types that could result in further levels of specificity.

Adhesion to Matrix Proteins

After migration through the endothelium, the eosinophil comes into contact with the proteins of the extracellular matrix. This is not simply a mesh in which the leucocytes are supported, but a complex network of large fibrillar proteins that have a profound influence on cellular function, mainly through adhesive contacts with integrin receptors. Eosinophils need to be adherent to a surface for optimal mediator release. For example, eosinophils in suspension cannot release superoxide or granule proteins when physiologically stimulated but do so when adherent to albumin-coated plastic or other adhesive surfaces. This priming effect seems to be mediated largely by CD18 [79]. Dri et al. [80] studied the production of superoxide by eosinophils resting on different surfaces including endothelial cells and a number of matrix proteins after stimulation with soluble mediators. They found that the nature of the surface influenced the amount of superoxide produced with for example endothelial cells inhibiting superoxide production and fibrinogen priming eosinophils for enhanced superoxide generation after stimulation with fMLP. Anwar et al. [81] demonstrated enhancement of calcium ionophore-stimulated leukotriene C_4 generation by eosinophils adhering to fibronectin when compared with BSA-coated surfaces, and Neeley et al. [82] have reported that VLA-4-mediated interaction with fibronectin resulted in increased fMLP-induced eosinophil degranulation. In contrast, Kita et al. [83] found that adherence to fibronectin and laminin inhibited EDN release stimulated by PAF, C5a and IL-5 but not by PMA. The secretogogue used and the mediator measured is obviously important in determining the effects of matrix proteins on eosinophil degranulation. When eosinophils were cultured for several days on plasma fibronectin they had increased survival compared to eosinophils cultured on BSA or plastic as a result of autocrine generation of GM-CSF and IL-3. Cytokine release and survival was inhibited by anti-VLA-4 mAb [84]. We extended these observations to show that tissue fibronectin was considerably more effective than plasma fibronectin at supporting eosinophil survival, presumably because tissue fibronectin contains more VLA-4 binding sites [85]. Eosinophils can adhere to laminin through $\alpha6\beta1$ [86], and laminin also promotes eosinophil survival [87]. As well as being important to eosinophil mediator generation in disease, the interaction between eosinophils and matrix proteins may be a homeostatic mechanism by which eosinophils survive for prolonged periods in tissue.

Adhesion to Epithelium

The pathology of asthma is characterized by an intense mucosal inflammation with infiltration of the airways by activated eosinophils and mononuclear cells in association with epithelial desquamation [88]. Epithelial damage in asthma is thought to be primarily mediated by the highly basic eosinophil granule proteins, such as major basic protein (MBP), which have been shown to be toxic for airway epithelium in vitro [89]. Indeed this observation forms one of the major pillars of the hypothesis that eosinophils and their mediators are responsible for much of the pathological and physiological abnormalities characteristic of asthma [discussed in 90]. By analogy with the way in which eosinophils kill helminthic parasites in which the first event is adhesion to the larval tegument, epithelial cytotoxicity of eosinophils is likely to require adhesion as an initial step. Godding et al. [91] investigated adhesion of eosinophils to A549 cells, an immortalized alveolar type 2 lung epithelial cell line, as well as commercially obtained human bronchial epithelial cells. Treatment of eosinophils with PMA increased eosinophil adhesion to both unstimulated and cytokine-stimulated epithelial cells. Interestingly, no increase in adhesion of unstimulated eosinophils to TNF-α or IL-1-stimulated epithelial cells was observed despite enhanced expression of ICAM-1. Consistent with this observation, enhanced adhesion was CD18 but not ICAM-1 dependent. Infecting A549 cells with RSV also enhanced eosinophil adhesion although, unlike neutrophils, only if the eosinophils were first stimulated with PMA. Enhanced adhesion in this model was inhibited by anti-ICAM-1 as well as anti-CD18 [92]. Co-culture of eosinophils and BEAS-2B cells (an SV-40-transformed bronchial epithelial cell line) resulted in enhanced eosinophil degranulation and adhesion when the eosinophils were treated with IL-5 and the epithelial cells with TNF-α for 16 h. Adhesion was partially blocked by anti-CD18, but not anti-ICAM-1 mAbs [93]. Recently bronchial epithelial cells were shown to express mRNA and protein for VCAM-1 and an antibody against VCAM-1, but not ICAM-1, inhibited eosinophil adhesion to TNF-α-stimulated BEAS-2B cells [94]. This was in contrast to a previous report that could find no VCAM-1 expression on BEAS-2B cells [95]. In previous studies, eosinophils have generally required stimulation with PMA for enhancement of adhesion to epithelial cells to be observed. The physiological stimuli promoting eosinophil adhesion to epithelium have not been investigated in detail although eosinophil adhesion to unstimulated HUVEC was increased by PAF and IL-5 [96, 97]. In addition, eotaxin, though not RANTES, enhanced eosinophil adhesion to lung vascular endothelial cells [98]. We have characterized eosinophil adhesion to A549 cells and BEAS-2B cells [99]. Stimulation of A549 cells with TNF-α, IFN-γ or a combination of 50 ng/ml of TNF-α, IFN-γ and IL-1 (cytomix) did not effect eosinophil binding despite an increase in ICAM-1 expression. Similarly, stimulation of eosinophils with PAF or IL-5 had no effect on eosinophil binding to medium- or cytokine-treated A549 cells. In contrast, stimulation of BEAS-2B cells with cytomix caused a significant increase in eosinophil adhesion. This was associated with an increase in expression of ICAM-1 and induced expression of VCAM-1. Treatment of eosinophils with Mn^{2+} and IL-5 but not eotaxin, RANTES or PAF also significantly enhanced eosinophil adhesion to medium-treated BEAS-2B cells. Using blocking mAbs, we were able to demonstrate that the increased adhesion resulting from stimulation of eosinophils or BEAS-2B cells was in both cases mediated by a combination of CD18 and α4 integrins. This study demonstrates a selective role for IL-5 in mediating integrin-dependent eosinophil adhesion to airway epithelium and once again emphasizes the importance of this cytokine in controlling eosinophil activation in diseases such as asthma.

In summary: Adhesion events are central to the proper functioning of eosinophils. They are required for maturation and release into the peripheral blood, for transmigration into tissue, for the priming and triggering of mediator release in the tissues and for their effector function both in host defence against helminthic parasites and in eosinophilic inflammatory diseases such as asthma. As with neutrophils, the CD18 integrins are involved in most of these events. However, unlike neutrophils, eosinophils express β1 integrins that can mediate adhesion to endothelium and epithelium as well as laminin and fibronectin which amongst other effects can lead to transmigration and prolonged survival in tissue, both of which can result in selective tissue accumulation. In addition, there are important differences between eosinophils and other leucocytes in their selectin-mediated adhesion in that they bind P-selectin avidly but E-selectin only weakly. This may also control selective eosinophil migration in Th2-mediated inflammation. Inhibition of eosinophil adhesion, particularly through the use of VLA-4 antagonists, but also antagonists of P-selectin/ PSGl-1, offer new directions for the treatment of asthma and related diseases.

References

1   Rosen SD: Cell surface lectins in the immune system. Semin Immunol 1993;5:237–247.
2   Picker LJ, Kishimoto TK, Smith CW, Warnock RA, Butcher EC: ELAM-1 is an adhesion molecule for skin-homing T cells. Nature 1991;349:796.
3   Maly P, Thall AD, Petryniak B, Rogers CE, Smith PL, Marks RM, Kelly RJ, Gersten KM, Cheng G, Saunders TL, Camper SA, Camphausen RT, Sullivan FX, Isogai Y, Hindsgaul O, Von Andrian UH, Lowe JB: The α(1,3)fucosyltransferase Fuc-TV11 controls leukocyte trafficking through an essential role in L-, E- and P-selectin ligand biosynthesis. Cell 1996;86:643–653.

4   Fuhlbrigge RC, Kieffer JD, Armerding D, Kupper TS: Cutaneous lymphocyte antigen is a specialized form of PSGL-1 expressed on skin homing T cells. Nature 1997;389:978–981.

5   Yao L, Pan J, Setiadi H, Patel KD, McEver RP: Interleukin-4 or oncostatin induces and prolonged increase in P-selectin mRNA and protein in human endothelial cells. J Exp Med 1996;184: 81–92.

6   Sako D, Comess KM, Barone KM, Camphausen RT, Cumming DA, Shaw GD: A sulfated peptide segment at the amino terminus of PSGL-1 is critical for P-selectin binding. Cell 1995;83:323–331.

7   Frenette PS, Mayadas TN, Rayburn H, Hynes RO, Wagner DD: Susceptibility to infection and altered hematopoiesis in mice deficient in both P- and E-selectins. Cell 1996;84:563–574.

8   Hynes RO: Integrins: Versatility, modulation and signalling in cell adhesion. Cell 1992;69:11–25.

9   Elices MJ, Osbourn L, Takada Y, Crouse C, Luhowskyj S, Hemler ME, Lobb RR: VCAM-1 on activated endothelium interacts with the leukocyte integrin VLA-4 at a site distinct from the VLA-4/fibronectin binding site. Cell 1990;60:577–584.

10   Erle DJ, Briskin MJ, Butcher ED, Garcia-Pardo A, Lazarovits AI, Tidswell M: Expression and function of the MAdCAM-1 receptor integrin a4/b7 on human leukocytes. J Immunol 1994;153: 517–528.

11   Cepek KL, Shaw SK, Parker CM, Russell GJ, Morrow JS, Rimm DL, Brenner MB: Adhesion between epithelial cells and T lymphocytes mediated by E-cadherin and the αEb7 integrin. Nature 1994;372:190–193.

12   Savill J, Dransfield I, Hogg N, Haslett C: Vitronectin receptor-mediated phagocytosis of cells undergoing apoptosis. Nature (Lond) 1990;343:170–173.

13   Liao F, Huynh HK, Eiroa A, Greene T, Polizzi E, Muller WA: Migration of monocytes across endothelium and passage through extracellular matrix involve separate molecular domains of PECAM-1. J Exp Med 1995;182:1337–1343.

14   Berlin C, Bargatze RF, Campbell JJ, von Adrian UH, Szabo MC, Hasslen SR, Nelson RD, Berg EL, Erlandsen SL, Butcher EC: α4 integrin mediates lymphocyte attachment and rolling under physiologic flow. Cell 1995;80:413–422.

15   Kyan-Aung U, Haskard DO, Poston RN, Thornhill MH, Lee TH: Endothelial leukocyte adhesion molecule-1 and intercellular adhesion molecule-1 mediated the adhesion of eosinophils to endothelial cells in vitro and are expressed by endothelium in allergic cutaneous inflammation in vivo. J Immunol 1991;146:521–528.

16   Leung YM, Pober JS, Cotran RS: Expression of endothelial-leukocyte adhesion molecule-1 in elicited late phase allergic reactions. J Clin Invest 1991;87:1805–1809.

17   Montefort S, Gratziou C, Goulding D, Polosa R, Haskard DO, Howart PH, Holgate ST, Carroll MP: Upregulation of leukocyte-endothelial cell adhesion molecules 6 hours after local allergen challenge of sensitised asthmatic airways. J Clin Invest 1993;93:1411–1421.

18   Bentley AM, Durham SR, Robinson DS, Menz G, Storz C, Cromwell O, Kay AB, Wardlaw AJ: Expression of endothelial and leukocyte adhesion molecules, intercellular adhesion molecule-1, E-selectin and vascular cell adhesion molecule-1 in the bronchial mucosa in steady state and allergen induced asthma. J Allergy Clin Immunol 1993;92:857–868.

19   Hirata N, Kohrogi H, Iwagoe H, Goto E, Hamamoto J, Fujii K, Yamaguchi T, Kawano O, Ando M: Allergen exposure induces the expression of endothelial adhesion molecules in passively sensitized human bronchus: Time course and the role of cytokines. Am J Respir Cell Mol Biol 1998;18:12–20.

20   Montefort S, Roche WR, Howarth PH, Djukanovic R, Gratziou C, Carroll M, Smith I, Britten KM, Haskard D, Lee TH: Intercellular adhesion molecule-1 and endothelial leucocyte adhesion molecule-1 expression in the bronchial mucosa of normals and asthmatic subjects. Eur Respir J 1992;5:815–823.

21   Gosset P, Tillie-Leblond I, Janin A, Marquette CH, Copin MC, Wallaert B, Tonnel AB: Expression of E-selectin, ICAM-1 and VCAM-1 on bronchial biopsies from allergic and non-allergic asthmatic patients. Int Arch Allergy Appl Immunol 1995;106:69–77.

22   Ohkawara Y, Yamauchi K, Maruyama N, Hoshi H, Ohno I, Honma M, Tanno Y, Tamura G, Shirato K, Ohtani H: In situ expression of the cell adhesion molecules in bronchial tissues from asthmatics with air flow limitation: In vivo evidence of VCAM-1/VLA-4 interaction in selective eosinophil infiltration. Am J Respir Cell Mol Biol 1995;12:4–12.

23 Fukuda T, Fukushima Y, Numao T, Ando N, Arima M, Nakajima H, Sagara H, Adachi T, Motojima S, Makino S: Role of interleukin-4 and vascular cell adhesion molecule-1 in selective eosinophil migration into the airways in allergic asthma. Am J Respir Cell Mol Biol 1996;14:84–94.

24 Montefort S, Feather IH, Wilson SJ, Haskard DO, Lee TH, Holgate ST, Howarth PH: The expression of leukocyte endothelial adhesion molecules is increased in perennial allergic rhinitis. Am J Respir Cell Mol Biol 1992;7:393–398.

25 Vignola AM, Campbell AM, Chanez P, Bousquet J, Lacoste P, Michel FB, Godard P: HLA-DR and ICAM-1 expression on bronchial epithelial cells in asthma and chronic bronchitis. Am Rev Respir Dis 1993;147:529–534.

26 Manolitsas ND, Trigg CJ, McAulay AE, Wang JH, Jordan SE, D'Ardenne AJ, Davies RJ: The expression of intercellular adhesion molecule-1 and the β1-integrins in asthma. Eur Respir J 1994; 7:1439–1444.

27 Ciprandi G, Pronzato C, Ricca V, Passalacqua G, Bagnasco M, Canonica GW: Allergen specific challenge induces intercellular adhesion molecule-1 (ICAM-1/CD54) expression on nasal epithelial cells in allergic subjects. Relationship with early and late inflammatory phenomena. Am J Respir Crit Care Med 1994;150:1653–1659.

28 Ciprandi G, Buscaglia S, Pesce GP, Villaggio B, Bagnesco M, Canonica GW: Allergic subjects express intracellular adhesion molecule 1 (ICAM-1 or CD54) on epithelial cells of conjunctiva after allergen challenge. J Allergy Clin Immunol 1993;91:783–792.

29 Lackie PM, Baker JE, Gunthert U, Holgate ST: Expression of CD44 isoforms is increased in the airway epithelium of asthmatic subjects. Am J Respir Cell Mol Biol 1997;16:14–22.

30 Montefort S, Lai CKW, Kapahi P, Leung J, Lai KN, Chan HS, Haskard DO, Howarth PH, Holgate ST: Circulating adhesion molecules in asthma. Am J Respir Crit Care Med 1994;149:1149–1152.

31 Kobayashi T, Hashimoto S, Imai K, Amemiya E, Yamaguchi M, Yachi A, Horie T: Elevation of serum-soluble intercellular adhesion molecule-1 and sE-selectin levels in bronchial asthma. Clin Exp Immunol 1994;96:110–115.

32 Koizumi A, Hashimoto S, Kobayashi T, Imai K, Yachi A, Horie T: Elevation of serum-soluble vascular cell adhesion molecule-1 levels in bronchial asthma. Clin Exp Immunol 1995;101:468–473.

33 Georas SN, Liu MC, Newman W, Beall LD, Stealey BA, Bochner BS: Altered adhesion molecule expression and endothelial cell activation accompany the recruitment of human granulocytes to the lung after segmental antigen challenge. Am J Respir Cell Mol Biol 1992;7:261–269.

34 Takahashi N, Liu MC, Proud D, Yu XY, Hasegawa S, Spannhake EW: Soluble intercellular adhesion molecule-1 in bronchoalveolar lavage fluid of allergic subjects following segmental antigen challenge. Am J Respir Crit Care Med 1994;150:704–709.

35 Zangrilli JG, Shaver JR, Cirelli RA, Cho SK, Garlisi CG, Falcone A, Cuss FM, Fish JE, Peters SP: sVCAM-1 levels after segmental allergen challenge correlates with eosinophil influx, IL-4 and IL-5 production and the late phase response. Am J Respir Crit Care Med 1995;151:1346–1353.

36 Azzawi M, Bradley B, Jeffery PK, Frew J, Wardlaw AJ, Assoufi B, Collins JV, Durham S, Kay AB: Identification of activated T lymphocytes and eosinophils in bronchial biopsies in stable atopic asthma. Am Rev Respir Dis 1990;142:1407–1413.

37 Kay AB, Stechschulte DJ, Austen KF: An eosinophil leukocyte chemotactic factor of anaphylaxis. J Exp Med 1971;133:602–619.

38 Sehmi R, Cromwell O, Taylor GW, Kay AB: Identification of guinea pig eosinophil chemotactic factor of anaphylaxis as leukotriene B₄ and 18(S),15(S)-dihydroxy-5,9,11,13(Z,E,Z,E)eicosatetraenoic acid. J Immunol 1991;147:2276–2283.

39 Goetzl EJ, Austen KF: Purification and synthesis of eosinophilotactic tetrapeptides of human lung. Identification as eosinophil chemotactic factor of anaphylaxis. Proc Natl Acad Sci USA 1975;72: 4123–4127.

40 Wardlaw AJ, Moqbel R, Cromwell O, Kay AB: Platelet-activating factor is a potent chemotactic and chemokinetic factor for human eosinophils. J Clin Invest 1986;78:1701–1706.

41 Wardlaw AJ: Molecular basis for eosinophil trafficking in asthma: A multistep paradigm. J Allergy Clin Immunol 1999;104:917–926.

42 Collins PD, Marleau S, Griffiths-Johnson DA, Jose PJ, Williams TJ: Cooperation between interleukin-5 and the chemokine eotaxin to induce eosinophil accumulation in vivo. J Exp Med 1995;182:1169–1174.

43 Palframan RT, Collins PD, Williams TJ, Rankin SM: Eotaxin induces a rapid release of eosinophils and their progenitors from the bone marrow. Blood 1998;91:2240–2248.

44 Palframan RT, Collins PD, Severs NJ, Rothery S, Williams TJ, Rankin SM: Mechanisms of acute eosinophil mobilization from the bone marrow stimulated by interleukin-5: The role of specific adhesion molecules and phosphatidylinositol 3-kinase. J Exp Med 1998;188:1621–1632.

45 Wardlaw AJ: Adhesion molecules; in Barnes P, Roger I, Thompson N (eds): Asthma: Basic Mechanisms and Clinical Management, ed 3, chapt 13. London, Academic Press, 1998, pp 239–251.

46 Grayson MH, Van der Vieren M, Sterbinsky SA, Gallatin MW, Hoffman PA, Staunton DE, Bochner BS: Alpha- and beta-2 integrin is expressed on human eosinophils and functions as an alternative ligand for vascular cell adhesion molecule 1. J Exp Med 1998;188:2187.

47 Yamamoto H, Sedgwick JB, Busse WW: Differential regulation of eosinophil adhesion and transmigration by pulmonary microvasular endothelial cells. J Immunol 1998;161:971–977.

48 Blease K, Seybold J, Adcock IM, Hellewell PG, Burke-Gaffney A: Interleukin-4 and lipopolysaccharide synergize to induce vascular cell adhesion molecule-1 expression in human lung microvascular endothelial cells. Am J Respir Cell Mol Biol 1998;18:620–630.

49 Fukuda T, Fukushima Y, Numao T, Ando N, Arima M, Nakajima H, Sagara H, Adachi T, Motojima S, Makino S: Role of interleukin-4 and vascular cell adhesion molecule-1 in selective eosinophil migration into the airways in allergic asthma. Am J Respir Cell Mol Biol 1996;14:84–94.

50 Beck LA, Stellato C, Beall LD, Schall TJ, Leopold D, Bickel CA, Baroody F, Bochner BS, Schleimer RP: Detection of the chemokine RANTES and endothelial adhesion molecules in nasal polyps. J Allergy Clin Immunol 1996;98:766–780.

51 Matsumoto K, Sterbinsky SA, Bickel CA, Zhou DF, Kovach NL, Bochner BS: Regulation of α4 integrin-mediated adhesion of human eosinophils to fibronectin and vascular cell adhesion molecule-1. J Allergy Clin Imunol 1997;99:648–656.

52 Sriramarao P, Von Adrian UH, Butcher EC, Bourdon MA, Broide DH: L-selectin and very late antigen-4 integrin promote eosinophil rolling at physiological shear stress rates in vivo. J Immunol 1994;152:4238.

53 Kitayama J, Fuhlbrigge RC, Puri KD, Springer TA: P-selectin, L-selectin and α4 integrin have distinct roles in eosinophil tethering and arrest on vascular endothelial cells under physiological flow conditions. J Immunol 1997;159:3929.

54 Ulfman LH, Kuijper PH, van der Linden JA, Lammers JW, Zwaginga JJ, Koenderman L: Characterisation of eosinophil adhesion to TNF-α-activated endothelium under flow conditions: α4 integrins mediate initial attachment and E-selectin mediates rolling. J Immunol 1999;163:343–350.

55 Richards IM, Kolbasa KP, Hatfield CA, Winterrowd GE, Vonderfecht SL, Fidler SF, Griffin RL, Brashier JR, Krzesicki RF, Sly LM, Ready KA, Staite ND, Chin JE: Role of VLA-4 in the antigen-induced accumulation of eosinophils and lymphocytes in the lungs and airway of sensitized brown Norway rats. Am J Respir Cell Mol Biol 1996;15:172–183.

56 Henderson WR, Chi EY, Albert RK, Chu SJ, Lamm WJ, Rochon Y, Jonas M, Christie PE, Harlan JM: Blockade of CD49d (α4 integrin) on intrapulmonary but not circulating leukocytes inhibits airway inflammation and hyperresponsiveness in a mouse model of asthma. J Clin Invest 1997;100:3083–3092.

57 Symon FA, Lawrence MB, Walsh GM, Watson SR, Wardlaw AJ: Characterisation of the eosinophil P-selectin ligand. J Immunol 1996;157:1711–1719.

58 Khew-Goodall Y, Wadham C, Stein BN, Gamble JR, Vadas MA: STAT-6 activation is essential for interleukin-4 induction of P-selectin transcription in human umbilical vein endothelial cells. Arterioscler Thromb Vasc Biol 1999;19:1421–1429.

59 Woltmann G, McNulty CA, Dewson G, Symon FA, Wardlaw AJ: PSGL-1 mediates the adhesion of eosinophils, but not neutrophils, to IL-13 stimulated HUVEC under flow. Blood 2000;95:3146–3152.

60 Patel KD: Eosinophil tethering to interleukin-4-activated endothelial cells requires both P-selectin and vascular cell adhesion molecule-1. Blood 1998;92:3904–3911.

61 Symon FA, Walsh GM, Watson S, Wardlaw AJ: Eosinophil adhesion to nasal polyp endothelium is P-selectin dependent. J Exp Med 1994;180:371.

62 Hamilos DL, Thawley SE, Kramper MA, Kamil A, Hamid QA: Effect of intranasal fluticasone on cellular infiltration, endothelial adhesion molecule expression, and proinflammatory cytokine mRNA in nasal polyp disease. J Allergy Clin Imunol 1999;103:79–87.

63   Broide DH, Humber D, Sullivan S, Sriramarao P: Inhibition of eosinophil rolling and recruitment in P-selectin and intercellular adhesion molecule-1-deficient mice. Blood 1998;91:2847–2856.

64   Broide DH, Sullivan S, Gifford T, Sriramarao P: Inhibition of pulmonary eosinophilia in P-selectin and ICAM-1-deficient mice. Am J Respir Cell Mol Biol 1998;18:218–225.

65   De Sanctis GT, Wolyniec WW, Green FHY, Qin S, Jiao A, Finn PW, Noonan T, Joetham AA, Gelfand E, Doerschuk CM, Drazen JM: Reduction of allergic airway responses in P-selectin-deficient mice. J Appl Physiol 1997;83:681–687.

66   Henriques GM, Miotla OJM, Cordeiro RSB, Wolitzky BA, Woolley ST, Hellewell PG: Selectins mediate eosinophil recruitment in vivo. A comparison with their role in neutrophil influx. Blood 1996;87:5297.

67   Sriramarao P, Norton CR, Borgstrom P, DiScipio RG, Wolitsky BA, Broide DH: E-selectin preferentially supports neutrophil but not eosinophil rolling under conditions of flow in vitro and in vivo. J Immunol 1996;157:4672–4680.

68   Teixeira MM, Hellewell PG: Contribution of endothelial selectins and α4 integrins to eosinophil trafficking in allergic and non-allergic inflammatory reactions in skin. J Immunol 1998;161:2516–2523.

69   Yang J, Furie BC, Furie B: The biology of P-selectin glycoprotein ligand-1: Its role as a selectin counterreceptor in leucocyte-endothelial leukocyte-platelet interaction. Thromb Haemost 1999;81: 1–7.

70   Butcher EC, Picker LJ: Lymphocyte homing and homeostasis. Science 1996;272:60–66.

71   Zimmerman GA, McIntyre TM, Prescott SM: Adhesion and signalling in vascular cell-cell interactions. J Clin Invest 1997;100:S3–S5.

72   Burke-Gaffney A, Hellewell PG: Eotaxin stimulates eosinophil adhesion to human lung microvascular endothelial cells. Biochem Biophys Res Commun 1996;227:35–40.

73   Weber C, Kitayama J, Springer TA: Differential regulation of β1 and β2 integrin avidity by chemoattractants in eosinophils. Proc Natl Acad Sci USA 1996;93:10939–10944.

74   DiScipio RG, Daffern PJ, Jagels MA, Broide DH, Sriramarao P: A comparison of C3a and C5a-mediated stable adhesion of rolling eosinophils in post-capillary venules and transendothelial migration in vitro and in vivo. J Immunol 1999;162:1127–1136.

75   Kitayama J, Mackay CR, Ponath PD, Springer TA: The C-C chemokine receptor CCR3 participates in stimulation of eosinophil arrest on inflammatory endothelium under flow. J Clin Invest 1998; 101:2017–2024.

76   McNulty C, Symon FA, Wardlaw AJ: Characterisation of the integrin and activation steps in human eosinophil and neutrophil adhesion to endothelium in a model of chronic eosinophilic inflammation. Am J Respir Cell Mol Biol 1999;20:1251–1259.

77   Chin JE, Winterrowd GE, Hatfield CA, Brashler JR, Griffin RL, Vonderfecht SL, Kolbasa KP, Fidler SF, Shull KL, Krzesicki RF, Read KA, Dunn CJ, Sly LM, Staite ND, Richards IM: Involvement of intercellular adhesion molecule-1 in the antigen-induced infiltration of eosinophils and lymphocytes into the airways in a murine model of pulmonary inflammation. Am J Respir Crit Care Med 1998; 18:158–167.

78   Gerwin N, Gonzalo JA, Lloyd C, Coyle AJ, Reiss Y, Banu N, Wang B, Xu H, Avrahim H, Engelhardt B, Springer TA, Gutierrez-Ramos JC: Prolonged eosinophil accumulation in allergic lung interstitium of ICAM-2-deficient mice results in extended hyperresponsiveness. Immunity 1999;10:9–19.

79   Kaneko M, Horie S, Kato M, Gleich GJ, Kita H: A crucial role for β2 integrin in the activation of eosinophils stimulated by IgG. J Immunol 1995;155:2631–2641.

80   Dri P, Cramer R, Spessotto P, Romano M, Patriarca P: Eosinophil activation on biologic surfaces. J Immunol 1991;147:613–620.

81   Anwar ARE, Cromwell O, Walsh GW, Kay AB, Wardlaw AJ: Adhesion to fibronectin primes eosinophils via α4/β1. Immunology 1994;82:222–228.

82   Neeley SP, Hamann KJ, Dowling TL, McAllister KT, White SR, Leff AR: Augmentation of stimulated eosinophil degranulation by VLA-4 (CD49d) mediated adhesion to fibronectin. Am J Respir Cell Mol Biol 1994;82:222–228.

83   Kita H, Horie S, Gleich GJ: Extracellular matrix proteins attenuate activation and degranulation of stimulated eosinophils. J Immunol 1996;156:1174–1181.

84 Anwar ARE, Cromwell O, Walsh GM, Kay AB, Wardlaw AJ: Adhesion to fibronectin prolongs eosinophil survival. J Exp Med 1993;177:839–843.
85 Walsh GM, Symon FA, Wardlaw AJ: Human eosinophils preferentially survive on tissue compared with plasma fibronectin. Clin Exp Allergy 1995;25:1128–1136.
86 Georas SN, McIntyre WB, Ebisawa M, Bednarczyk JL, Sterbinsky SA, Schlemier RP, Bochner BS: Expression of a functional laminin receptor a6b1 (very late activation antigen-6] on human eosinophils. Blood 1993;82:2872–2879.
87 Walsh GM, Wardlaw AJ: Dexamethasone inhibits prolonged survival and autocrine GM-CSF production by human eosinophils cultured on laminin and tissue fibronectin. J Allergy Clin Immunol 1997;100:208–215.
88 Jeffery PK: Airway pathology in asthma; in Barnes P, Rodger I, Thomson N (eds): Asthma: Basic Mechanisms and Clinical Management, ed 3, chapt 3. London, Academic Press, 1998, pp 33–38.
89 Hastie AT, Loegering DA, Gleich GJ, Kueppers F: The effect of purified human eosinophil major basic protein on mammalian ciliary activity. Am Rev Respir Dis 1987;135:848.
90 Wardlaw AJ, Moqbel R, Kay AB: Eosinophils: Biology and role in disease. Adv Immunol 1995; 60:151–266.
91 Godding V, Stark JM, Sedgwick JB, Busse WB: Adhesion of activated eosinophils to respiratory epithelial cells is enhanced by tumor necrosis factor-α and interleukin-1β. Am J Respir Cell Mol Biol 1995;13:555–562.
92 Stark JM, Godding V, Sedgwick JB, Busse WW: Respiratory syncytial virus infection enhances neutrophil and eosinophil adhesion to cultured respiratory epithelial cells. J Immunol 1996;156: 4774–4782.
93 Takafuji S, Ohtoshi T, Takizawa H, Tadokoro K, Ito K: Eosinophil degranulation in the presence of bronchial epithelial cells. Effect of cytokines and role of adhesion. J.Immunol.1996;156:3980–3985.
94 Atsuta J, Sterbinsky SA, Plitt J, Schwiebert LM, Bochner BS, Schleimer RP: Phenotyping and cytokine regulation of the BEAS-2B human bronchial epithelial cell: Demonstration of inducible expression of the adhesion molecules VCAM-1 and ICAM-1. Am J Respir Cell Mol Biol 1997;17: 571–582.
95 Bloemen PGM, van den Tweel MC, Henricks PAJ, Engels F, Wagenaar SS, Rutten AAJJL, Nijkamp FP: Expression and modulation of adhesion molecules on human bronchial epithelial cells. Am J Respir Cell Mol Biol 1993;9:586–593.
96 Kimani G, Tonnensen MG, Henson PM: Stimulation of eosinophil adherence to human vascular endothelial cell in vitro by platelet-activating factor. J Immunol 1988;140:3161.
97 Walsh GM, Hartnell A, Wardlaw AJ, Kurihara K, Sanderson CJ, Kay AB: IL-5 enhances the in vitro adhesion of human eosinophils, but not neutrophils in a leucocyte integrin (CD11/18)-dependent manner. Immunology 1990;71:258–265.
98 Burke-Gaffney A, Hellewell PG: Eotaxin stimulates eosinophil adhesion to human lung microvascular endothelial cell. Biochem Biophys Res Commun 1996;227:35–40.
99 Sanmugalingham D, de Vries E, Gauntlett R, Symon FA, Bradding P, Wardlaw AJ: IL-5 enhances eosinophil adhesion to bronchial epithelial cells. Clin Exp Allergy 2000;30:255–263.

Andrew J. Wardlaw, Professor of Respiratory Medicine, Division of Respiratory Medicine,
Clinical Sciences Building University of Leicester Medical School, Glenfield Hospital,
Groby Road, Leicester LE3 9QP (UK)
Tel. +44 116 256 3734, Fax +44 116 236 7768, E-Mail aw24@le.ac.uk

Robinson DS (ed): Immunological Mechanisms in Asthma and Allergic Diseases.
Chem Immunol. Basel, Karger, 2000, vol 78, pp 112–123

....

Proposing Th2 DTH Relevant to Asthma: Cutaneous Basophil Hypersensitivity Then and Now

Philip W. Askenase

Section of Allergy and Clinical Immunology, Department Internal Medicine,
Yale University School of Medicine, New Haven, Conn., USA

Cutaneous Basophil Hypersensitivity in Former Times

Delayed-type hypersensitivity (DTH) can be defined as a delayed-time-course tissue inflammation due to local recruitment of different kinds of effector T cells (Th1, Th2, Tc1 Tc2) out of blood vessels and into tissues, to bind appropriate antigen presenting cells (APC), and thus be activated to produce cytokines that mediate inflammation by recruiting and activating various leukocytes, such as monocytes, basophils, eosinophils, and neutrophils, depending on the profile of T-cell-secreted cytokines. The subset of DTH known as cutaneous basophil hypersensitivity (CBH) was discovered in the late 1960s by the Dvoraks [1, 2] employing plastic embedded thin tissue sections. This revealed large basophil infiltrates in a variety DTH responses, but notably not in the classical tuberculin reaction. With hindsight, now knowing that the tuberculin reaction is a classical Th1 response, and also knowing that the immunization procedures used to induce CBH are known to induce Th2 cells, it is easy to see that CBH might now be redesignated as a form of Th2 DTH. Using more routine histological techniques that allowed quantitative survey of larger pieces of tissue, we showed that B cells and antibodies could also mediate CBH [3, 4], and this was confirmed by others [5] and by Dvorak [6]. In guinea pigs, the antibodies were IgG1 [7] and IgE [8] mast-cell-sensitizing isotypes, that mediated basophil-rich CBH late-phase responses (LPR). Recent work in humans has confirmed that allergen-induced cutaneous LPR, that probably are due to overlapping allergen-specific IgE and Th2 cells, similarly contain basophils [9], confirming that Th2 cellular and Th2 humoral responses can lead to CBH.

Besides allergies, such as contact dermatitis, atopic dermatitis, allergic rhinitis and conjunctivitis [10], the strongest CBH responses are to parasites invading the surfaces, like the skin and intestine [11]. These parasite-induced CBH responses can be associated with immune resistance and rejection of the parasites, and thereby provide an example of the biological usefulness of allergic disease tissue inflammation, and provide reason for the preservation of seemingly deleterious allergic responses in the genome throughout vertebrates. Thus an allergy-like Th2 DTH response in the tissues, which contains basophils and eosinophils, can participate in the rejection of complex multicellular parasites [12]. Further, depletion of basophils or eosinophils with specific antibodies, showed that both cells are involved in parasite rejection [13]. In the case of rejection of ectoparasitic arthropod ticks from the skin of guinea pigs, basophils play a predominant role, and in fact are largely responsible for recruiting the eosinophils, suggesting that tick antigen-specific Th2 cells and IgE/IgG1 lead to CBH recruitment of basophils [14], that then might produce CC chemokines to recruit eosinophils. The relevant point is that these basophil- and eosinophil-rich parasite CBH reactions, driven by Th2 cells and Th2 antibodies, also occur in various allergic disease tissue responses, and are proposed herein to be a subset of a broader category of reactivity that is defined as Th2 DTH.

CBH Responses Today

Study of CBH today is focused on analyses with new specific anti-human basophil monoclonal antibodies (mAb), that for the first time allow definitive quantitative identification of basophils in tissues. Following the lead of Irani and Schwartz [15] in Virginia, Andrew Walls [16] in Southampton described the BB1 mAb that specifically binds a granule protein of basophils, and identifies basophils in human biopsies [9]. Sun Ying and Barry Kay [9] in a study of human cutaneous LPR to challenge with grass pollen allergen, have identified basophil infiltrates peaking at 24 h, and in contrast noted that eosinophils peak earlier at 6 h, and are more numerous (3:1). This suggests different mechanisms for basophil vs. eosinophil recruitment, even though both cells express CCR3, the Th2-associated eotaxin and CC-chemokine receptor [17].

Different mechanisms for recruitment were confirmed when correlating basophil vs. eosinophil numbers with expression of five different CC chemokines (eotaxin-1, eotaxin-2, MCP-3, MCP-4 and RANTES) in the allergen LPR, and with the chemokine receptor CCR3, that is principally responsible for eosinophil recruitment, but also is found on basophils, and importantly on Th2 cells, but not on Th1 cells [17]. Eosinophil recruitment in allergen-induced LPR of humans correlated with eotaxin-1 at 6 h, and with eotaxin-2 and MCP-4 while declining at 24 h, and also with CCR3 expression, determined by mAb and in situ mRNA expression [9]. However, basophil infiltrates did not correlate with any of the five CC chemokines, nor with CCR3 expression [9]. These findings in the cutaneous LPR suggest that early-acting IgE and late-acting Th2 DTH responses to allergen challenge, lead to CC chemokines that mediate eosinophil recruitment, but are not responsible for simultaneous basophil recruitment. The idea that allergen-induced LPR can largely be due to Th2 DTH is supported by recent demonstration by Haselden, Oldfield, Larche, and Kay that cat allergen T-cell peptides, that do not bind IgE, can elicit similar responses [unpubl. observations]. The cutaneous LPR findings concerning basophils vs. eosinophils could be explained in two ways. Either other chemokine receptors such as CCR1, CCR2, or CCR4, all of which are known to be expressed on basophils [18], are important in basophil recruitment, or the local tissues produce more specific basophil chemokines, that act on basophils preferentially, or synergize with CC chemokines acting on CCR3, to specifically attract basophils.

Restriction of Th2 CBH to Organs at Surfaces, Like Skin and Intestine

The above concerned chemokine participation in CBH, as an aspect of Th2 DTH responses, that are restricted to the skin. In contrast, eosinophils participate in Th2 DTH in all tissues. A vivid example of this dichotomy is in the parasitical disease schistosomiasis. Here, skin penetration in a sensitized host with larvae acquired in fresh water, produces strong CBH responses, called 'swimmers itch' [19]. These contain both basophils and eosinophils, while simultaneous liver lesions to schistosome eggs embolized from portal veins are florid Th2 eosinophil-rich granulomas [20], with no basophils. Further, eggs caught in the intestinal mucosa elicit basophils and eosinophils, and similar CBH-like mucosal responses occur in the intestines of guinea pigs infested with helminths [20, 21], or in intestinal contact sensitivity [22]. In addition, when isolated eggs are used as particulate antigens for challenge in the skin of schistosome-infested animals, CBH again is obtained, while if the eggs are given intravenously and embolize to the lungs, an eosinophilic granuloma develops, without basophils. Thus, surface organs like the skin and intestine manifest Th2 DTH responses expressing a basophil component, along with eosinophils, while the deep organs, like liver and lung, manifest predominant eosinophilic Th2 DTH, with few basophils. This suggests that tissue cells of the skin and intestine, such as keratinocytes and epithelial cells respectively, may produce a special basophil-directed chemokine.

Differential basophil vs. eosinophil recruitment in Th2 DTH in various tissues fits with additional recent findings made in the Kay laboratory using the BB1 antibasophil mAb of Walls [16]. Alison Macfarlane [23] studied bronchial biopsies following airway challenge with allergen to elicit bronchial LPR in atopic asthmatics. Again, there was a 6-hour eosinophil-rich response, while basophil increases again peaked at 24 h, but were quite modest, and much less than in the skin. Thus, in the allergen-induced cutaneous LPR, the ratio of eosinophils to basophils at peak of each response (6 vs. 24 h, respectively) was 3:1, while in the airways the ratio of eosinophils to basophils at 24 h was 10:1 [23]. Nasreen Khan [24] confirmed the weaker basophil component of Th2 DTH in asthma, and further, in a study of airway LPR in atopic asthmatics treated with cyclosporin, extended findings suggesting that basophils and eosinophils are attracted differently. Cyclosporin strongly inhibited eosinophil infiltrates in bronchial biopsies, along with IL-5, GM-CSF and eotaxin levels, but had no effect on the basophils. Since cyclosporin is thought to act mainly by inhibiting transcription of the Th2 cytokines, this finding suggests that different Th2 cytokines, or the production of particular basophil-specific chemokines, is less sensitive to cyclosporin treatment. Alternatively, mast cell release of mediators and cytokines can also be inhibited by cyclosporin [25], and perhaps there is less sensitivity to cyclosporin inhibition of mast cell release of basophil attractants.

Initiation of Th2 DTH in Asthma

It is therefore proposed that the delayed eosinophil-rich inflammatory T-cell aspect of allergic tissue responses, particularly in asthma, represent examples of Th2 DTH. Other examples of Th2 DTH already in the literature include: the classic example schistosome hepatic egg granuloma [26], and also: epicutaneous protein-induced immune inflammation [27], intradermal KLH in guinea pigs [28], and Jones Mote Reactions in man [29]; contact sensitivity (CS) in mice to TMA, aldehyde [30], DNCB [31] and chronic TNCB [32]; DTH transfer with Th2 [33], and Tc2 clones [34], Th2 cutaneous drug-induced hypersensitivity [35], transplant responses [36, 37], oxazolone and TNBSA-induced experimental colitis [38, 39], and tumor immune responses [40]. Thus, there are numerous examples of Th2 DTH, to which we now have added CBH, and also the Th2 aspect of LPR in skin, and in the lungs in asthma.

In studies of classical cutaneous Th1 DTH in CS of mice, we recently found that B-1 B cells produce specific IgM antibodies that are responsible for an early initiation process required for recruitment of the Th1 cells into the tissues [41]. We call this overall process 'DTH initiation'. IgM is produced by B-1 cells at the time of immunization, is present in the tissues at the time of Ag challenge to elicit CS, and binds Ag to activate complement (C′) to generate C5a [42]. We detected locally generated C5a, in skin extracts with a chemotactic assay [43]. However, besides acting as a chemotactic factor for the T cells [44], C5a may also act indirectly by binding C5a receptors on local mast cells [45, 46], and platelets [47, 48], to activate production of vasoactive serotonin [49, 50], and TNF-α that induce expression of endothelial adhesion molecules, like ICAM-1 and VCAM-1 [51], to bind circulating T cells, to aid in their recruitment into the tissues. Thus, in proposing Th2 DTH asthma, we need to postulate what initiating processes are involved to mediate early recruitment of Th2 cells into airway tissues.

Possible Role of IgE Antibody in Initiation of Th2 DTH in Asthma

We hypothesize that allergen-specific IgE antibody is a likely candidate for mediating the initiation of Th2 DTH in asthma. We propose that initiating the elicitation of Th2 DTH in asthma may be a function of the IgE-dependent LPR, since allergen-induced IgE activation of mast cells occurs uniformly in asthma, and likely precedes infiltration of Th2 DTH cells to then mediate airway inflammation (fig. 1). Thus, following natural environmental airway challenge with allergen, or laboratory challenge, specific IgE produced previously via atopic gene-dependent Th2-helper cell mechanisms, and sensitizing airway luminal and mucosal mast cells, triggers release of immediate-acting mediators, like histamine and leukotrienes, and also mediates subsequent LPR due to delayed synthesis and release of a Th2 profile of cytokines like IL-4, IL-5 and IL-13, and chemokines [52]. Some are CC chemokines, like eotaxin, MCP-2,3,4, and RANTES, that may act specifically on circulating Th2 cells, which preferentially express CCR3 that bind these ligands [17]. In addition, IgE-mast cell-CC chemokine-attracted Th2 cells may adhere to local endothelium because simultaneous mast cell-derived TNF-α and IL-4 have unregulated expression of endothelial adhesion molecules, such as ICAM-1 and VCAM-1. Thus the Th2 cells probably are not recruited via antigen-specific B-1 cell-derived IgM antibody mechanisms, as occurs in Th1 DTH/CS [41–43, 53]. Instead, in asthma, initiation of Th2 recruitment to then mediate Th2 DTH in the airways, may proceed via the relatively Th2-specific chemokine receptor CCR3 (fig. 1). IgE need not always be involved in Th2 cell recruitment across the vessels, since mast cells can be activated by other mechanisms, such as via C5a [42, 43]. In fact, local cells other than mast cells may provide needed vasoactivating cytokines, or in some instances the Th2 cells may be sufficiently preactivated to not need additional factors to allow adequate binding to constitutively expressed endothelial adhesion molecules, thereby allowing direct entry into the airway tissues.

Once in the tissues, those few recruited Th2 CCR3 + cells, that are specific for allergens, then bind to allergen-derived peptides complexed with MHC class II molecules on local airway tissue APC (fig. 2). It is pertinent to point out that as few as only one Ag-specific T cell may be sufficient to elicit such a DTH response [54]. This peptide/MHC binding and additional costimulation via

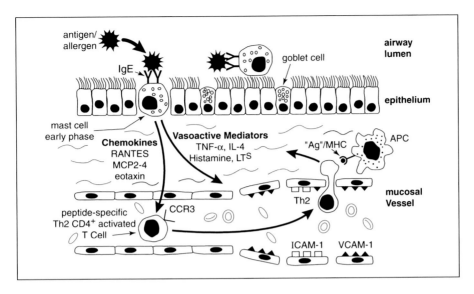

Fig. 1. IgE and mast cells may initiate Th2 DTH in asthma. Figure shows postulated initiation processes, via IgE and mast cell activation, for recruitment out of vessels into airway tissues of Th2 DTH asthma effector Th2 cells. Starting at the top left, the inhaled native allergen molecules cross-link specific IgE antibodies bound to FcεR1 on the surface of mast cells in the lumen and in the epithelium of the airways. This causes release of mast cell-derived vasoactive mediators, such as TNF-α, IL-4, histamine, and leukotrienes, and also release of CCR3-activating chemokines; possibly RANTES, MCP-2, MCP-3 and MCP-4, and/or eotaxin. Together these IgE mast cell-dependent Th2 DTH-initiating mediators activate the local vasculature for increased permeability, and also for expression of surface adhesion molecules like ICAM-1 and VCAM-1, and also these attract circulating allergen-peptide-specific Th2 CD4+ T cells expressing surface CCR3, resulting in the recruitment across the local endothelium of Th2 T cells with multiple Ag specificities, at the middle right.

CD28:B7 and CD40:CD40L, stimulates these few T cells to produce characteristic Th2 cytokines like IL-4, IL-5, IL-9 and IL-13 [52, 55, 56]. These Th2 cytokines then stimulate local tissue cells; like epithelial, goblet, macrophage and smooth muscle cells, to produce chemokines, such as eotaxin, to preferentially attract CCR3+ eosinophils [57]. Together the Th2 cytokines, CC chemokines and the activated eosinophils of Th2 inflammation alter these local tissue cells to produce the asthmatic state (fig. 2). Consistent with the formulation outlined above is the recent finding that treatment with anti-IgE, that lowers serum levels of IgE, and expression of FcεR1 on mast cells, inhibits not only the early mast cell-dependent asthmatic response, but also the late response due to local recruitment of T cells, in both humans [58] and in mice [59].

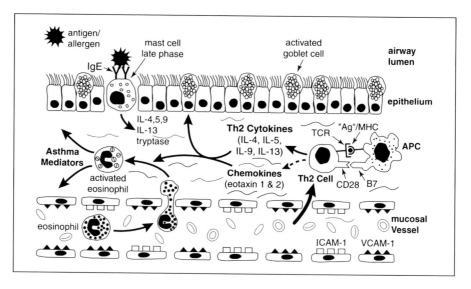

Fig. 2. Late-phase recruitment of Th2 DTH T cells to mediate asthma, following IgE/ mast cell initiation. Starting at the right middle of the figure, Th2 DTH T cells of diverse allergen specificities are recruited into the extravascular tissues in part because of their surface CCR3. In the tissues, the few among these that have surface αβ-TCR that are specific for allergen peptides that are expressed in complexes with MHC class II molecules on local APC, are then specifically activated via these αβ-TCR and via costimulation provided by CD28:B7 etc., to produce Th2 cytokines produce in the local airway tissues, such as IL-4, IL-5, IL-9 and IL-13, as well as causing local tissue cells, like epithelial cells, to release relevant CC chemokines such as eotaxin-1 and -2, that together locally recruit and then activate inflammatory cells such as eosinophils, from the circulation into the tissues, as well as cause epithelial goblet cell differentiation and discharge, and smooth muscle reactivity changes, that together constitute the asthmatic response.

Evidence That IgE Antibody Can Initiate DTH

Our Th2 DTH hypothesis for asthma postulates further that an airway IgE-mast cell-LPR serves an initiating function to recruit the Th2 asthma-promoting effector cells into the extravascular tissues. In fact, there already is evidence that IgE antibody can mediate DTH recruitment of T cells, as we are proposing, but in another system. In prior studies of Th1 DTH initiation in CS responses of mice, we showed that isolated CS effector Th1 cells, which had contaminating CS-initiating B-1 cells removed prior to intravenous transfer, could not on their own mediate 24-hour CS responses [60]. However, addition of quite small amounts of IgE (or IgG1) mast-cell-sensitizing mAb, of the same antigen specificity as the CS effector Th1 cells, allowed T-cell recruitment into the tissues to mediate 24-hour CS responses. In fact, very low systemic doses of IgE sufficed, even below those needed to cause detectable LPR, or macroscopic immediate responses. Thus, as little as 1 ng of Ag-specific IgE per mouse sufficed to mediate Th1 DTH initiation, and 10–100 ng per mouse was optimal [60]. We think these findings could apply to Th2 DTH in asthma, since by definition, all atopic allergic asthmatics have raised levels of IgE specific for conformational determinants of the same inhalant allergens to which Th2 cells have specificity for peptide determinants.

Possible Th2 DTH in Nonatopic Asthma

If the mouse Th1 DTH skin analogy of specific IgE mediating recruitment of effector T cells holds, then very low amounts of IgE could suffice in Th2 DTH asthma. Atopic allergic asthmatics have diverse allergen-specific IgE to many environmental allergens, and IgE is a profoundly powerful immunoreactant, with very small doses known to mediate quite powerful biological effects. Compared to atopic allergic asthmatics, the nonatopic 'intrinsic' asthmatics have nearly identical Th2 eosinophil-rich immunopatholological findings in their airways [61–63]. This suggests similar Th2 DTH pathogenesis as allergic asthma, but the nonatopics have no elevated serum IgE, or only mildly elevated but still normal IgE, and have negative immediate wheal and flare skin test responses to typical inhalant environmental allergens. However, perhaps low levels of IgE antibodies specific for known allergens, or for unknown substances in the environment, could suffice to initiate recruitment of Th2 T cells in nonatopic asthmatics with αβ-TCR specific for these same substances, producing similar eosinophil-rich inflammatory responses due to Th2 DTH mechanisms. Thus, it is of interest that recent evaluation of local expression of IgE mRNA transcripts in nonatopic bronchial mucosae has shown levels equal to that in atopic asthmatics [64].

Thus, perhaps in evaluating asthma, we are wrong to apply the quantitative IgE requirements, and wheal and flare skin test responsiveness of allergic rhinitis, which are more indicative of atopic allergic disease due to IgE/mast mechanisms. In contrast, asthma may be a very different, but related allergic disease, in which there is less need for large amounts of IgE to produce dramatic mast cell-dependent immediate responses, but instead requires far smaller amounts of IgE to initiate lower airway recruitment of the dominant Th2 DTH effect. Thus, if low levels of specific IgE to unknown environmental substances are crucial to Th2 DTH in nonatopic asthma, then these patients may be improved by treatment with anti-IgE antibody that strongly lowers IgE levels, and lowers expression of IgE FcεIR on mast cells, and has been shown to inhibit the early mast cell and late T-cell recruitment phases of atopic asthma in man [58], and allergic airway inflammation in mice [59]. Such a therapeutic response in nonatopic asthma would contribute to verifying the ideas we have put forward concerning the possibility of IgE leading to Th2 DTH, and playing a role not only in allergic atopic asthma, but also in nonatopic asthma.

Conclusion

We propose that the dominant T-cell aspect of allergic tissue responses like those occurring in asthma, are manifestations of newly designated Th2 DTH. Such Th2 DTH is related to diverse previously described other examples that now are included under this overall heading of Th2 DTH, including the Jones Mote Reaction, and CBH responses to allergens and parasites. These particular examples of Th2 DTH have a basophil-rich aspect that occurs in certain species, and in certain tissues, and can participate strongly in responses to multicellular parasites at body surfaces, such as the skin and intestine. The basophil aspect probably depends on special Th2-dependent basophil-specific chemokines, that perhaps are produced by epithelial cells at the surfaces. Initial recruitment of Th2 effector cells for initiation of Th2 DTH in asthma may involve early IgE/mast cell triggering by allergen to produce an LPR, in which mast cell-derived TNF-α and IL-4 activate the vasculature, and simultaneously CC chemokines recruit CCR3+ Th2 cells, of various allergen specificities. Then the greater expression of $\alpha\beta$-TCR specific for allergens on recruited Th2 cells leads to activation of just a few recruited Th2 cells by appropriate allergen-derived peptides, complexed with class II molecules on local APC in the lung, activating production of Th2 cytokines, like IL-4, IL-5, IL-9 and IL-13, that orchestrate tissue changes in goblet, epithelial, macrophage and airway smooth muscle cells in the tissues, that along with eosinophils recruited via IL-5 and eotaxin, produce the asthma diathesis. Work is now ongoing to examine these hypotheses experimentally.

Acknowledgments

The author is indebted to Mark Larche and Fan Chung for thorough review and critique of the manuscript. PWA was supported by a Travel Fellowship from the Wellcome Foundation and by grants from the NIH (AI-43371 and SCORP50 HL-56389).

References

1   Dvorak HF, Dvorak AM, Simpson BA, Richerson HB, Leskowitz S, Karnovsky MJ: Cutaneous basophil hypersensitivity. II. A light and electron microscopic description. J Exp Med 1970;132: 558–582.
2   Dvorak HF, Simpson BA, Bast RC Jr, Leskowitz S: Cutaneous basophil hypersensitivity. 3. Participation of the basophil in hypersensitivity to antigen-antibody complexes, delayed hypersensitivity and contact allergy. Passive transfer. J Immunol 1971;107:138–148.
3   Askenase PW: Cutaneous basophil hypersensitivity in contact-sensitized guinea pigs. I. Transfer with immune serum. J Exp Med 1973;138:1144–1155.
4   Askenase PW, Haynes JD, Hayden BJ: Antibody-mediated basophil accumulations in cutaneous hypersensitivity reactions of guinea pigs. J Immunol 1976;117:216–224.

5   Stashenko PP, Bhan AK, Schlossman SF, McCluskey RT: Local transfer of delayed hypersensitivity and cutaneous basophil hypersensitivity. J Immunol 1977;119:1987–93.

6   Askenase PW, Dvorak HD: Confirmation that antibodies transfer CBH. Unpublished results 1984.

7   Haynes JD, Rosenstein RW, Askenase PW: A newly described activity of guinea pig IgG1 antibodies: Transfer of cutaneous basophil reactions. J Immunol 1978;120:886–894.

8   Graziano FM, Gunderson L, Larson L, Askenase PW: IgE antibody-mediated cutaneous basophil hypersensitivity reactions in guinea pigs. J Immunol 1983; 131:2675–2681.

9   Ying S, Robinson DS, Meng Q, Barata L, McEuen AR, Buckley MG, Walls AF, Askenase PW, Kay AB: C-C chemokines in allergen-induced late phase cutaneous responses in atopic subjects: Association of eotaxin with early 6 hr eosinophils, and eotaxin-2 and MCP-4 with the later 24 hr tissue eosinophilia, and relationship to basophils and other C-C chemokines. J Allergy Clin Immunol 1999;103:S54 (abstr 207).

10 Mitchell EB, Askenase PW: Basophils in human disease. Clin Rev Allergy 1983;1:427–448.

11 Askenase PW: The role of basophils, mast cells and vasoamines in hypersensitivity reactions with a delayed time course. Prog Allergy 1977;23:199–320.

12 Askenase PW: Immunopathology of parasitic diseases: Involvement of basophils and mast cells. Springer Semin Immunopathol 1980;2:417–442.

13 Brown SJ, Galli SJ, Gleich GJ, Askenase PW: Ablation of immunity to *Amblyomma americanum* by anti-basophil serum: Cooperation between basophils and eosinophils in expression of immunity to ectoparasites (ticks) in guinea pigs. J Immunol 1982;129:790–796.

14 Brown SJ, Askenase PW: Immune rejection of ectoparasites (ticks) by T cell and IgG1 antibody recruitment of basophils and eosinophils. Fed Proc 1983;42:1744–1749.

15 Irani AMA, Huang C, Xia HZ, Kepley C, Nafie A, Fouda ED, Craig S, Zweiman B, Schwartz L: Immunohistochemical detection of human basophils in late-phase skin resections. J Allergy Clin Immunol 1998;101:354–362.

16 McEuen AR, Buckley MG, Compton SJ, Walls AF: Development and characterization of a monoclonal antibody specific for human basophils and the identification of a unique secretory product of basophil activation. Lab Invest 1999;79:27–38.

17 Sallusto F, Lanzavecchia A, Mackay CR: Chemokines and chemokine receptors in T-cell priming and Th1/Th2-mediated responses. Immunol Today 1998;19:568.

18 Uguccioni M, Mackay CR, Ochensberger B, Loetscher P, Rhis S, LaRosa GJ, Rao P, Ponath PD, Baggiolini M, Dahinden CA: High expression of the chemokine receptor CCR3 in human blood basophils. Role in activation by eotaxin, MCP-4, and other chemokines. J Clin Invest 1997;100:1137–1143.

19 Askenase PW, Higashi GI: Cutaneous basophil hypersensitivity and macrophage migration inhibition in guinea pigs with schistosomiasis. Clin Exp Immunol 1976;23:318–327.

20 Askenase PW: Role of basophils, mast cells, and vasoamines in hypersensitivity reactions with a delayed time course. Prog Allergy 1977;23:199–320.

21 Rothwell TLW: Studies of the responses of basophil and eosinophil leucocytes and mast cells to the nematode *Trichostrongylus colubriformis*. I. Observations during expulsion of first and second infections by guinea pits. J Pathol 1975;116:15.

22 Askenase PW, Boone WT, Binder HJ: Colonic basophil hypersensitivity. J Immunol 1978;120:198–301.

23 Macfarlane AJ, Zeibecoglou K, Kahn N, Haselden BM, Ying S, Robinson DS, McEuen AR, Buckley MG, Walls AF, Barnes NC, Kay AB: Elevated numbers of basophils in baseline atopic asthma compared to rhinitic and normal controls, and after allergen challenge. J Allergy Clin Immunol 1999;103:S192(abstr 738).

24 Khan LN, Ying S, Macfarlane AJB, Barnes NC, Kay AB: The effects of cyclosporin A on allergen-induced infiltration of EG2+ eosinophils, BB1+ basophils, and eotaxin+ cells in bronchial biopsies from mild atopic asthmatics. J Allergy Clin Immunol 1999;103:S47(abstr 178).

25 Draberova L: Cyclosporin A inhibits rat mast cell activation. Eur J Immunol 1990;20:1469–1473.

26 Kaplan MH, Whitfield JR, Boros DL, Grusby MJ: Th2 cells are required for the *Schistosoma mansoni* egg-induced granulomatous response. J Immunol 1998;160:1850–1856.

27 Spergel JM, Mizoguchi E, Oettgen H, Bhan AK, Geha RS: Roles of Th1 and Th2 cytokines in a murine model of allergic dermatitis. J Clin Invest 1999;103:1103–1111.

28 Askenase PW, Haynes JD, Tauben D, De Bernardo R: Specific basophil hypersensitivity induced by skin testing and transferred using immune serum. Nature 1975;256:52–54.

29 Askenase PW, Atwood JE. Basophils in tuberculin and 'Jones-Mote' delayed reactions of humans. J Clin Invest 1976;58:1145–1154.

30 Dearman RJ, Basketter DA, Evans P, Kimber I: Comparison of cytokine secretion profiles provoked in mice by glutaraldehyde and formaldehyde. Clin Exp Allergy 1999;29:124–132.

31 Traidl C, Jugert F, Kreig T, Merk H, Hunzelmann N: Inhibition of allergic contact dermatitis to DNCB but not to oxazolone in interleukin-4-deficient mice. J Invest Dermatol 1999;112:476–482.

32 Kitagaki H, Ono N, Hayakawa K, Kitazawa T, Watanabe K, Shiohara T: Repeated elicitation of contact hypersensitivity induces a shift in cutaneous cytokine milieu from a T-helper cell type 1 to a T-helper cell type 2 profile. J Immunol 1997;159:2484–2491.

33 Muller KM, Jaunin F, Masouye I, Saurat JH, Hauser C: Th2 cells mediate IL-4-dependent local tissue inflammation. J Immunol 1993;150:5576–5584.

34 Li L, Sad S, Kagi D, Mosmann TR: CD8Tc1 and Tc2 cells secrete distinct cytokine patterns in vitro and in vivo but induce similar inflammatory reactions. J Immunol 1997;158:4152–4161.

35 Hertl M, Merk HF: Lymphocyte activation in cutaneous drug reactions. J Invest Dermatol 1995; 105:95S–98S.

36 Matesic D, Valujskikh A, Pearlman E, Higgins AW, Gillman AC, Heeger PS: Type 2 immune deviation has differential effects on alloreactive CD4 + and CD8 + T cells. J Immunol 1998;161:5236–5244.

37 Zelenika D, Adams E, Mellor A, Simpson E, Chandler P, Stockinger B, Waldmann H, Cobbold SP: Rejection of H-Y disparate skin grafts my monospcific CD4 + Th1 and Th2 cells: No requirement for CD8 + T cells or B cells. J Immunol 1998;161:1868–1874.

38 Boirivant M, Fuss IJ, Chu A, Strober W: Oxazolone colitis: A murine model of T-helper cell type 2 colitis treatable with antibodies to interleukin 4. J Exp Med 1998;188:1929–1939.

39 Dohi T, Fujijashi K, Rennert PD, Iwatani K, Kiyono H, McGee JR: Hapten-induced colitis is associated with colonic patch hypertrophy and T-helper cell 2-type responses. J Exp Med 1999;189: 1169–1179.

40 Hung K, Hayashi R, Lafond-Walker A, Lowenstein C, Pardoll D, Levitsky H: The central role of CD4 + T cells in the anti-tumor immune response. J Exp Med 1998;188:2357–2368.

41 Askenase PW, Kawikova I, Paliwal V, Akahira-Azuma M, Gerard C, Hugli T, Tsuji R: A new paradigm of T cell allergy: Requirement for the B-1 cell subset. Int Arch Allergy Appl Immunol 1999;118:145–149.

42 Tsuji RF, Geba GP, Wang Y, Kawamoto K, Matis LA, Askenase PW: Required early complement activation in contact sensitivity with generation of local C5-dependent chemotactic activity, and late T cell interferon-gamma: A possible initiating role of B cells. J Exp Med 1997;186:1015–1026.

43 Tsuji RF, Kawikova I, Ramabhadran R, Akahira-Azuma M, Taub D, Hugli TE, Gerard C, Askenasse PW: Early local generation of C5a initiates the elicitation of contact sensitivity by leading to early T cell recruitment. J Immunol 2000;165:1588–1598.

44 Nataf S, Daavoust N, Amer RS, Barnum SR: Human T cells express the C5a receptor and are chemoattracted to C5a. J Immunol 1999;162:4018–4023.

45 Kops SK, Van Loveren H, Rosenstein RW, Ptak W, Askenase PW: Mast cell activation and vascular alterations in immediate hypersensitivity-like reactions induced by a T-cell-derived antigen-binding factor. Lab Invest 1984;50:421–434.

46 Van Loveren H, Kraeuter-Kops S, Askenase PW: Different mechanisms of release of vasoactive amines by mast cells occur in T-cell-dependent compared to IgE-dependent cutaneous hypersensitivity responses. Eur J Immunol 1984;14:40–47.

47 Geba GP, Ptak W, Anderson GM, Paliwal V, Ratzlaff RE, Levin J, Askenase PW: Delayed-type hypersensitivity in mast cell-deficient mice: Dependence on platelets for expression of contact sensitivity. J Immunol 1996;157:557–565.

48 Matsuda H, Ushio H, Geba GP, Askenase PW: Human platelets can initiate T-cell-dependent contact sensitivity through local serotonin release mediated by IgE antibodies. J Immunol 1997; 158:2891–2897.

49   Askenase PW, Bursztajn S, Gershon MD, Gershon RK: T-cell-dependent mast cell degranulation and release of serotonin in murine delayed-type hypersensitivity. J Exp Med 1980;152:1358–1374.

50   Ameisen JC, Meade R, Askenase PW: A new interpretation of the involvement of serotonin in delayed-type hypersensitivity. Serotonin-2 receptor antagonists inhibit contact sensitivity by an effect on T cells. J Immunol 1989;142:3171–3179.

51   McHale J, Harari OA, Marshall D, Haskard DO: Vascular endothelial cell expression of ICAM-1 and VCAM-1 at the onset of eliciting contact hypersensitivity in mice: Evidence for a dominant role of TNF-α. J Immunol 1999;162:1648–1655.

52   Robinson DSH, Ying S, Tsicopoulos A, Barkans J, Bentley AM, Corrigan C, Durham SR, Kay AB: Predominant TH2-like bronchoalveolar T-lymphocyte population in atopic asthma. N Engl J Med 1992;326:298.

53   Askenase PW, Tsuji RF: B-1 B cell IgM antibody initiates T cell elicitation of contact sensitivity. Current Topics in Microbiology and Immunology, in press.

54   Marchal G, Seman M, Milon G, Truffa-Bachi P, Zilberfarb V: Local adoptive transfer of skin delayed-type hypersensitivity initiated by a single T lymphocyte. J Immunol 1982;129:954–958.

55   Corry DB, Folkesson HG, Warnock ML, Erle DJ, Matthay MA, Wiener JP, Kronish X, Locksley RM: Interleukin-4, but not interleukin-5 or eosinophils, is required in a murine model of acute airway hyperreactivity. J Exp Med 1996;183:109.

56   Wills-Karp M, Luyimbazi J, Xu X, Schofield B, Neben TY, Karp CL, Donaldson DD: Interleukin-13: Central mediator of allergic asthma. Science 1998;282:2258–2261.

57   Brown JR, Kleimberg J, Marini M, Sun G, Bellini A, Mattoli S: Kinetics of eotaxin expression and its relationship to eosinophil accumulation and activation in bronchial biopsies and bronchoalveolar lavage of asthmatic patients after allergen inhalation. Clin Exp Immunol 1998;114:137–146.

58   Fahy JV, Fleming HE, Wong HH, Liu JT, Su JQ, Reimann J, Fick RB Jr, Boushey HA: The effect of an anti-IgE monoclonal antibody on the early- and late-phase responses to allergen inhalation in asthmatic subjects. Am J Respir Crit Care Med 1997;155:1828–1834.

59   Coyle AJ, Wagner K, Bertrand C, Tsuyuki S, Bews J, Heusser C: Central role of immunoglobulin (Ig) E in the induction of lung eosinophil infiltration and T-helper 2 cell cytokine production: Inhibition by a non-anaphylactogenic anti-IgE antibody. J Exp Med 1996;183:1303–1310.

60   Ptak W, Geba GP, Askenase PW: Initiation of delayed-type hypersensitivity by low doses of monoclonal IgE antibody. Mediation by serotonin and inhibition by histamine. J Immunol 1991;146:3929–3936.

61   Ying SH, Barkans J, Corrigan C, Pfister R, Menz G, Larche MR, Durham SR, Kay AB: Expression of IL-4 and IL-5 mRNA and protein product by CD4 + and CD8 + T cells, eosinophils, and mast cells in bronchial biopsies obtained from atopic and nonatopic (intrinsic) asthmatics. J Immunol 1977;158:3539–3544.

62   Humbert M, Durham S, Ying S, Kimmitt P, Barkans J, Assoufi B, Pfister R, Menz G, Robinson D, Kay AB, Corrigan C: IL-4 and IL-5 mRNA and protein in bronchial biopsies from patients with atopic and nonatopic asthma: Evidence against 'intrinsic' asthma being a distinct immunopathologic entity. Am J Respir Crit Care Med 1996;154:1497–1504.

63   Humbert MY, Ying S, Corrigan C, Menz G, Barkans J, Pfister R, Meng Q, Van Damme J, Opdenakker SR, Durham SRK, Kay AB: Bronchial mucosal expression of the genes encoding chemokines RANTES and MCP-3 in symptomatic atopic and nonatopic asthmatics: Relationship to the eosinophil-active cytokines interleukin (IL)-5, granulocyte macrophage-colony-stimulating factor and IL-3. Am J Respir Cell Mol Biol 1997;16:1–8.

64   Durham SR, Ying S, Meng Q, Humbert M, Gould H, Kay AB: Local expression of germ-line gene transcripts (Iε) and RNA for the heavy chain of IgE (Cε) in the bronchial mucosae in aopic and non-atopic asthma. J Allergy Clin Immunol 1998;101:S162.

Philip W. Askenase, MD, Professor and Head, Section of Allergy and Clinical Immunology,
Department of Internal Medicine, Yale University School of Medicine,
333 Cedar Street, New Haven, CT 06520-8012 (USA)
Tel. +1 203 785 4143, Fax +1 203 785 3229, E-Mail philip.askenase@yale.edu

Robinson DS (ed): Immunological Mechanisms in Asthma and Allergic Diseases.
Chem Immunol. Basel, Karger, 2000, vol 78, pp 124–134

....

Novel Immunosuppressants in Asthma

O. M. Kon

Chest and Allergy Clinic, St Mary's Hospital, London, UK

Introduction

The use of inhaled corticosteroids is now established in international and national guidelines on asthma management. Although this has significantly reduced the number of patients who require long-term oral corticosteroids, approximately 1% of the asthmatic population still require such treatment ('steroid-dependent' asthmatics). Many such patients will suffer from side effects of the corticosteroids (such as diabetes, hypertension and osteoporosis) and also from poorly controlled disease. In addition, there are patients who have corticosteroid-resistant asthma and who may therefore require alternative anti-inflammatory treatment. Given these reasons and the accumulating evidence for an inflammatory basis to the pathogenesis of chronic asthma, there has been interest in the use of immunosuppressive therapy which may enable the reduction or elimination of the need for oral corticosteroids and improved asthma control.

The best studied agents to date have been methotrexate, gold and cyclosporin A. All of the immunosuppressants that have been investigated in asthma have potentially serious side effects and no controlled study has proceeded for more than 1 year. Furthermore, no study has yet compared the relative effects of different corticosteroid-sparing agents. At present the use of these drugs should either be in clinical trials or on an individual patient basis with the clinician attempting to weigh up the relative benefits and risks of treatment.

Methotrexate

The most widely used and studied immunosuppressant in asthma is methotrexate. Methotrexate is an antimetabolite that antagonizes folate metabolism. It competitively inhibits dihydrofolate reductase and therefore impairs thymidilate and DNA synthesis [1]. As a result of these properties, methotrexate is capable of acting on all dividing cells. It has an established role as a corticosteroid-sparing agent and anti-inflammatory drug in rheumatoid arthritis. It has actions on neutrophil recruitment and responses to inflammation [2] and has been noted to reduce wheal and flare responses to skin prick testing [3, 4]. Basophil release of histamine [5] and macrophage secretion of interleukin(IL)-1 [6] has also been demonstrated to be inhibited by methotrexate. In addition, methotrexate appears to antagonize the effects of IL-1 on monocytes although it has minimal effects on other humoral and cellular responses [7]. More recently, there is evidence that methotrexate may also inhibit T-cell function [8].

Mullarkey et al. [9] demonstrated in a randomized double-blind crossover trial in corticosteroid-dependent asthmatics that there was a significant decrease in the requirement for oral corticosteroids. While taking 15 mg of methotrexate per week patients were able to reduce their requirement to a mean of 15.2 mg/day as compared to a mean dose of 26.1 mg/day in the placebo arm. Since then, a number of other studies of methotrexate have been performed. The largest and best controlled was by Shiner et al. [10]. This was a parallel-group study in 68 corticosteroid-dependent asthmatics, who received either oral methotrexate 15 mg/week or placebo for 24 weeks. In the first 10 weeks of the study, there was no difference in oral steroid requirement, but by the end of this treatment period there was a significant benefit to the methotrexate group with a 50% decrease in oral steroid requirement in the active treatment group compared with 14% decrease in the placebo group. There was no improvement in lung function but there was a significant decrease in exacerbations requiring an increased dose of steroids in the methotrexate group. Three further crossover design studies have also been performed which have demonstrated a reduction in requirement for oral steroids [11–13]. However, these results have not been reproduced in other randomized controlled trials of methotrexate in severe asthma. Three were with oral methotrexate [14–16] and one assessed the effect of intramuscular administration [17].

A meta-analysis of placebo-controlled, randomized studies from 1985 to 1995 [18] was only able to detect a beneficial effect in the parallel-group design studies and postulated that the crossover design studies may have been confounded by carryover effects. A further meta-analysis by Marin [19] showed that methotrexate treatment resulted in a decrease in steroid requirements by an average of 4.37 mg (or of 23.7% of the original dose) and that this effect was greatest in patients in which there was an attempt to reduce baseline steroid usage and in whom treatment was given for 24 weeks.

The main side effects of methotrexate are of abnormalities of liver enzymes and hepatic fibrosis. Views about the risk of this complication are variable with some authorities suggesting liver biopsies after a cumulative dose of 1.5 g or every 3 years while on treatment [20]. However, in guidelines published in 1994 [21], routine liver biopsies were not advocated for patients on low-dose methotrexate for rheumatoid arthritis unless there was significant elevation of liver enzymes or alcohol abuse. Methotrexate has been reported to cause opportunistic lung infections in both rheumatoid arthritis [22, 23] and asthma [24, 25] and there have been cases of fatal varicella infections in asthmatic subjects receiving methotrexate [26, 27]. In addition, there have been case reports of methotrexate possibly causing asthma and increasing bronchial hyperresponsiveness [28, 29]. Pneumonitis occurring in a patient with asthma following 3 months of methotrexate treatment has also been described [30].

At present, methotrexate should only be used in patients requiring long-term oral steroids in spite of high-dose inhaled corticosteroids. A trial of treatment for at least 3 months is needed to see if there is any beneficial effect. If no decrease in steroid requirement is seen at this time, methotrexate should be discontinued.

Gold

Gold has been used as a steroid-sparing and disease-modifying agent in rheumatoid arthritis for many years. The mechanism of action of gold is not clear. It has been demonstrated to inhibit mediator release following anti-IgE stimulation from basophils and mast cells [31, 32] inhibit mediator-induced smooth muscle contraction [33], affect leukotriene production from polymorphonuclear leukocytes [32, 34] and their response to such mediators [35]. Notably it has also been shown to selectively inhibit IL-5-mediated eosinophil survival [36].

Studies have been performed of both intramuscular and oral gold. The largest study of intramuscular gold involved 79 asthmatic patients who did not require long-term steroids [37]. After 30 weeks of treatment, the actively treated group had fewer symptoms and required less medication. A significant number of patients dropped out of the study with side effects such as dermatitis, stomatitis or proteinuria. In a small study of 10 steroid-dependent asthmatics treated with intramuscular gold, there was a reduction in prednisolone dosage but this did not achieve statistical significance [38]. Nierop et al. [39] performed a double-blind parallel-group study in 32 patients dependent on long-term oral corticosteroids where treatment with oral gold caused a small but statistically significant decrease in steroid dosage, an increase in forced expiratory volume in 1 s (FEV_1), a decrease in asthma exacerbations and reduced symptoms. Side effects were minor. In a large placebo-controlled, parallel-group multicentre study of 3 mg twice daily of oral gold, Bernstein et al. [40] were also able to demonstrate that a significant number of subjects (41.2%) were able to reduce their oral steroid requirement to < 50% of baseline after a mean of 16.5 weeks on treatment. There was no improvement in symptoms or lung function and there was a significant incidence of gastrointestinal and dermatological side effects. Side effects of gold treatment include diarrhoea, mouth ulcers, skin rashes, proteinuria and blood disorders.

Cyclosporin A (CsA)

CsA is a lipophilic cyclic undecapeptide derived from the fungus *Tolypocladium inflatum Gams*. CsA (complexed to its immunophilin, cyclophilin), inhibits calcineurin phosphatase activity which in turn is required for translocation of the cytoplasmic component of the nuclear factor of activated T cells (NFAT) to the nucleus. It therefore arrests T-lymphocyte division in the G0 or early G1 phase of the cell cycle and inhibits activation by decreasing IL-2 and IL-2 receptor expression [41]. It is of paramount importance in organ transplantation and there is extensive experience in using low-dose CsA in autoimmune diseases and inflammatory conditions where the activated T lymphocyte appears to be involved, particularly psoriasis, atopic dermatitis, Crohn's disease and rheumatoid arthritis. CsA suppresses IL-5 and GM-CSF mRNA transcription and translation by CD4+ T lymphocytes in asthmatic subjects [42, 43]. Although the predominant effect of CsA is on the T lymphocyte, it also has effects on the rapid release of preformed and de novo synthesized mediators from human mast cell in vitro and basophils ex vivo. In addition, it affects the production of cytokines from eosinophils, mast cells and monocytes and has been demonstrated to affect antigen-presenting cell function.

Three controlled clinical trials of CsA have been reported in severe asthma. In a placebo-controlled crossover study of oral corticosteroid-dependent asthmatics, Alexander et al. [44] demonstrated an improvement in morning peak expiratory flow rate of 12% and FEV_1 of 18% in patients on 5 mg/kg/day of CsA over placebo. There was also a decrease in the number of exacerbations of asthma requiring a boost in the dose of oral corticosteroids in patients treated with CsA. In a follow-up study, the same group [45] demonstrated in a parallel-group design study of 39 subjects that the same dose of CsA allowed a significant decrease in oral corticosteroid requirement over the course of 36 weeks (median reduction of 62%) with an increase in lung function and a trend towards less disease exacerbations. Interestingly, during the washout period, corticosteroid requirements returned to baseline values. Nizankowska et al. [46] have shown a smaller decrease in oral corticosteroid requirement over the trial period in a parallel-group design study. Although the final corticosteroid dose reduction when compared to placebo was not significantly different, they were able to demonstrate a significant reduction in night-time symptoms and inhaled β-agonist use. In a small open study of corticosteroid-dependent asthmatics, Fukuda et al. [47] demonstrated a decrease in bronchial hyperresponsiveness and T-cell activation markers following CsA therapy and therefore provided further evidence to implicate the mode of action of CsA in severe asthmatics as being primarily on the T lymphocyte. More recently, a double-blind, placebo-controlled study by Sihra et al. [48], demonstrated a 50% reduction (by pretreatment with two doses of CsA) in the late asthmatic reaction with no effect on the early phase response using an allergen challenge model in mild asthmatics. This is likely to reflect the predominant effect of CsA on the T lymphocyte rather than on mast cell degranulation.

Side effects in the studies in asthma were those predictable for CsA with an increase in diastolic blood pressure and decrease in renal function. Other side effects include hepatic dysfunction, hypertrichosis, tremor, gingival hyperplasia and paraesthesia. De novo malignancies secondary to CsA and the occurrence of lymphoproliferative disorders is rare in low-dose treatment. Inhalation of drugs in asthma improves the therapeutic index by allowing the drug to act locally within the lung but preventing systemic toxicity. Studies have demonstrated that in the short term, inhaled CsA is tolerated and effective in lung transplantation [49] and therefore administration of CsA by this route may be of potential use in asthma.

Other Potential Novel Immunosuppressants

New immunosuppressive agents continue to be assessed, particularly in the field of transplantation medicine, with view to achieving more effective immunosuppression but with less toxic effects. Some of these novel compounds may also serve as effective corticosteroid-sparing agents in severe asthma.

Anti-CD4 mAb therapy has been used in other diseases associated with activated T lymphocytes such as organ transplantation rejection, rheumatoid arthritis, nephritis, systemic lupus erythematosus, psoriasis, inflammatory bowel disease and Wegener's granulomatosis. The effects of a single intravenous infusion of a chimeric anti-CD4 monoclonal antibody (mAb) in severe corticosteroid-dependent asthma has been recently reported [50]. In a small randomized placebo-controlled, double-blind, dose-ranging study, patients receiving 3.0 mg/kg had a significant increase from baseline in morning and evening peak expiratory flow rate (PEFR) from day 1–14 (fig. 1). There was also a

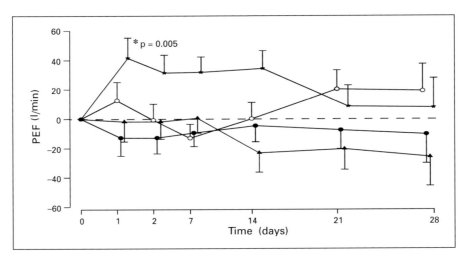

Fig. 1. Changes from baseline in morning peak expiratory flow (PEF) following infusion with an anti-CD4 mAb, keliximab, in chronic severe corticosteroid-dependent asthmatics. Error bars = SE. The area under curve of change from baseline for days 1–14 in the 3.0 mg/kg group was significantly different from placebo (p = 0.0174).

trend to an improvement in symptom scores in the 3.0 mg/kg cohort. There were significant transient reductions in CD4 counts in all three active dosing cohorts (0.5, 1.5 and 3.0 mg/kg) but with the highest dosing cohort appearing to have a longer period of decrease in CD4 counts. There were no serious adverse effects related to treatment. In this study a single infusion was used and it may be that repeated doses may have a more prolonged beneficial effect. Previous studies of anti-CD4 mAb in rheumatoid arthritis, even with prolonged depletion of CD4 + lymphocytes and in combination with other immunosuppressant therapy, have not demonstrated any significant increase in the risk of opportunistic infections or neoplasms. However, the use of these agents in asthma should still be regarded as being experimental and will require further large trials to substantiate if anti-CD4 therapy may be a safe and effective adjunctive treatment in severe asthmatics.

FK506 (tacrolimus), a macrolide produced from *Streptomyces tsukubaensis*, is already being employed in transplantation medicine and has a similar mode of action to CsA by binding to the immunophilin FKBP, thereby blocking cytokine gene transcription. In lung transplantation, FK506 may be more effective than CsA in reducing persistent rejection [51]. It has inhibitory effects on the transcription of IL-2, IL-3, IL-4, IL-5, GM-CSF, IFN-γ and TNF-α from both mononuclear cells and mast cells and is capable of inhibiting

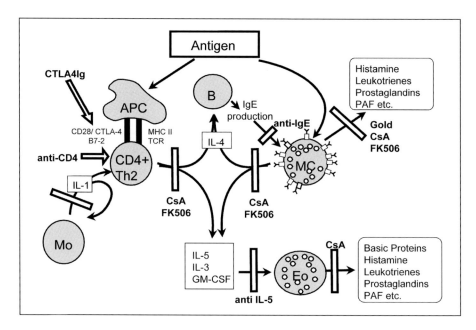

Fig. 2. Diagrammatic representation of the inflammatory cells and the cytokine networks involved in episodic and chronic asthma with possible sites of action of some immunosuppressives and novel agents. Eo = Eosinophil; APC = antigen-presenting cell; Th2 = T-helper type 2 cell; Mo = monocyte; B = B-cell; MC = mast cell.

IgE-dependent histamine release from basophils and mast cells and may therefore have a role in asthma.

Rapamycin, another macrolide derived from *Streptomyces hygroscopius*, inhibits signal transduction mediated by IL-2 and other cytokines and therefore only targets cells late in the G1 phase of cell cycle [52]. This allows it to inhibit cells already activated and therefore is likely to have a more rapid immunomodulatory effect. It has inhibitory properties on immunoglobulin synthesis. Because of its binding to FKBP it also offers the possibility of synergism with CsA. There is also in vitro evidence that it inhibits IL-5-induced eosinophil survival and degranulation [53]. Similarly, leflunomide [54], through its metabolite A77 1726, functions as a protein tyrosine kinase inhibitor and inhibits T- and B-cell responses to IL-2. It inhibits a crucial step in pyrimidine synthesis through its effect on dihydroorotate dehydrogenase. Because of the resultant inhibition of T- and B-cell proliferation, immunoglobulin production and smooth muscle proliferation, leflunomide is a potentially useful agent in asthma and has already been studied in animal models of allergic disease with promising results [55]. Although stimulation of the T cell through the CD28 pathway is insensitive to CsA and FK506, rapamycin and leflunomide are capable of blocking this.

Mycophenolate mofetil limits de novo purine synthesis through inhibition of inosine monophosphate dehydrogenase and therefore selectively inhibits proliferation of activated T and B lymphocytes. It has been assessed in preventing acute rejection in transplants in combination with CsA with promising results and a relatively good toxicity profile [56]. Similarly, brequinar sodium also inhibits de novo pyrimidine synthesis. Deoxysperguanolin, a semisynthetic polyamine, appears to have effects on the differentiation and proliferation of T lymphocytes but also inhibits antigen-presenting cells and B cells.

Fusion proteins have been developed that can interact with a variety of target molecules. For example, CTLA4-Ig (a CD28 receptor analogue), whose counter-ligand is the B7 family of molecules on antigen presenting cells involved in the co-stimulatory pathway of T-lymphocyte activation, has been successfully used in inducing antigen-specific hyporesponsiveness in rodent models [57].

A diagrammatic representation of possible sites of action of some immunosuppressants and novel agents on the inflammatory cells and the cytokine networks involved in episodic and chronic asthma are shown in figure 2.

In summary: Studies of methotrexate, gold and CsA have demonstrated some clinical efficacy in severe corticosteroid-dependent asthmatics. A small trial of an anti-CD4 monoclonal antibody has also produced promising improvements in this group of difficult patients. However, there are still significant potential toxicities associated with such therapy and therefore other safer and more specific T-cell-directed treatment may be useful additional treatment in asthmatics. Further development and clinical trials of such compounds in asthma are warranted.

References

1   Kremer JM: The mechanism of action of methotrexate in rheumatoid arthritis: The search continues. J Rheumatol 1994;21:1–5.
2   Suarez CR, Pickett WC, Bell DH, McClintock DK, Oronsky AL, Kerwar SS: Effect of low-dose methotrexate on neutrophil chemotaxis induced by leukotriene B_4 and complement C5a. J Rheumatol 1987;14:9–11.
3   Cream JJ, Pole DS: The effect of methotrexate and hydroxyurea on neutrophil chemotaxis. Br J Dermatol 1980;102:557–563.
4   Ternowitz T, Bjerring P, Andersen PH, Schroder JM, Kragballe K: Methotrexate inhibits the human C5a-induced skin response in patients with psoriasis. J Invest Dermatol 1987;89:192–196.
5   Nolte H, Stahl SP: Inhibition of basophil histamine release by methotrexate. Agents Actions 1988; 23:173–176.
6   Hu SK, Mitcho YL, Oronsky AL, Kerwar SS: Studies on the effect of methotrexate on macrophage function. J Rheumatol 1988;15:206–209.

7   Segal R, Yaron M, Tartakovsky B: Methotrexate: Mechanism of action in rheumatoid arthritis. Semin Arthritis Rheum 1990;20:190–200.

8   Wascher TC, Hermann J, Brezinschek HP, Brezinschek R, Wilders Truschnig M, Rainer F, Krejs GJ: Cell-type specific response of peripheral blood lymphocytes to methotrexate in the treatment of rheumatoid arthritis. Clin Invest 1994;72:535–540.

9   Mullarkey MF, Blumenstein BA, Andrade WP, Bailey GA, Olason I, Wetzel CE: Methotrexate in the treatment of corticosteroid-dependent asthma. A double-blind crossover study. N Engl J Med 1988;318:603–607.

10 Shiner RJ, Nunn AJ, Chung KF, Geddes DM: Randomised, double-blind, placebo-controlled trial of methotrexate in steroid-dependent asthma. Lancet 1990;336:137–140.

11 Dyer PD, Vaughan TR, Weber RW: Methotrexate in the treatment of steroid-dependent asthma. J Allergy Clin Immunol 1991;88:208–212.

12 Stewart GE, Diaz JD, Lockey RF, Seleznick MJ, Trudeau WL, Ledford DK: Comparison of oral pulse methotrexate with placebo in the treatment of severe glucocorticosteroid-dependent asthma. J Allergy Clin Immunol 1994;94:482–489.

13 Hedman J, Seideman P, Albertioni F, Stenius-Aarniala B: Controlled trial of methotrexate in patients with severe chronic asthma. Eur J Clin Pharmacol 1996;49:347–349.

14 Coffey MJ, Sanders G, Eschenbacher WL, Tsien A, Ramesh S, Weber RW, Toews GB, McCune WJ: The role of methotrexate in the management of steroid-dependent asthma. Chest 1994;105:117–121.

15 Trigg CJ, Davies RJ: Comparison of methotrexate 30 mg per week with placebo in chronic steroid-dependent asthma: A 12-week double-blind, cross-over study. Respir Med 1993;87:211–216.

16 Taylor DR, Flannery EM, Herbison GP. Methotrexate in the management of severe steroid-dependent asthma. NZ Med J 1993;106:409–411.

17 Erzurum SC, Leff JA, Cochran JE, Ackerson LM, Szefler SJ, Martin RJ, Cott GR: Lack of benefit of methotrexate in severe, steroid-dependent asthma. A double-blind, placebo-controlled study. Ann Intern Med 1991;114:353–360.

18 Wong E, Lacasse Y, Guyatt GH, et al: Is methotrexate effective as a steroid-sparing agent in steroid-dependent asthmatics? A meta-analysis. Am J Respir Crit Care Med 1996;153:A801.

19 Marin MG: Low-dose methotrexate spares steroid usage in steroid-dependent asthmatic patients: A meta-analysis. Chest 1997;112:29–33.

20 Lewis JH, Schiff E: Methotrexate-induced chronic liver injury: Guidelines for detection and prevention. The ACG Committee on FDA-Related Matters. American College of Gastroenterology. Am J Gastroenterol 1988;83:1337–1345.

21 Kremer JM, Alarcon GS, Lightfoot RW Jr, Willkens RF, Furst DE, Williams HJ, Dent PB, Weinblatt ME: Methotrexate for rheumatoid arthritis. Suggested guidelines for monitoring liver toxicity. American College of Rheumatology. Arthritis Rheum 1994;37:316–328.

22 LeMense GP, Sahn SA: Opportunistic infection during treatment with low-dose methotrexate. Am J Respir Crit Care Med 1994;150:258–260.

23 Wollner A, Mohle Boetani J, Lambert RE, Perruquet JL, Raffin TA, McGuire JL: *Pneumocystis carinii* pneumonia complicating low-dose methotrexate treatment for rheumatoid arthritis. Thorax 1991;46:205–207.

24 Kuitert LM, Harrison AC: *Pneumocystis carinii* pneumonia as a complication of methotrexate treatment of asthma. Thorax 1991;46:936–937.

25 Vallerand H, Cossart C, Milosevic D, Lavaud F, Leone J: Fatal pneumocystis pneumonia in asthmatic patient treated with methotrexate. Lancet 1992;339:1551.

26 Gatnash AA, Connolly CK: Fatal chickenpox pneumonia in an asthmatic patient on oral steroids and methotrexate. Thorax 1995;50:422–423.

27 Morice AH, Lai WK: Fatal varicella zoster infection in a severe steroid-dependent asthmatic patient receiving methotrexate. Thorax 1995;50:1221–1222.

28 Jones G, Mierins E, Karsh J: Methotrexate-induced asthma. Am Rev Respir Dis 1991;143:179–181.

29 Fertel D, Wanner A: Methotrexate: Does it treat or induce asthma? Am Rev Respir Dis 1991;143:1–2.

30 Tsai JJ, Shin JF, Chen CH, Wang SR: Methotrexate pneumonitis in bronchial asthma. Int Arch Allergy Appl Immunol 1993;100:287–290.

31   Marone G, Columbo M, Galeone D, Guidi G, Kagey Sobotka A, Lichtenstein LM: Modulation of the release of histamine and arachidonic acid metabolites from human basophils and mast cells by auranofin. Agents Actions 1986;18:100–102.

32   Wojtecka-Lukasik E, Sopata I, Maslinski S: Auranofin modulates mast cell histamine and polymorphonuclear leukocyte collagenase release. Agents Actions 1986;18:68–70.

33   Malo PE, Wasserman M, Parris D, Pfeiffer D: Inhibition by auranofin of pharmacologic and antigen-induced contractions of the isolated guinea pig trachea. J Allergy Clin Immunol 1986;77: 371–376.

34   Parente JE, Wong K, Davis P, Burka JF, Percy JS: Effects of gold compounds on leukotriene B$_4$, leukotriene C$_4$ and prostaglandin E$_2$ production by polymorphonuclear leukocytes. J Rheumatol 1986;13:47–51.

35   Hafstrom I, Ringertz B, Palmblad J, Malmsten C: Effects of auranofin on leukotriene production and leukotriene-stimulated neutrophil function. Agents Actions 1984;15:551–555.

36   Suzuki S, Okubo M, Kaise S, Ohara M, Kasukawa R: Gold sodium thiomalate selectivity inhibits interleukin-5-mediated eosinophil survival. J Allergy Clin Immunol 1995;96:251–256.

37   Muranaka M, Miyamoto T, Shida T, Kabe J, Makino S, Okumura H, Takeda K, Suzuki S, Horiuchi Y: Gold salt in the treatment of bronchial asthma – A double-blind study. Ann Allergy 1978;40: 132–137.

38   Klaustermeyer WB, Noritake DT, Kwong FK: Chrysotherapy in the treatment of corticosteroid-dependent asthma. J Allergy Clin Immunol 1987;79:720–725.

39   Nierop G, Gijzel WP, Bel EH, Zwinderman AH, Dijkman JH: Auranofin in the treatment of steroid dependent asthma: A double-blind study. Thorax 1992;47:349–354.

40   Bernstein IL, Bernstein DI, Dubb JW, Faiferman I, Wallin B: A placebo-controlled multicenter study of auranofin in the treatment of patients with corticosteroid-dependent asthma. Auranofin Multicenter Drug Trial. J Allergy Clin Immunol 1996;98:317–324.

41   Kahan BD: Cyclosporine. N Engl J Med 1989;321:1725–1738.

42   Mori A, Suko M, Nishizaki Y, Kaminuma O, Kobayashi S, Matsuzaki G, Yamamoto K, Ito K, Tsuruoka N, Okudaira H: IL-5 production by CD4 + T cells of asthmatic patients is suppressed by glucocorticoids and the immunosuppressants FK506 and cyclosporin A. Int Immunol 1995;7: 449–457.

43   Sano T, Nakamura Y, Matsunaga Y, Takahashi T, Azuma M, Okano Y, Shimizu E, Ogushi F, Sone S, Ogura T: FK506 and cyclosporin A inhibit granulocyte/macrophage colony-stimulating factor production by mononuclear cells in asthma. Eur Respir J 1995;8:1473–1478.

44   Alexander AG, Barnes NC, Kay AB: Trial of cyclosporin in corticosteroid-dependent chronic severe asthma. Lancet 1992;339:324–328.

45   Lock SH, Kay AB, Barnes NC: Double-blind, placebo-controlled study of cyclosporin A as a corticosteroid-sparing agent in corticosteroid-dependent asthma. Am J Respir Crit Care Med 1996; 153:509–514.

46   Nizankowska E, Soja J, Pinis G, Bochenek G, Sladek K, Domagala B, Pajak A, Szczeklik A: Treatment of steroid-dependent bronchial asthma with cyclosporin. Eur Respir J 1995;8:1091–1099.

47   Fukuda T, Asakawa J, Motojima J, Makino S: Cyclosporine A reduces T lymphocyte activity and improves airway hyperresponsiveness in corticosteroid-dependent chronic severe asthma. Ann Allergy Asthma Immunol 1995;75:65–72.

48   Sihra BS, Kon OM, Durham SR, Walker S, Barnes NC, Kay AB: Effect of cyclosporin A on the allergen-induced late asthmatic reaction. Thorax 1997;52:447–452.

49   O'Riordan TG, Iacono A, Keenan RJ, Duncan SR, Burckart GJ, Griffith BP, Smaldone GC: Delivery and distribution of aerosolized cyclosporine in lung allograft recipients. Am J Respir Crit Care Med 1995;151:516–521.

50   Kon OM, Sihra BS, Compton CH, Leonard TB, Kay AB, Barnes NC: Randomised, dose-ranging, placebo-controlled study of chimeric antibody to CD4 (keliximab) in chronic severe asthma. Lancet 1998;352:1109–1113.

51   Keenan RJ, Konishi H, Kawai A, Paradis IL, Nunley DR, Iacono AT, Hardesty RL, Weyant RJ, Griffith BP: Clinical trial of tacrolimus versus cyclosporine in lung transplantation. Ann Thorac Surg 1995;60:580–585.

52 Bonham CA, Thomson AW, Kay AB (eds): Allergy and Allergic Diseases, vol 36. Immuno-suppressants (Drugs and Monoclonal Antibodies). Oxford, Blackwell Science, 1997, pp 642–666.
53 Meng Q, Ying S, Corrigan CJ, Wakelin M, Assoufi B, Moqbel R, Kay AB: Effects of rapamycin, cyclosporin A, and dexamethasone on interleukin-5-induced eosinophil degranulation and prolonged survival. Allergy 1997;52:1095–1101.
54 Fox RI: Mechanism of action of leflunomide in rheumatoid arthritis. J Rheumatol Suppl 1998;53: 20–26.
55 Eber E, Uhlig T, McMenamin C, Sly PD: Leflunomide, a novel immunomodulating agent, prevents the development of allergic sensitization in an animal model of allergic asthma. Clin Exp Allergy 1998;28:376–384.
56 Sollinger HW: Update on preclinical and clinical experience with mycophenolate mofetil. Transplant Proc 1996;28:24–29.
57 Bolling SF, Lin H, Wei RQ, Turka LA: Preventing allograft rejection with CTLA4IG: Effect of donor-specific transfusion route or timing. J Heart Lung Transplant 1996;15:928–935.

Dr. Onn Min Kon, Chest and Allergy Clinic, St Mary's Hospital,
Praed Street, London W2 1NY (UK)
Tel. +44 171 886 1613, Fax +44 171 886 1344, E-Mail onn.kon@sm.stmarys-tr.nthames.nhs.uk

Robinson DS (ed): Immunological Mechanisms in Asthma and Allergic Diseases.
Chem Immunol. Basel, Karger, 2000, vol 78, pp 135–147

....

T-Cell Recruitment and Specificity in Allergic Inflammation

A.J. Frew

University Department of Medical Specialities, University of Southampton, UK

In 1985, when I first became interested in airways inflammation and started to think about the research that I might undertake in the Department of Allergy and Clinical Immunology, the role of T cells in allergic inflammation was not at all well defined. It had been known for many years that T cells were critical to the regulation of IgE production, but the prevailing view was that IgER provided the trigger for inflammation, which was then expressed through the activation of mast cells and eosinophils. However, around that time, Patricia Diaz and Barry Kay [1] performed studies looking at the recruitment of CD4+ and CD8+ cells into BAL. These studies suggested that late asthmatic reactions were associated with a relative increase in CD4+ cells in BAL, while subjects who only showed early responses had similar proportions of CD4+ and CD8+ cells in BAL and in blood.

During my 3 years at the department, a T-cell research programme was established to address three distinct questions relevant to the role of T cells in allergic inflammation. My work asked whether T cells were recruited into sites of allergic inflammation [2]. Robyn O'Hehir [3] investigated whether there were T cells recognizing house dust mites in the blood of patients with allergic rhinitis and Chris Corrigan [4] looked for evidence of T-cell activation in clinical asthma. The results of these studies provided a platform for research that continues in the department and elsewhere. After leaving the NHLI and completing clinical training I moved to Southampton where we have embarked on a series of studies designed to address the antigen specificity and function of T cells in the airways of asthmatic human subjects.

Introduction

It is now generally agreed that asthma is an inflammatory disorder in which a special form of chronic inflammation affects the airways. This inflammation is considered to be responsible for the symptoms and disordered physiology found in clinical asthma. Several lines of evidence indicate that T lymphocytes orchestrate this inflammatory response [2–19]. Many T cells can be found in the bronchial mucosa of asthmatics [5, 6], with many expressing markers of activation [7, 8]. A positive correlation was found between the extent of T-cell activation and the level of bronchial hyperresponsiveness [6]. Increased numbers of activated T cells are found in the peripheral blood during acute episodes of asthma and their numbers decrease as the acute episode resolves [4]. Conversely, treatment with inhaled corticosteroids leads to a dramatic decrease in the mucosal content of mast cells and eosinophils in parallel with reduced expression of markers of T-cell activation [9]. When asthmatic airways are challenged locally with allergen, T cells, neutrophils and eosinophils are recruited into the bronchial epithelium and submucosa, in parallel with an upregulation of endothelial adhesion molecules [10]. In situ hybridization studies have shown expression of mRNA encoding IL-5, IL-4 and GM-CSF in asthmatic mucosal biopsies and in BAL T cells, both in cross-sectional studies and after allergen challenge [11, 12]. These observations suggest that the T cells present in asthmatic airways and those recruited during the late-phase reaction belong to the human homologue of the murine Th2 CD4+ T-cell subset [12, 13].

T lymphocytes are intimately involved in the generation of allergic responses: following the uptake and presentation of allergens by antigen presenting cells, helper T (Th) cells become activated and produce an array of soluble messengers (cytokines) which stimulate surrounding cells. In particular, IL-4 and IL-13 promote the switching of B cells from IgM to IgE production [14] while IL-3, IL-5 and GM-CSF promote the development and activation of eosinophils [15]. Moreover, IL-13 has recently been linked to several other features of the pathology of asthma, including subepithelial fibrosis, mucus hypersecretion and eotaxin production [16]. In order to explore this, several groups have used T-cell cloning techniques to clone individual T cells and assess their functional phenotype. This approach has demonstrated an increased proportion of Th2-like cells in the blood of atopic individuals [17] and in the conjunctiva of patients with vernal conjunctivitis [18]. T cells have also been cloned from bronchial biopsies obtained after challenge with pollen or toluene diisocyanate [19, 20]. We therefore set out to assess the cytokine profiles of T cells from asthmatic airways before and after allergen challenge and went on to clone T cells from BAL samples in order to address functional heterogeneity among the T cells present in the lavage samples [21].

T-Cell Cytokines

Asthmatic subjects were recruited by advertising for volunteers. At the time of enrolment all subjects had stable pulmonary function with a forced expiratory volume in 1 s (FEV_1) within 15% of that predicted for their age and height. They all had allergic asthma with hyperreactive airways to inhaled histamine and positive skin tests to common airborne allergens. None of the subjects had experienced an upper respiratory tract infection within 6 weeks of investigation. None had been treated with oral corticosteroids, sodium cromoglycate, or theophylline for at least 6 weeks prior to their participation in this study.

Local bronchial challenge was performed with a dose of allergen chosen on the basis of a skin test titration series. BAL samples were obtained from a control segment prior to challenge; post-challenge samples were obtained 4 or 24 h after challenge.

Unstimulated bulk samples of BAL T cells, obtained 10 min after allergen or saline challenge, expressed IFN-γ (5/6 cases), IL-13 (4/6), and TNF-α (5/6). IL-4 mRNA and IL-5 mRNA were found in a minority of cases. No IL-3 mRNA was detected. Overnight stimulation with PHA increased the expression of IL-3, IL-4 and IL-5 in 4/6 samples. Within individuals, the samples from the allergen and saline 10-min sites showed almost identical patterns of mRNA expression. The pattern of cytokine mRNA expression varied in BAL cells obtained 24 h after saline challenge, with IL-3 and IL-4 in 2/5 samples, IFN-γ, IL-5 and IL-13 in 3/5. After overnight PHA stimulation, IFN-γ and TNF-α were found in all 5 samples, IL-3 and IL-4 in 3/5 and IL-5 and IL-13 in 4/5. Although the cell numbers were equivalent, the BAL T-cell samples from the allergen-challenged sites gave weaker PCR signals than those from saline-challenged sites.

When stimulated in vitro by PHA, similar concentrations of immunoreactive IL-4 were generated by cells obtained from the allergen and saline sites after 10 min (mean 13.5 vs. 9.9 pg/ml respectively). Slightly more IFN-γ protein was generated by the BAL cells obtained at 10 min from the allergen site (mean 439 vs. 348.8 pg/ml). When BAL cells obtained 24 h after challenge were cultured with PHA, there was more IL-4 production by cells from the allergen site compared to the saline sites (mean 162.3 vs. 31.9 pg/ml; p = NS) but less IFN-γ (mean 221.1 vs. 403.7 pg/ml).

T-Cell Cloning

In order to assess the cytokine profile of individual T cells, enriched BAL T cells were plated out at 100, 30, 10, 3, 1 and 0.3 T cells per well in 96-well flat-bottomed microtitre plates with the mitogen PHA and irradiated autologous feeder cells. The cells were fed with IL-2 on day 5 and examined for positive growth on day 14. Wells with a high probability of being mono-clonal were selected for subculture and expanded into 48- and 24-well plates with weekly feeds of PHA and irradiated feeder cells, and twice weekly IL-2. After 6–8 weeks, sufficient cells were available for clones to be phenotyped by flow cytometry and for cytokine profiles to be obtained by RT-PCR and ELISA.

The proportion of BAL T cells that could be cloned with PHA was about 1/40 for both the allergen- and saline-challenged sites. There was no difference in the frequency of obtaining clones between the allergen and saline sites. A total of 72 T-cell clones survived in subculture for up to 6–8 weeks. These represent the progeny of 7 of the initial 17 panels. Of the 72 clones phenotyped, 50 were CD4 +, and 22 were CD8 +.

Cytokine analysis was performed on T-cell clones from 2 subjects. Clones derived from baseline lavages and from a lavage 4 h after challenge with saline showed strong expression of mRNA for IL-13. In addition, substantial mRNA signals for TNF-α, IFN-γ, IL-3 and GM-CSF were detected. IL-2 mRNA was found in the saline-challenged 4-hour site but not in the baseline clones. There were weaker mRNA signals for IL-4 and IL-5. IL-5 mRNA was weakly detectable in 7/11 clones from the baseline ST lavage, but IL-6 and IL-10 were not detected. Consistent with the RT-PCR profiles, the IL-4 concentrations in the DF clone supernatants ranged from 0 to 64 pg/ml while IFN-γ concentrations were between 0 and 49 pg/ml. In keeping with the stronger IL-4 mRNA signal, the baseline ST clones produced more IL-4 protein. The cytokine profiles of T-cell clones derived from the 24-hour post-allergen challenge seg-ment showed strong expression of mRNA for IL-3, IL-4, IL-5, IL-13 and GM-CSF. There was no expression of IL-2 or IL-10 in any of these clones, and TNF-α, IFN-γ and IL-6 were only weakly expressed. Clones from the saline site showed a similar cytokine profile to the clones from the allergen site.

The supernatants from the clones derived 24 h post-challenge contained larger amounts of IL-4 protein than those from the 4-hour saline site. This was true for both the allergen-challenged site (range 14–1,701 pg/ml) and the saline-challenged site (0–1,122 pg/ml). Some of the clones showed a 10-fold increase in IL-4 production compared to the bulk T-cell overnight cultures. Most clones that had strong IL-4 mRNA signals also had large amounts of

IL-4 in their supernatants but there was a wide scatter in the amount of IL-4 produced from clones with apparently similar amounts of mRNA. Interestingly, several of the T-cell clones from subject ST were CD8+ rather than CD4+, and yet produced large amounts of IL-4, in keeping with the recently described Tc2 phenotype [21]. IFN-γ production was more modest. Compared to clones derived from the baseline lavages in this subject, there was an increase in the relative production of IL-4 protein (IL-4/IFN-γ ratio rising from a mean of 9.7 to 19.7).

Thus the airways of patients with mild atopic asthma contained T cells which basally expressed mRNA for the cytokines IFN-γ , TNF-α, IL-13 and GM-CSF. mRNA for IL-3 and IL-4 was not basally expressed but could be induced by mitogen stimulation. 24 h after local allergen challenge, there was a shift in cytokine repertoire towards a Th2-like pattern, with less mRNA for TNF-α or IFN-γ and increased expression of the type 2 cytokines IL-3, IL-4 and IL-5. This pattern was enhanced after PHA stimulation. Using T-cell cloning techniques we were able to show that this general pattern reflects considerable heterogeneity among the airways T cells, with little evidence of 'pure' Th1- or Th2-pattern T cells. Moreover, there was wide variation in the amount of IL-4 produced by cloned T cells which appeared similar when judged by RT-PCR mRNA profiles. These results emphasize the importance of using several techniques to address the question of cytokine production by human airways cells and particularly the need to study protein and mRNA together to arrive at useful and valid conclusions.

Only a limited number of studies have addressed cytokine production by BAL cells before and after allergen challenge. Most have relied on in situ hybridization to assess cytokine expression rather than protein production. Robinson et al. [12] found increased expression of mRNA for IL-2, IL-3, IL-4, IL-5 and GM-CSF in BAL T cells from asthmatics as compared with control subjects. Inhalation allergen challenge led to a further increase in the proportions of BAL cells expressing mRNA for IL-4, IL-5 and GM-CSF but no change in IL-3, IL-2 or IFN-γ mRNA expression [6]. However, when cytokine proteins were measured in BAL from patients with asthma, significantly elevated concentrations were found for TNF, GM-CSF and IL-6 but not IL-4 or IL-1α, and when symptomatic airways were compared with asymptomatic asthmatic airways, only IL-1β and IL-2 showed increases associated with symptoms [22]. Eighteen hours after inhalation challenge, increased concentrations of IL-1, IL-2, IL-5, IL-6, IL-8 and TNF-α but no increase in IL-4 or IFN-γ were found in BAL fluid [23]. Others have reported increased concentrations of IL-4 and IL-5 in concentrated BAL fluid 24 h after local allergen challenge, which was also associated with eosinophil influx and the release of soluble VCAM-1 [24]. Other cytokines were either not measured or not reported in that study. In contrast, Huang et al. [25] found marked increases in IL-13 but relatively little IL-4 or IL-5 protein 18–24 h after segmental allergen challenge, and identified the cellular source of the IL-13 as the mononuclear cell fraction. Another recent study has also measured IL-13 in human asthma [26], and taken together, these studies suggest that IL-13 may be quantitatively more important than IL-4 in the local regulation of IgE switching in asthmatic airways. Moreover, while the actions of IL-4 and IL-13 on B cells are similar, it is now clear that IL-13 has several additional properties that may be directly relevant to the pathophysiology of asthma [16].

This study also demonstrated that T cells can be cloned directly from human airways (without an initial bulk culture) and that sufficient cell numbers could be derived for phenotypic and functional analysis. Both CD4+ and CD8+ clones were derived. However, several of the panels of clones could not be expanded, which limits the general applicability of the technique and results. With this proviso, the majority of T cells which could be cloned expressed mRNA for cytokines of the Th2 T-cell subtype, consistent with previous reports using in situ hybridization [11, 12], but there was a considerable degree of functional heterogeneity between clones from the same site.

Another major concern about using T-cell cloning to assess functional phenotype is the possible influence of culture conditions on the eventual phenotype of the clone. Proliferation of particular T-cell subtypes may be favoured by the presence of various cytokines. Thus Th2 cells proliferate better in the presence of IL-4 or IL-10, while the growth of Th1-type cells is enhanced in the presence of IL-2, IL-12 and IFN-γ [27, 28]. In addition, the culture conditions may bias pluripotential precursor cells towards Th1 or Th2 phenotype, e.g. IL-4 encouraging differentiation to a Th2 pattern and TGF-β to a Th1 pattern [29]. However, our data indicate that cloned airways T cells still show a considerable heterogeneity of cytokine expression after 6–8 weeks' culture, and this presumably reflects their initial cytokine profile. Further confirmation comes from the bulk BAL T-cell cultures, which represent the integrated response of many T cells, but nevertheless indicate a Th2 pattern at the allergen sites from which the Th2-type T-cell clones were subsequently derived.

Intracellular Cytokine Staining

To address the ability of peripheral blood and BAL cells to generate IL-2, IL-4 or IFN-γ, we developed a flow cytometric method which allows analysis of cytokine production at the single cell level within 5 h of obtaining the cell sample. When stimulated with phorbol myristic acetate (PMA) and ionomycin, there was a greatly increased proportion of IFN-γ-producing cells among BAL T cells from the subjects with asthma as compared to the atopic and nonatopic control subjects. The proportion of BAL T cells producing IL-4 was small (median 1.7% in the asthmatic group). In all three groups, the proportion of BAL T cells producing IL-2 or IFN-γ was increased compared to T cells from peripheral blood. These findings showed firstly that IL-4 production was confined to a relatively small proportion of T cells and secondly that there is a selective enhancement of IFN-γ production by airway T cells in asthma [30].

We also used this method to assess the functional significance of the activation marker expression seen in BAL T cells, and to examine cytokine production in relation to T-cell subset markers (CD4 and CD8). A higher percentage of peripheral blood CD4 + cells produced IL-2 compared to IFN-γ (24 vs. 7%) and, conversely, a higher percentage of blood CD8 + T cells produced IFN-γ compared to IL-2 (29 vs. 7%). There was no difference in the percentages of CD4 + BAL T cells expressing IL-2 or IFN-γ (46 vs. 51%), but more BAL CD8 + T cells produced IFN-γ than produced IL-2 (63 vs. 23%). We did not find any association between CD25 expression and cytokine production in either blood or BAL T cells. HLA-DR expression was associated with IFN-γ and IL-2 production by BAL T cells but not blood T cells. CD69 expression correlated much more closely with cytokine production in both compartments. Thus both CD4 + and CD8 + T cells contribute to the increased production of IFN-γ in BAL T cells in asthma. CD25 expression by BAL T cells is not congruent with the ability to produce cytokines upon stimulation, but CD69 expression seems to be a more relevant marker of the ability of BAL T cells to produce cytokines.

Thus it emerged that that IFN-γ and IL-2 are produced by both CD4 + T cells and CD8 + T cells in both blood and BAL. Similar proportions of BAL CD4 + cells produced both cytokines, but a 3-fold greater proportion of BAL CD8 + T cells produced IFN-γ. In both compartments, cytokine production was associated with expression of the early activation marker CD69. Neither of the later activation markers, CD25 and HLA-DR, was associated with cytokine production in blood-derived T cells while cytokine production was linked to HLA-DR but not to CD25 in BAL T cells.

These results obtained using whole blood are similar to those found in other studies in which isolated CD4 + and CD8 + T-cell subsets were cultured and their supernatants analysed for cytokine production [19, 31, 32]. Although both subsets expressed IL-2 and IFN-γ, the majority of IFN-γ-producing T cells were of the CD8 + subset and the majority of IL-2-producing T cells were of the CD4 + subset. In BAL T cells however, there was no difference in the percentage of CD4 + cells expressing IFN-γ compared to IL-2 and the majority of both IL-2- and IFN-γ-producing cells were CD4+ compared to CD8+. This indicates that CD4+ T cells play a greater role in Th1 cytokine production in the asthmatic lung compared to their CD8+ counterparts. The initial study found an increase of IFN-γ-producing BAL T cells in asthmatics compared to normal controls [30], and it now looks as if the bulk of this increase in asthma is due to increased expression of IFN-γ by CD4+ BAL T cells. It has been suggested recently that IL-4-producing blood T cells may be identified by CD30 expression, and therefore that CD30 might be used to detect Th2 cells [33]. Although CD30 is expressed on only 1–2% of blood T cells, a similar percentage to the proportion of IL-4+ T cells in the present study, no cells stained simultaneously for CD30 and IL-4, suggesting that CD30 is not a useful marker for IL-4-producing cells in these cell populations.

CD69 is an early T-cell activation marker which was originally described as a fibronectin receptor and is expressed within 5 h of activation, whereas CD25 and HLA-DR are not expressed until 24–72 h after T-cell activation [34–37]. Therefore, CD69 expression presumably indicates that the T cells have been activated during the 5-hour in vitro culture with PMA and ionomycin while CD25 and HLA-DR expression are more likely to indicate previous activation in vivo. We were initially surprised that we did not find any association between CD25 expression and cytokine production by either blood or BAL T cells for any of the four cytokines studied. This lack of association may be due to preactivated T cells needing a period of recuperation before they can be reactivated, i.e. they may be in a temporary anergic state [38]. This could be explored further by separating cells on the basis of CD25 expression and then stimulating CD25+ and CD25– populations independently. HLA-DR expression was associated with production of both IFN-γ and IL-2 in BAL T cells where the percentages of cytokine-positive cells were similar for CD69 and HLA-DR. HLA-DR expression after T-cell activation occurs later than expression of CD25 and it may be that by the time that HLA-DR is expressed alone, sufficient time has elapsed after initial activation (in vivo) to allow reactivation by PMA and ionomycin in vitro. However, it has also been suggested that T cells from different biological compartments have different kinetics of HLA-DR expression, and that cytokine and surface marker kinetics are at least partly stimulus-dependent [39–41], so this difference in cytokine production by HLA-DR+ T cells from blood and BAL could reflect a difference in HLA-DR kinetics between T cells from different biological compartments. Alternatively, it may indicate a faster reactivation time after in vivo stimulation for BAL T cells compared to blood T cells.

Therefore, while we remain convinced that T cells play a critical role in orchestrating the allergic response, our data suggest that CD25 expression by

BAL T cells cannot be taken as unequivocal evidence of T-cell activation. Rather it appears that CD25 may identify a population of T cells that have been activated recently and are currently incapable of responding to stimulation. In the context of the human airway, T-cell unresponsiveness is probably a desirable state, in that active responses are not always desirable at mucosal surfaces, in contrast to the need for the immune system to respond vigorously to agents that cross the mucosal or skin barriers. Further work on the significance of activation marker expression might be achievable by cell sorting and appropriate ex vivo stimulation.

T-Cell Receptor Analysis

In the final part of this work we have tried to assess the nature of the T-cell contribution to allergic inflammation by studying the T-cell receptor (TCR) repertoire in normal and asthmatic airways. T lymphocytes recognize antigens through a receptor structure, TCR, which is strictly associated with the γ, δ, ε and ζ chains of the CD3 molecule which serves as a signal transducer to the T-cell interior. TCRs are heterodimers comprising either α/β or γ/δ chains each encoded (just like immunoglobulins on B cells) by variable (V), diversity (D), joining (J) and constant (C) gene segments that undergo somatic rearrangement during T-cell development [42]. The CD3 components show no amino acid variability in different T cells and thus do not influence the diversity associated with TCRs. The $V\alpha$ and $V\beta$ gene segments can be clustered into families based upon nucleotide sequence similarities and their protein products can be identified by family-specific monoclonal antibodies. To date, 30 $V\alpha$ and 24 $V\beta$ families have been identified in man. The diversity created by the random pairing of $V\alpha$ and $V\beta$ genes thus allows 720 possible combinations. This is further augmented by junctional flexibility (the imprecise joinings of the gene segments) and N-region diversity (the addition of nongenomic nucleotides at junction points) which occur during the somatic rearrangement process. The hypervariability of the V(D)J joining process leads to an almost innumerable range of possible amino acid sequences in the antigen-recognition site and hence the ability to recognize an almost infinite variety of antigens [42]. The TCR (and (chains each have three points of contact with the MHC molecule peptide. These are termed complementarity-determining regions (CDRs). The CDR1 and CDR2 regions bind to polymorphic framework regions of the MHC molecule, while the CDR3 region constitutes the antigen-combining site. Broadly speaking, the CDR1 and CDR2 regions are formed from the framework regions of the V segment, while the CDR3s are formed from the $V\alpha$-$J\alpha$ and $V\beta$-$D\beta$-$J\beta$ junction regions.

The T-cell response of an individual to antigens depends on the available T-cell repertoire, which is known to be influenced by the HLA haplotype of the individual, but is also affected by environmental factors such as exposure to antigens or superantigens [43]. With antigens that have a very restricted range of T-cell epitopes there may be an extremely restricted repertoire of TCRs which can recognize that antigen. In the human context, analysis of TCR family usage at sites of inflammation such as the airways can yield insight into the forces that drive the formation of the T-cell repertoire [44]. In peripheral blood the TCR repertoire within any given Vβ family is virtually always polyclonal, but clonal populations can be identified in airways' T-cell populations, both in health and disease [45–49]. This type of analysis has allowed us to detect clonal expansion within the airways in sarcoidosis [45, 46], in extrinsic allergic alveolitis [46, 47], and in asthma [48, 49], and makes it possible to assess whether the T-cell activation seen in asthmatic airways is a specific or a nonspecific event. Interestingly, it seems that allergen challenge of human airways can lead to the appearance of new, clonal T-cell subpopulations which are not present at baseline and are not seen after sham challenge with saline [49]. Our current work is focusing on the relationship between TCR usage and cytokine profile. To date it appears that expanded T-cell subsets can be identified, with cytokine profiles that are more similar to the Th2 phenotype than the background BAL T-cell population. Further work is needed to verify that the analytical protocols are appropriate and to establish whether there is any consistency between and within subjects.

Acknowledgments

All the studies described here were approved by the Southampton Hospitals and University Ethics Committee, and all subjects gave their written informed consent.

References

1   Gonzalez MC, Diaz P, Galleguilos FR, Ancic P, Cromwell O, Kay AB: Allergen-induced recruitment of bronchoalveolar helper (OKT4) and suppressor (OKT8) T-cells in asthma. Am Rev Respir Dis 1987;136:600–604.
2   Frew AJ, Kay AB: Eosinophils and T-lymphocytes in late phase allergic reactions. J Allergy Clin Immunol 1990;85:533–539.
3   O'Hehir RE, Garman RD, Greenstein JL, Lamb JR: The specificity and regulation of T-cell responsiveness to allergens. Annu Rev Immunol 1991;9:67–95.
4   Corrigan CJ, Kay AB: CD4 T lymphocyte activation in acute severe asthma: Relationship to disease severity and atopic status. Am Rev Respir Dis 1990;141:970–977.
5   Azzawi M, Bradley B, Jeffery PK, Frew AJ, Wardlaw AJ, Knowles G, Assoufi B, Collins JV, Durham SR, Kay AB: Identification of activated T lymphocytes and eosinophils in stable atopic asthma. Am Rev Respir Dis 1990;142:1407–1413.

6   Bradley BL, Azzawi M, Jacobson M, Assoufi B, Collins JV, Irani AA, Schwartz LB, Durham SR, Jeffery PK, Kay AB: Eosinophils, T-lymphocytes, mast cells, neutrophils, and macrophages in bronchial biopsy specimens from atopic subjects with asthma: Comparison with biopsy specimens from atopic subjects without asthma and normal control subjects and relationship to bronchial hyperresponsiveness. J Allergy Clin Immunol 1991;88:661–674.

7   Wilson JW, Djukanovic R, Howarth PH, Holgate ST: Lymphocyte activation in bronchoalveolar lavage and peripheral blood in atopic asthma. Am Rev Respir Dis 1992;145:958–960.

8   Djukanovic R, Roche WR, Wilson JW, Beasley CRW, Twentyman OP, Howarth PH, Holgate ST: Mucosal inflammation in asthma. Am Rev Respir Dis 1990;142:434–457.

9   Wilson JW, Djukanovic R, Howarth PH, Holgate ST: Inhaled beclomethasone dipropionate downregulates airway lymphocyte activation in atopic asthma. Am J Respir Crit Care Med 1994;149:86–90.

10   Montefort S, Gratziou C, Goulding D, Polosa R, Haskard DO, Howarth PH, Holgate ST, Carroll MP: Bronchial biopsy evidence for leukocyte infiltration and upregulation of leukocyte-endothelial cell adhesion molecules 6 hours after local allergen challenge of sensitized asthmatic airways. J Clin Invest 1994;93:1411–1421.

11   Hamid Q, Azzawi M, Ying S, Moqbel R, Wardlaw AJ, Corrigan CJ, Bradley B, Durham SR, Collins JV, Jeffery PK, Quint DJ, Kay AB: Expression of mRNA for interleukin-5 in mucosal bronchial biopsies from asthma. J Clin Invest 1991;87:1541–1546.

12   Robinson DS, Hamid Q, Ying S, Tsicopoulos A, Barkans J, Bentley AM, Corrigan CJ, Durham SR, Kay AB: Predominant 'TH2-like' bronchoalveolar lavage T-lymphocyte population in atopic asthma. N Engl J Med 1992;326:298–304.

13   Mosmann TR, Coffman RL: TH1 and TH2 cells: Different patterns of lymphokine secretion lead to different functional properties. Annu Rev Immunol 1989;7:145–173.

14   Punnonen J, Aversa G, Cocks BG, De Vries JE: Role of IL-4 and IL-13 in synthesis of IgE and expression of CD23 by human B-cells. Allergy 1994;49:576–586.

15   Saito H, Hatake K, Dvorak AM, Leiferman KM, Donnenberg AD, Arai N, Ishizaka K, Ishizaka T: Selective differentiation and proliferation of hematopoietic cells by recombinant human interleukins. Proc Natl Acad Sci USA 1988;85:2288–2292.

16   Zhu Z, Homer RJ, Wang Z, Chen Q, Geba GP, Wang J, Zhang Y, Elias JA: Pulmonary expression of IL-13 causes inflammation, mucus hypersecretion, subepithelial fibrosis, physiologic abnormalities and eotaxin production. J Clin Invest 1999;103:779–788.

17   Wierenga EA, Snoek M, De Groot C, Chrétien I, Bos JD, Jansen HM, Kapsenberg ML: Evidence for compartmentalization of functional subsets of CD4 + T lymphocytes in atopic patients. J Immunol 1990;144:4651–4656.

18   Maggi E, Biswas P, DelPrete G, Parronchi P, Macchia D, Simonelli C, Emmi L, De Carli M, Tiri A, Ricci M, Romagnani S: Accumulation of Th2-like helper cells in the conjunctiva of patients with vernal conjunctivitis. J Immunol 1991;146:1169–1174.

19   Pène J, Lagier B, Rivier A, Chanez P, Vendrell JP, Bousquet J: Phenotype of T-cell clones obtained from bronchial biopsies and peripheral blood from three asthmatics. Cell Biol Int 1993;17:353–357.

20   Maestrelli P, Del Prete GF, de Carli M, Saetta M, Di Stefano A, Ricci M, Romagnani S, Fabbri LM: Activated CD8 T lymphocytes producing interferon-γ and interleukin-5 in bronchial mucosa of subjects sensitised to toluene diisocyanate. Scand J Work Environ Health 1994;20:376–381.

21   Bodey KJ, Semper AE, Redington AE, Madden J, Teran LM, Holgate ST, Frew AJ: Cytokine profiles of BAL T-cells and T-cell clones obtained from human asthmatic airways after local allergen challenge. Allergy 1999;54:1083–1094.

22   Broide DH, Lotz M, Cuomo AJ, Coburn DA, Federman EC, Wasserman SI: Cytokines in symptomatic asthma airways. J Allergy Clin Immunol 1992;89:958–67.

23   Virchow JC, Walker C, Hafner D, Kortsik C, Werner P, Matthys H, Kroegel C: T-cells and cytokines in BAL fluid after segmental allergen provocation in atopic asthma. Am J Respir Crit Care Med 1995;151:960–968.

24   Zangrilli JG, Shaver JR, Cirelli RA, Cho SK, Garlisi CG, Falcone A, Cuss FM, Fish JE, Peters SP: sVCAM-1 levels after segmental allergen challenge correlate with eosinophil influx, IL-4 and IL-5 production, and the late phase response. Am J Respir Crit Care Med 1995;151:1346–1353.

25   Huang SH, Xiao HQ, Kleine-Tebbe J, Paciotti G, Marsh DG, Lichtenstein LM, Liu MC: IL-13 expression at the sites of allergen challenge in patients with asthma. J Immunol 1995;155:2688–2694.

26   Kroegel C, Julius P, Matthys H, Virchow JC, Luttman W: Endobronchial secretion of IL-13 following local allergen challenge in atopic asthma: Relationship to IL-4 and eosinophil counts. Eur Respir J 1996;9:899–904.

27   Lederer JA, Liou JS, Todd MD, Glimcher LH, Lichtman AH: Regulation of cytokine gene expression in T helper subsets. J Immunol 1994;152:77–86.

28   Trinchieri G: Interleukin-12 and its role in the generation of TH1 cells. Immunol Today 1993;14:335–338.

29   Sad S, Mosmann TR: Single IL-2-secreting precursor CD4 T-cell can develop into either Th1 or Th2 cytokine-secreting phenotype. J Immunol 1994;153:3514–3522.

30   Krug N, Madden J, Redington AE, Lackie P, Djukanovic R, Schauer U, Holgate AT, Frew AJ, Howarth PH: T-cell cytokine profile evaluated at the single cell level in BAL and blood in allergic asthma. Am J Respir Cell Mol Biol 1996;14:319–326.

31   Krouwels FH, Hol BE, Bruinier B, Lutter R, Jansen HM, Out TA: Cytokine production by T-cell clones from bronchoalveolar lavage fluid of patients with asthma and healthy subjects. Eur Respir J Suppl 1996:22;95s–103s.

32   Mori A, Suko M, Tsuruoka N, Kaminuma O, Ohmura T, Nishizaki Y, Ito K, Okudaira H: Allergen-specific human T cell clones produce interleukin-5 upon stimulation with the TH1 cytokine interleukin-2. Int Arch Allergy Immunol 1995:107;220–222.

33   Romagnani S, del Prete G, Maggi E, Caligaris Cappio F, Pizzolo G: CD30 and type-2 T helper responses [cf. erratum: J Leukoc Biol 1995;57:978]. J Leukoc Biol 1995;57:726–730.

34   Cotner T, Williams JM, Christenson L, Shapiro HM, Strom TB, Strominger J: Simultaneous flow cytometric analysis of human T cell activation antigen expression and DNA content. J Exp Med 1983;157:461–72.

35   Cantrell DA, Smith KA: Transient expression of interleukin-2 receptors. Consequences for T-cell growth. J Exp Med 1983;158:1895–1911.

36   Risso A, Smilovich D, Capra MC, Baldissarro I, Tan G, Bargellesi A, Cosulich ME: CD69 in resting and activated T lymphocytes. Its association with a GTP binding protein and biochemical requirements for its expression. J Immunol 1991;146:4105–4114.

37   Werfel T, Boeker M, Kapp A: Rapid expression of the CD69 antigen on T cells and natural killer cells upon antigenic stimulation of peripheral blood mononuclear cell suspensions. Allergy 1997;52:465–469.

38   Schall TJ, O'Hehir RE, Goeddel DV, Lamb JR: Uncoupling of cytokine mRNA expression and protein secretion during the induction phase of T-cell anergy. J Immunol 1992;148:381–387.

39   Lee SC, Liu W, Dickson DW, Brosnan CF, Berman JW: Cytokine production by human foetal microglia and astrocytes. Differential induction by lipopolysaccharide and IL-1β. J Immunol 1993;150:2659–2667.

40   Riccioli A, Filippini A, de Cesaris P, Barbacci E, Stefanini M, Starace G, Ziparro E: Inflammatory mediators increase surface expression of integrin ligands, adhesion to lymphocytes and secretion of interleukin-6 in mouse Sertoli cells. Proc Natl Acad Sci USA 1995;2:5808–5812.

41   Hartung T, Sauer A, Wendal A: Testing of immunomodulatory properties in vitro. Dev Biol Stand. Basel, Karger, 1996, vol 86, pp 85–96.

42   Alt FW, Oltz EM, Young F, Gorman J, Taccioli G, Chen J: VDJ recombination. Immunol Today 1992;13:306–314.

43   Akolkar PN, Gulwani-Akolkar B, Pergolizzi R, Bigler RD, Silver J: Influence of HLA genes on T cell receptor V segment frequencies and expression levels in peripheral blood lymphocytes. J Immunol 1993;150:2761–2773.

44   Pannetier C, Even J, Kourilsky P: T-cell repertoire diversity and clonal expansions in normal and clinical samples. Immunol Today 1995;16:176–181.

45   Grunewald J, Janson CH, Eklund A, Ohrn M, Olerup O, Persson U, Wigzell H: Restricted Vα2.3 gene usage by CD4+ T lymphocytes in bronchoalveolar lavage fluid from sarcoidosis patients correlates with HLA-DR3. Eur J Immunol 1992;22:129–133.

46 Trentin L, Zambello R, Facco M, Tassinari C, Sancetta R, Siviero M, Carutti A, Cipriani A, Marcer G, Majori M, Pesci A, Agostini C, Semenzato G: Selection of T-lymphocytes bearing limited TCR-Vβ regions in the lung of hypersensitivity pneumonitis and sarcoidosis. Am J Respir Crit Care Med 1997;155:587–596.

47 Wahlström J, Berlin M, Lundgren R, Olerup O, Wigzell H, Eklund A, Grunewald J: Lung and blood T-cell receptor repertoire in extrinsic allergic alveolitis. Eur Respir J 1997;10:772–777.

48 Gelder CM, Peters MJ, O'Connor BJ, Adcock IM, Barnes PJ, Chung KF, Morrison JFJ: Restriction of endobronchial T-cell Vα gene usage in atopic asthma. Thorax 1993;48:458P.

49 Dasmahapatra J, Hodges E, Smith JL, Lanham S, Krishna MT, Holgate ST, Frew AJ: T-cell receptor Vβ gene usage in bronchoalveolar lavage and peripheral blood T-cells from asthmatic and normal subjects. Clin Exp Immunol 1998;112:363–374.

A.J. Frew, Reader in Medicine & Head of University Department of Medical Specialities,
University of Southampton, Mailpoint 810, Southampton General Hospital,
Southampton SO16 6YD (UK)
Tel. +44 23 8079 4069, Fax +44 23 8077 7996, E-Mail ajf1@soton.ac.uk

Robinson DS (ed): Immunological Mechanisms in Asthma and Allergic Diseases.
Chem Immunol. Basel, Karger, 2000, vol 78, pp 148–158

....

T Cells and Fibrosis

Ben G. Marshall, Rory J. Shaw

Department of Respiratory Medicine, National Heart and Lung Institute,
Imperial College School of Medicine, Hammersmith Campus, London, UK

Introduction

Fibrosis with associated scarring and irreversible tissue damage is the
final step of many pathological processes. Pulmonary fibrosis can complicate
diverse pulmonary and systemic pathologies. There is considerable literature
on the mechanisms by which wound healing, for example following surgical
incision, results in inflammation and fibrosis [1]. However, the exact relationship between the development of fibrosis and the early stages of an immune
or inflammatory process is unknown. Similarly, the time course linking these
events can be variable. We have little information to date on how the progression to fibrosis is regulated or on the optimal approaches to developing therapeutic interventions. When the inflammatory process is driven by an immune
response, the mechanisms are likely to be complex since subtle differences
in the numbers of different cellular subsets have the potential to affect the
progression to fibrosis. This difficulty is further compounded by the heterogeneity of cytokines and inflammatory mediators that can be observed in different
clinical situations. This diversity, however, may be important and help explain
the variation in the magnitude of scarring in different immune mediated diseases. Such diseases include schistosomiasis, sarcoidosis and asthma.

One of the difficulties of using these diseases as models is the poorly
understood immunological component of the pathophysiology. Mycobacterial
diseases are also associated with tissue fibrosis. By contrast, the immunology
in these diseases is well understood and recent advances in molecular biology
allow manipulation of the anti-mycobacterial immune response to enhance
further our understanding of pathogenetic mechanisms. Alternatively, by genetic manipulation of the mycobacterial genome, we are now able to allow

the expression by mycobacteria of key mammalian proteins involved in the host immune response. Using these useful experimental tools, it has been shown to be possible to dissect out the role of individual immune factors on host inflammatory and fibrotic response. For this reason, the present review will focus on experimental data derived from mycobacterial studies.

Immunologically Mediated Diseases Associated with Tissue Fibrosis

One of the best characterized immunological diseases associated with fibrosis is schistosomiasis. In this disease the pathogenic hallmark of the immune response is chronic granulomatous inflammation, dominated by Th2 cells and recruited eosinophils, and there is progression to local fibrosis. Previous work has shown that induction of schistosome egg granulomas requires an intact T-cell response [2], specific orchestration of both T-cell- and macrophage-derived cytokines [3] and induction of chemotactic factors [4]. These immune mediators may regulate recruitment of inflammatory cells to the site of the trapped egg and induce collagen synthesis, leading to reactive fibrosis [5].

By contrast, asthma, which is recognized to be associated with marked activation of Th2 lymphocytes, is not associated with gross pulmonary fibrosis, although there is clear evidence of activation of myofibroblasts within the airway [6], and fibrosis confined to the airway subepithelium [7]. Myofibroblasts are cells which contribute to the fibrotic process and may be associated with a progression from reversible to irreversible airways obstruction. Although some studies suggest that at least one feature of this airway wall remodelling associated with asthma, i.e. subepithelial fibrosis, is reversible and thus by acting early enough, either with preventive measures or with anti-inflammatory treatment it is possible to prevent airway remodelling [8]. Many interstitial lung diseases are associated with immune cell activation, in particular sarcoidosis and hypersensitivity pneumonitis (extrinsic allergic alveolitis) [9]. Progression to fibrosis in sarcoidosis is very variable, even in the presence of marked lymphocyte activation [10]. This may relate to lymphocyte subtype since the lymphocytes in sarcoidosis appear to be predominately of the Th1 subtype and high levels of interferon-γ (IFN-γ) have been identified [11]. Similarly, hypersensitivity pneumonitis is associated with cellular infiltration (monocytes, lymphocytes of both CD4 and CD8 subtypes and plasma cells) and with continued exposure this is accompanied by progressive fibrosis in the lung interstitium and alveolar spaces which may become extensive [12].

Tuberculosis has long been recognized to be associated with fibrosis. Indeed, in the skin the presence of scarring is used clinically to differentiate lupus vulgaris from lupus pernio. In the lung, contraction and loss of lung

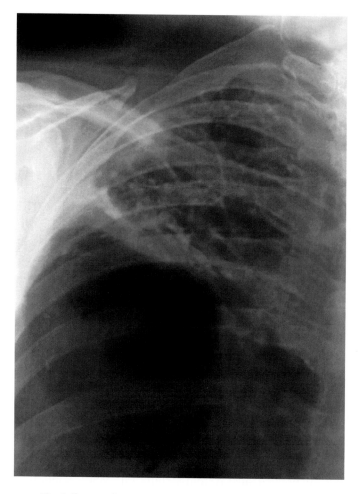

Fig. 1. Progressive upper zone fibrosis following treatment for pulmonary tuberculosis.

volume are pathognomonic features (as illustrated in figure 1). Consequently these events serve as a paradigm for understanding fibrotic pathways in other diseases and for the development of therapeutic interventions.

Mycobacterial Disease as a Model for Progression to Tissue Fibrosis

Intracellular bacteria, such as *Mycobacterium tuberculosis*, induce strong T-cell and macrophage responses, resulting in the formation of granulomas and fibrosis, due to the production of cytokines that stimulate fibroblast prolif-

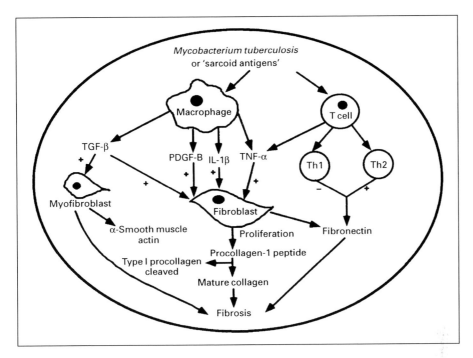

Fig. 2. Diagram of interrelationship between T cells and fibrosis in myocobacterial disease.

eration and collagen synthesis (fig. 2). In addition to clinical evidence from patients of fibrosis and scarring associated with *M. tuberculosis* infection, there is data from laboratory studies. In human, rabbit and guinea pigs, progression of tuberculosis is associated with liquefaction of solid caseous tuberculous lesions with cavitation [13]. The walls of these cavities consist of an external zone of collagen, hyalinized capsule containing granulation tissue rich in capillaries, fibroblasts, macrophages and lymphocytes. The concept has been extended to suggest that the host's delayed-type hypersensitivity (DTH) response contributes to host defence by stimulating the process to wall off sites of infection and thus prevent dissemination and reactivation of disease [14]. Many of the respiratory sequelae associated with pulmonary tuberculosis are caused by replacement of normal lung architecture with scar tissue.

In a study comparing human cutaneous forms of tuberculosis with sarcoidosis we performed immunochemistry on skin biopsies from affected individuals [15]. The biopsies from both diseases were shown to contain granulomas, which exhibited marked staining by antibodies to fibronectin, transforming growth factor-β (TGF-β) and type 1 procollagen. Type 1 procollagen is a marker of newly formed collagen since it is identified by antibodies directed at the ends of the collagen type 1 precursor membrane which are lost as mature collagen forms in the tissues. Accentuated staining of extracellular matrix was seen both in the granulomas and in the perigranulomatous regions. When the granulomas in the skin of patients with tuberculosis and sarcoidosis were compared, there were important differences. In tuberculosis there were numerous fibroblasts throughout the granuloma staining for type 1 procollagen. In sarcoidosis there was less type 1 procollagen staining within the granulomas. In both diseases there was evidence of matrix proteins surrounding the granulomas.

BCG Studies

Evidence of tissue fibrosis following local infections with *Mycobacterium bovis* BCG is well recognized in man. Indeed the presence of scarring over the ensuing years has been taken as evidence of BCG immunization [16], although recent work refuted this contention and found no relationship to scar size and vaccine-induced protective immunity [17]. In a murine footpad model of BCG inoculation, we have confirmed the presence of a fibrotic reaction in the footpad injected with BCG, by demonstrating the expression of inflammatory cytokines and de novo synthesis of extracellular matrix proteins, when compared to the opposite footpad injected with control medium [18]. We have also demonstrated in an in vitro model, that local expression at the site of infection of the anti-inflammatory cytokine interleukin (IL)-10 by a recombinant strain of mycobacterium, can significantly reduce the levels of two host macrophage products, tumor necrosis factor-α (TNF-α) and nitric oxide (NO). Both potentially harmful inflammatory T-cell products which may be associated with the fibrotic response in mycobacterial disease [19]. This might have implications for attempts to modulate the immunological potential of recombinant mycobacterial vaccines as well as approaches in immunotherapy of immune mediated fibrotic diseases. Finally, recent work in our laboratory has confirmed that host immunopathology to mycobacterial infection can be abrogated, using a strategy to inhibit the host fibrotic response by engineering BCG to express a naturally occurring cytokine antagonist latency-associated peptide (LAP). LAP serves to downregulate TGF-β induction in infected organs, thus reducing collagen deposition and improving the host-protective immune response [Marshall et al., manuscript in preparation].

Studies Following PPD Inoculation

Evidence that there is a clear link between the immune response and a fibrotic reaction in the context of mycobacterial infection was provided by performing immunohistochemical analysis of human skin biopsies taken following intradermal injection of the mycobacterial peptide preparation, PPD [15, 20]. Biopsies performed on individuals at different times following the tuberculin test (Heaf test) and compared with controlled biopsies were studied by immunohistochemistry using antibodies to key inflammatory profibrotic cytokines and extracellular matrix proteins, with absolute counts of positive staining cells per cm^2. Over a 14-day time course there was progressive increase in the cells in both the dermis and the perivascular area which stained positively for type 1 procollagen, whereas there was no change observed in controls. These results were associated with a time-dependent increase in myofibroblasts in the skin biopsy as identified by α smooth muscle actin staining and a persistent increase in staining for fibronectin, TNF-α and IL-1β.

Contribution of Nonspecific Inflammatory Mediators to Fibrosis

A fibrotic response may occur in response to unremitting inflammation in an immune mediated response, with tissue injury from the local release of reactive oxygen and nitrogen species, proteases and lysosomal products from phagocytic cells in the presence of inflammatory cytokines. TNF-α is a proinflammatory cytokine produced by macrophages stimulated by agents such as lipopolysaccharide. The role of TNF-α in human tuberculosis is paradoxical, because although there is much evidence for a protective role, there is also increasing evidence that TNF-α plays a role in the immunopathology and tissue damage that characterizes the human disease. TNF-α appears to be essential for host immunity but overproduction of this cytokine may have serious pathological consequences. Rook and co-workers [21, 22] suggest that several properties of *M. tuberculosis* may 'pervert' the normal protective function of TNF-α by rendering the host's tissues exquisitely sensitive to the toxic effects of TNF. The resulting tissue-damaging response is unlikely to play a protective role, and may actually be detrimental to the host by allowing spread of the organisms to other tissues.

The production of NO and other reactive nitrogen intermediates by cytokine-activated cells is an important component of antimicrobial responses [23]. The potential role of NO as a cytopathic molecule in mycobacterial infection, which might contribute to tissue damage and scarring, is unclear, but experimental evidence implicates NO as a relevant mediator in the development of an inflammatory reaction in other pathological processes [24–27]. However, iNOS knockout mice exhibit delayed wound healing, and the reversal of this impairment by gene transfer of iNOS DNA establishes a key role for iNOS in wound repair [28]. We have shown the presence of increased expression of iNOS in BCG-infected murine footpads. Mice infected with live BCG show enhanced levels of iNOS compared to those infected with killed BCG. This leads to elaboration of excess collagen deposition locally [18].

Chemokines are likely to play an important role in the early stages of the host immune response to tuberculosis, especially in the recruitment of monocyte and lymphocyte populations to the site of infection and the initiation of a granuloma [29, 30]. The induction of a number of different chemokines has been demonstrated to occur following phagocytosis of *M. tuberculosis* in humans [31–33] and mice [34]. It seems most likely in human tuberculosis that proinflammatory cytokines and chemokines act as part of a cascade of mediators that play roles in mobilizing and activating cellular immune responses, contributing to granuloma formation and together determining the type of immunological response, ultimately leading to disease progression and fibrotic tissue damage, or resolution. The liquefaction process in tuberculous infection, which precedes fibrosis, is associated with the presence of mature macrophages containing high concentrations of proteinases, which hydrolyse solid caseous material [35]. This is likely to be an indirect consequence of upregulation of the activity of certain inflammatory cytokines such as IL-1 and TNF-α and may contribute to the overall progression to fibrosis and scarring in this disease.

The Role of T-Cell Subsets

Tuberculosis is the prototype infection that requires cellular immune responses for its control. Collaboration between T cells and macrophages is critical in the acquired protective immune response to *M. tuberculosis* and is associated with a proinflammatory cytokine environment. A complex series of events ensues and is believed to involve a variety of T-cell subsets manifesting themselves in the performance of numerous functions, including the induction of DTH, cytolysis, protection and memory immunity [36]. This cell-mediated response to mycobacteria is orchestrated by the CD4 T cell through the release of specific cytokines. In the mouse model, two distinct populations of CD4 T cells, distinguished by the profile of cytokines they secrete, contribute to this response [37]. T-helper 1 T cells (Th1 cells) mediate DTH responses through the secretion of interferon-γ and IL-2 [38], whereas T-helper 2 T cells (Th2 cells) enhance B-cell differentiation and therefore antibody production, by the elaboration of IL-4, IL-5 and IL-10. The striking contribution of these two subpopulations to outcomes of infection is exemplified by infection with other intracellular pathogens, such as *Leishmania* [39], *Schistosoma* [40] and *M. leprae* [41], in which Th1 cells producing IFN-γ contribute to control and elimination of infection, whereas Th2 cells producing IL-4 result in progressive, tissue-damaging disease. By manipulating this axis, it may be possible to inhibit an immune-mediated fibrotic response through the upregulation of Th1 T-cell synthesized cytokines. In a murine model of mycobacterial induced fibrosis, we have observed a more rapid clearance of mycobacteria in mice infected with a recombinant BCG strain expressing IFN-γ (BCG-IFN) [42]. Importantly, this effect was not associated with enhancement in any of the markers of tissue pathology. Granuloma formation, iNOS expression, and fibrosis were all lower in mice infected with BCG-IFN than in mice infected with a control BCG strain. This can be explained by one or both of the following mechanisms: either the local expression of recombinant IFN-γ triggers early activation of a protective type 1 T-cell response, promoting bacterial killing in the absence of fibrosis and reducing the number of organisms capable of inducing subsequent pathology; alternatively, an increase in the level of IFN-γ in host tissues may be directly responsible for preventing fibrosis. A similar approach was taken in a murine model designed to develop an antipathology vaccine for schistosomiasis [43]. It was clearly demonstrated that IL-12 has potential for modulating fibrosis in this disease by acting as an adjuvant to a conventional vaccine, enhancing cell-mediated immunity and suppressing both granuloma formation and fibrosis in infected organs. IL-12 is known to favour the priming of Th1 rather than Th2 cells and the effects on fibrosis are accompanied by replacement of Th2-dominated pattern of cytokine expression characteristic of schistosomal infection with one dominated by Th1 cytokines. An analogous approach which dampened Th2 responses directly by using antibodies to Th2 cytokines also served to inhibit the acute granulomatous and fibrotic responses in schistosoma-infected mice [44].

Interestingly, other experimental work suggests that when a Th2 response is superimposed upon a pre-existing Th1 response, the resulting cell-mediated inflammatory site may become exquisitely sensitive to cytokine-mediated tissue damage [45], thus exacerbating local tissue damage [46]. We have recently shown in an experimental model of granulomatous lung disease, using transgenic technology, that the presence of Th2 lymphocytes is specifically associated with fibrosis. A prior injection of murine splenocytes cultured ex vivo differentiated towards a Th2 population induced a more profound pulmonary fibrotic response to peptide-coated Sepharose beads than occurred in mice injected with Th1 polarized T lymphocytes [Arun Wangoo et al., manuscript in preparation]. Idiopathic pulmonary fibrosis, a disease characterized by a destructive fibroproliferative response, is associated with an overexuberant Th2 T-cell immune response [47] and impaired IFN-γ production [48]. Studies in both mice [49] and humans [50] have demonstrated beneficial outcomes in response to therapeutic trials of IFN-γ. It is apparent from all these studies that a fibrotic response can be manipulated by utilizing the Th1/Th2 subset antagonism with potentially beneficial results in the amelioration of fibrotic pathology.

Conclusion

Tissue fibrosis is a common outcome of many chronic inflammatory diseases. It is characterized by an increase in extracellular matrix proteins such as collagen. Many of the cellular mechanisms leading to fibrosis appear to be shared, irrespective of the initiating cause. In this chapter, we have chosen to highlight our experimental work on the mammalian host response to myco-bacterial infection to illustrate the complexities of a chronic inflammatory disease mediated by an enhanced T-cell response, which ultimately progresses to disabling tissue fibrosis. Consequently, these events serve as a paradigm for understanding fibrotic pathways in other diseases affecting different tissues and for the development of therapeutic interventions.

References

1   Wangoo A, Laban C, Cook HT, Glenville B, Shaw RJ: IL-10 and corticosteroid-induced reduction in type 1 procollagen in a human ex vivo culture. Int J Exp Pathol 1997;78:33–41.
2   Byram JE, von Lichtenberg F: Altered schistosome granuloma formation in nude mice. Am J Trop Med Hyg 1977;26:944.
3   Chensue SW, Warmington K, Ruth J, Lincoln P, Kuo MC, Kunkel SL: Cytokine responses during mycobacterial and schistosomal antigen-induced pulmonary granuloma formation. Am J Pathol 1994;145:1105–1113.
4   Lukacs NW, Kunkel SL, Strieter RM, Chensue SW: The role of chemokines in *Schistosoma mansoni* granuloma formation. Parasitol Today 1994;10:322.
5   Wynn TA, Eltoum I, Oswald IP, Cheever AW, Sher A: Endogenous interleukin-12 regulates granu-loma formation induced by eggs of *Schistosoma mansoni* and exogenous IL-12 both inhibits and prophylactically immunises against egg pathology. J Exp Med 1994;179:1551.
6   Brewster CEP, Howarth PH, Djukanovic R, Wilson J, Holgate ST, Roche WR: Myofibroblasts and subepithelial fibrosis in bronchial asthma. Am J Respir Cel Mol Biol 1990;3:507–511.
7   Roche WR, Beasley R, Williams JR, Holgate ST: Subepithelial fibrosis in the bronchi of asthmatics. Lancet 1989;i:520–524.
8   Chetta A, Foresi A, Del Donno M, et al: Airways remodelling is a distinctive feature of asthma and is related to severity of disease. Chest 1997;111:852–857.
9   Suga M, Yamasaki H, Nakagawa K, Kohorogi H, Ando M: Mechanisms accounting for granu-lomatous responses in hypersensitivity pneumonitis. Sarcoidosis Vasc Diffuse Lung Dis 1997;14:131–138.
10 DeRemee RA, Anderson HA: Sarcoidosis: A correlation of dyspnoea with roentgenographic stage and pulmonary function changes. Mayo Clin Proc 1974;49:742–745.
11 Robinson BW, McLemore TL, Crystal RG: Gamma interferon is spontaneously released by alveolar macrophages and lung T lymphocytes in patients with pulmonary sarcoidosis. J Clin Invest 1985;75:1488–1495.
12 Reynolds HY: Hypersensitivity pneumonitis: Correlation of cellular and immunological changes with clinical phases of disease. Lung 1991;169:S109–S128.

13   Smith D, Harding G: Animal model of human disease: Experimental airborne tuberculosis in the guinea pig. Am J Pathol 1977;89:273–277.

14   Orme I: The immunopathogenesis of tuberculosis: A new working hypothesis. Trends Microbiol 1998;6:94–97.

15   Marshall BG, Wangoo A, Cook HT, Shaw RJ: Increased inflammatory cytokines and new collagen formation in cutaneous tuberculosis and sarcoidosis. Thorax 1996;51:1253–1261.

16   Fine PEM, Rodrigues LC: Modern vaccines: Mycobacterial diseases. Lancet 1990;335:1016–1020.

17   Sterne JAC, Fine PEM, Ponnighaus JM, Sibanda F, Munthali M, Glynn JR: Does bacille Calmette-Guérin scar size have implications for protection against tuberculosis or leprosy? Tubercle Lung Dis 1996;77:117–123.

18   Chambers M, Marshall B, Wangoo A, et al: Differential responses to challenge with live and dead Mycobacterium bovis bacillus Calmette-Guérin. J Immunol 1997;158:1742–1748.

19   Marshall BG, Chambers MA, Wangoo A, Shaw RJ, Young DB: Production of tumour necrosis factor and nitric oxide by macrophages infected with live and dead mycobacteria and their suppression by an interleukin-10-secreting recombinant. Infect Immun 1997;65:1931–1935.

20   Wangoo A, Cook HT, Taylor GM, Shaw RJ: Enhanced expression of type 1 procollagen and transforming growth factor-β in tuberculin-induced delayed-type hypersensitivity. J Clin Pathol 1995;48:339–345.

21   Al Attiyah R, Rosen H, Rook GAW: A model for the investigation of factors influencing haemorrhagic necrosis mediated by tumour necrosis factor in tissue sites primed with mycobacterial antigen preparations. Clin Exp Immunol 1992;88:537–542.

22   Filley EA, Bull HA, Dowd PM, Rook GAW: The effect of Mycobacterium tuberculosis on the susceptibility of human cells to the stimulatory and toxic effects of tumour necrosis factor. Immunology 1992;77:505–509.

23   Nathan CF, Hibbs JB Jr: Role of nitric oxide synthesis in macrophage antimicrobial activity. Curr Opin Immunol 1991;3:65–75.

24   Anderson SE, Kallstrom L, Malm M, Miller-Larsson A, Axelsson B: Inhibition of nitric oxide synthase reduces Sephadex-induced oedema formation in the rat lung: Dependence on intact adrenal function. Inflamm Res 1995;44:418.

25   Stefanovic-Racic M, Meyers K, Meschter C, Coffe JW, Hoffman RA, Evans CH: Ng-monomethyl-L-arginine suppresses development of adjuvant arthritis in rats; in The Biology of Nitric Oxide. London, Portland Press Proceedings, 1995, vol 4.

26   Heiss LN, Lancaster JR Jr, Corbett JA, Goldman WE: Epithelial autotoxicity of nitric oxide: Role in the respiratory cytopathology of pertussis. Proc Natl Acad Sci USA 1994;91:267–270.

27   Royall JA, Kooy NW, Beckman JS: Nitric oxide-related oxidants in acute lung injury. New Horiz 1995;3:113–122.

28   Yamasaki K, Edington HDJ, McClosky C, et al: Reversal of impaired wound repair in iNOS-deficient mice by topicasl adenoviral-mediated iNOS gene transfer. J Clin Invest 1998;101:967–971.

29   Boring L, Gosling J, Chensue S, Kunkel S, Farese R Jr, Broxmeyer H: Impaired monocyte migration and reduced type 1 (Th1) cytokine responses in C-C chemokine receptor 2 knockout mice. J Clin Invest 1997;100:2552–2561.

30   Lin Y, Gong J, Zhang M, Xue W, Barnes P: Production of monocyte chemoattractant protein 1 in tuberculosis patients. Infect Immun 1998;66:2319–2322.

31   Friedland J, Remick D, Shattock R, Griffin G: Secretion of interleukin-8 following phagocytosis of Mycobacterium tuberculosis by human monocytic cell lines. J Immunol 1992;22:1373–1378.

32   Kashahara K, Tobe T, Tomita M, et al: Selective expression of monocyte chemotactic and activating factor/monocyte chemoattractant protein 1 in human blood monocytes by Mycobacterium tuberculosis and its components. J Infect Dis 1994;170:1238–1247.

33   Antony V, Godbey S, Kunkel S, Hott J, Hartman D, Burdick M, Strieter RM: Recruitment of inflammatory cells to the pleoral space. Chemotactic cytokines, IL-8, and monocytic chemotactic peptide-1 in human pleural fluids. J Immunol 1993;151:7216–7223.

34   Rhoades E, Coope A, Orme I: Chemokine response in mice infected with Mycobacterium tuberculosis. Infect Immun 1995;63:3871–3877.

35 Chang J, Wysocki A, Tchou-Wong K, Moskowitz N, Zhang Y, Rom W: Effect of *Mycobacterium tuberculosis* and its release of matrix metalloproteinases. Thorax 1996;51:306–311.

36 Orme I: Characteristics and specificity of acquired immunological memory to *Mycobacterium tuberculosis* infection. J Immunol 1988;140:3589–3593.

37 Mosmann TR, Cherwinski H, Bond MW, Giedlin MA, Coffman RL: Two types of murine helper T cell clone. I. Definition according to profiles of lymphokine activities and secreted proteins. J Immunol 1986;136:2348–2357.

38 Cher D, Mosmann T: Two types of murine helper T cell clone. II. Delayed type hypersensitivity is mediated by TH1 clones. J Immunol 1987;138:3688–3694.

39 Heinzel F, Sadick M, Holaday B, Coffman R, Locksley R: Reciprocal expression of interferon-γ or interleukin-4 during the resolution or progression of murine leishmaniasis. Evidence for expansion of distinct helper T cell subsets. J Exp Med 1989;169:59–72.

40 Boros DL: The role of cytokines in the formation of the schistosome egg granuloma. Immunobiology 1994;191:441–450.

41 Bloom B, Modlin R, Salgame P: Stigma variations: Observations on suppressor T cells and leprosy. Annu Rev Immunol 1992;10:453–488.

42 Wangoo A, Brown I, Marshall BG, Young DB, Shaw RJ: BCG-associated inflammation and fibrosis: Modulation by recombinant BCG expressing interferon-γ. Clin Exp Immunol 2000;119:92–98.

43 Wynn TA, Cheever AW, Jankovic D, et al: An IL-12-based vaccination method for preventing fibrosis induced by schistosome infection. Nature 1995;376:594–596.

44 Boros DL, Whitfield JR: Enhanced Th1 and dampened Th2 responses synergise to inhibit acute granulomatous and fibrotic responses in murine schistosomiasis mansoni. Infect Immun 1999;67:1187–1193.

45 Rook G, Hernandez-Pando R: T-cell helper types and endocrines in the regulation of tissue damaging mechanisms in tuberculosis. Immunobiology 1994;191:478–492.

46 Hernandez-Pando R, Orocozcoe H, Samieri A, et al: Correlation between the kinetics of Th1/Th2 cells and the pathology in a murine model of experimental pulmonary tuberculosis. Immunology 1996;89:26–33.

47 Wallace WA, Ramage EA, Lamb D, Howie SE: A type 2 (Th2-like) pattern of immune response predominates in the pulmonary interstitium of patients with cryptogenic fibrosing alveolitis. Clin Exp Immunol 1995;101:436–441.

48 Prior C, Haslam PL: In vivo levels and in vitro production of interferon-γ in fibrosing lung diseases. Clin Exp Immunol 1992;88:280–287.

49 Gurujeyalakshmi G, Giri SN: Molecular mechanisms of antifibrotic effect of interferon γ in bleomycin-mouse model of lung fibrosis: Downregulation of TGF-β and procollagen I and III gene expression. Exp Lung Res 1995;21:791.

50 Ziesche R, Hofbauer E, Wittmann K, Petkov V, Block LH: A preliminary study of the long-term treatment with interferon γ-1b and low dose prednisolone in patients with idiopathic pulmonary fibrosis. N Engl J Med 1999;341:1246–1249.

Prof. Rory J. Shaw, Hammersmith Hospital NHS Trust, Hammersmith House,
Hammersmith Hospital, Du Cane Road, London, W12 0HS (UK)
Tel. +44 181 383 3370, Fax +44 181 393 3361, E-Mail r.shaw@ic.ac.uk

Robinson DS (ed): Immunological Mechanisms in Asthma and Allergic Diseases.
Chem Immunol. Basel, Karger, 2000, vol 78, pp 159–165

....

Molecular Pathology of Allergic Diseases

Pota Christodoulopoulos, Shigeo Muro, Qutayba Hamid

Meakins-Christie Laboratories, McGill University, Montreal, Canada

Introduction

Allergic diseases are characterized by the IgE-dependent release of mast cell-derived mediators and cellular infiltration particularly of activated eosinophils and T lymphocytes. The in situ detection of cytokines has provided valuable information on the mechanisms responsible for allergic inflammation as cytokines have been shown to be important biochemical mediators essential in allergic inflammatory reactions. Allergic diseases such as asthma and rhinitis are associated with persistent infiltration of the airways with inflammatory cells particularly exhibiting a Th2-like cytokine profile [1–3]. It is evident that Th2-type cytokines, particularly IL-4, IL-5 and IL-13, perform important regulatory roles in allergic inflammation since their gene expression has been localized in vivo at the level of the tissue. These cytokines have been shown to be the driving force behind IgE production, eosinophil activation, and stimulation of the endothelium to produce mediators important in the inflammatory response. Investigation beyond purely the presence of activated cells within the tissues, in situ localization has enabled both the cellular source and relative contribution of cytokines to be assessed, as well as indicating the possible pathways involved. While there is growing evidence to suggest that cytokines are playing an important role in initiating and maintaining inflammatory reactions associated with allergy, to confirm such a role it is essential to identify the expression of cytokine genes and gene products, and further, to localize cytokine receptors in vivo at the level of the tissue. The most widely used techniques to identify cytokine expression are in situ hybridization (ISH) and immunocytochemistry (ICC). Using labeled mRNA probes, ISH detects the synthesis of genes encoding for cytokines within a cell, and in a complementary fashion, ICC detects the presence of immunoreactive protein. Since each methodology tells us slightly different information regarding the synthesis and secretion of cytokines, a combination of these techniques may be necessary to determine their presence within the tissue.

Immunolocalization of Cytokines

ICC is used to detect the presence of immunoreactive protein within cells or tissue and thus provide evidence that translation from mRNA to protein has occurred by means of an antigen-antibody reaction. This technique allows the precise examination of many aspects of cell function and their relation to our perception of cell and tissue morphology, and as such has enhanced our understanding of disease processes. Given the rapid release of cytokines, their short half-life and the presence of high-affinity receptors, the technique of immunolocalizing cytokines with specific antibodies has been particularly informative in the pathogenesis of allergic diseases. ICC may also localize the secretion of cytokines from specialized storage granules which can occur in the absence of apparent mRNA production. For example, mast cells or eosinophils have the capacity to store cytokines intracellularly, and both acute release and storage of these mediators can be detected by ICC [4–6]. Many methods are available for immunocytochemistry, thus the major criteria for selecting a technique to detect a particular antigen includes the sensitivity, reliability, cost, versatility and safety of the methodology [7]. In general, the three principle methods available are direct, indirect, and unlabeled antibody enzymatic methods. The direct method is the simplest ICC method in which a label is directly conjugated to the antibody. While simple, this technique is not particularly sensitive, nor does it utilize the specificity of antibodies used in other methods. The indirect method consists of an unlabelled primary antibody whose binding is revealed by a labeled second antibody specific to the immunoglobulin of the species providing the primary antibody. Since at least two secondary antibody molecules can be bound to each primary antibody molecule, this method is more sensitive than the direct method. In the unlabeled antibody enzymatic methods, an unconjugated bridging secondary antibody is used between the primary antibody and the label detection reagent which is usually an enzyme-antienzyme complex or an avidin-biotin complex. Enzymatic methods include the peroxidase and antiperoxidase (PAP) and the alkaline phosphatase antialkaline phosphatase (APAAP) technique. Special reference is made to cytokine immunohistology using the APAAP methodology. This technique is especially suited to cytokine ICC since it is sensitive to detect low levels of secreted proteins and is suitable for use with monoclonal antibodies. Due to the similarity between cytokines in general, the use of monoclonal antibodies is essential to ensure the specificity of the reaction. The presence of cytokine immunoreactivity in a particular cell does not necessarily indicate that the cell actually synthesized the protein, some cells like macrophages and epithelial cells have the ability to endocytose protein from surrounding media.

The use of ICC to detect cytokine immunoreactivity requires an intrinsic understanding of the basic principles combined with an appreciation of cytokine biology. Given the appropriate reagents and conditions, ICC provides a powerful tool in aiding our awareness of immunoregulation

Confocal Microscopy

The confocal microscope utilizes laser to identify different wave light fluorescent signals, and has the ability to obtain multiple sequential pictures of the same image which allows the identification and subcellular localization of protein and mRNA. Confocal microscopy is of potential value to also examine the intracellular movement of protein in living cells. It has been used extensively for multiple staining using simultaneous ISH and ICC. It can identify up to five markers in a single cell. This microscope is also of potential value for signal quantification (ICC and ISH) and could be of great interest to investigate and to examine the relative expression of mRNA or immunoreactivity of particular proteins.

Multiple Staining Techniques

Initially, it was generally perceived that most cytokines in allergic inflammation were the products of activated T cells. However, it has recently been demonstrated that other inflammatory cells in man possess the capacity to produce certain cytokines under the appropriate stimulation. For example, eosinophils can produce GM-CSF, IL-3, IL-5, IL-6 and TGF-β [8–11], mast cells produce IL-3, IL-4, IL-5 and TNF-α [12–14], and other cell types such as basophils, macrophages, monocytes and epithelial cells are also capable of producing a wide variety of these cytokines. This has created the need to develop a number of techniques specifically to identify the phenotype of cells expressing cytokine mRNA in tissues obtained from the site of allergic inflammation which include simultaneous ICC and ISH. In addition, more than one cytokine might be produced by the same cell and in some instances it is important to confirm. The technique which can be utilized for this purpose is simultaneous ISH. ISH is usually used to detect more than one mRNA in the same cell, particularly in the case of multiple gene expression and alternative supplies. However, it could also be used to identify the phenotype of cells expressing a certain mRNA by combining two probes, one coding for an mRNA in question and the other for an mRNA known to be expressed specifically in one type of cell.

In Situ Detection of Cytokines

During the last few years we have been using various methods to identify the in situ expression of cytokines in tissues obtained from allergic individuals. ISH has been used extensively to localize cytokine mRNA in tissue sections and cytospin preparations from normal and diseased individuals [15–17].

This approach is valuable in cytokine research as there is in vitro evidence suggesting that cytokines are synthesized de novo and released very rapidly. In that case, the chances of detecting their immunoreactivity in lymphocytes or other cells are limited. For example, T cells in particular have a low capacity to store cytokines and generate cytokine mRNA readily upon the appropriate stimulation. As such, localization of cytokine production from T cells is more evident using ISH techniques. The localization of cytokine mRNA at the tissue level indicates the expression and activation of the gene and the potential ability of the cell to produce cytokines. ISH in general can be defined as the cellular localization of specific nucleic acid sequences, using a labeled complementary strand. The two nucleic acid forms, DNA and RNA, are found in both the nucleus and the cytoplasm and the technical approach to the demonstration of these molecules in each anatomical location is different. Although ISH was used initially for the localization of specific DNA sequences [18], more recently it has been applied to localize mRNA, the intermediate molecule in the transfer of genetic information from genomic DNA to functional polypeptide. The general principle of ISH is based on the fact that labeled single-stranded RNA or DNA containing complementary sequences are hybridized intracellularly to mRNA under appropriate conditions, thereby forming a stable hybrid. This will be detected according to the type of labeling of the probe. Different probes are available to detect mRNA including double- and single-stranded DNA, oligonucleotides and single-stranded RNA probes. Single-stranded RNA probes have been used extensively in recent years for the detection of cytokine mRNA by both isotopic and nonisotopic methods. The use of RNA probes has a number of advantages over other types of probes [19]. These include the ability to synthesize a probe of relatively constant size, the high stability and affinity of RNA hybrids and the ability of RNase to remove the unhybridized probe. All of these favor the high specificity and sensitivity of RNA probes. To construct a labeled RNA probe, the DNA sequences of interest are subcloned into a RNA expression vector (e.g. pGEM), transfected into *Escherichia coli* bacteria, extracted, and then linearized prior to the in vivo transcription. The regulation of gene expression through transcriptional activation and inactivation within a cell, is reflected by the cellular content and distribution of the specific message. The demonstration of mRNA within a cell provides valuable information about gene expression and indicates possible synthesis of the corresponding protein. In diseased states, it can be used for temporary studies in relation to physiological, pathological and developmental processes.

Quantification and Interpretation of Results

Many factors must be carefully considered and controlled if quantitative data are to be collected [20]. These include section thickness, nucleic acid retention, consistency of hybridization, length of exposure and development conditions. The inclusion of a known standard and the construction of a standard curve are essential. However even under optimal conditions, the quantification of cytokine mRNA at the ISH level is at best semiquantitative.

When interpreting ISH results it is essential to be convinced that the autoradiographic signal is really specific. For example, a number of inflammatory cells like eosinophils and macrophages have the capacity to bind probe nonspecifically, especially with ^{35}S-labeled probes [15]. Caution must be exercised in the interpretation of autoradiographic signal at the edge of the section (edge artefact). It is also important to take into consideration other factors like the formation of imperfect duplexes with nonhomologous nucleic acids, electrostatic interactions among charged groups, physical entrapment of probe in the three-dimensional lattice of the tissue section. A proper microscope with dark-field illumination and phase-contrast facilities is essential for proper interpretation of autoradiographic signals. It is essential to include a positive and negative control in each radioactive ISH experiment. Absence of autoradiographic hybridization signal does not necessarily indicate the absence of a particular mRNA and its translation product. mRNA could be expressed in low copy number which is beyond the sensitivity of the technique. Moreover, ISH determines the steady-state amount of hybridizable specific mRNA, whereas immunoreactive proteins are localized by immunocytochemistry. Despite the fact that the expression of the majority of genes is regulated by the amount of specific mRNA, conclusions drawn from double staining experiments, such as estimation of secretory activity, must be considered carefully. In addition, several other factors at the post-transcriptional and post-translational levels influence the amount and type of detectable gene expression products.

Explant Model

Our current understanding of the pathogenesis of allergic airway disease is derived primarily from studying the events which follow in vivo allergen exposure, either naturally or deliberately by allergen challenge, as well as the effects of culturing inflammatory cells with allergen and/or other mediators of allergy. Studying the inflammatory process subsequent to in vivo allergen exposure provides information on the natural course of disease, however, the relative contribution of resident versus infiltrating inflammatory cells cannot be determined. Although cell culture has greatly advanced our knowledge of the consequences of cell and cytokine interactions, the problem with using this technique is that it lacks important elements of the in vivo situation, like cell-cell and cell-matrix interactions as well as complex intercytokine networking. Based on recent work in which rat lung explants were cultured in allergen-treated medium [21], ex vivo techniques for culturing human nasal mucosal biopsies to study local events following ex vivo allergen challenge have recently been developed. In isolation from systemic variables, explanted tissue provides a useful system for delineating local inflammatory events while maintaining normal structural and cellular inter-relationships.

Conclusion

ISH and ICC are powerful tools being used in cytokine research and their applications have improved our understanding of the biology and molecular pathology of allergic diseases. Furthermore, they have potential for improving the diagnosis, the assessment of disease severity, as well as the response to treatment, which may thus lead to potential therapeutic interventions.

References

1   Robinson D, Hamid Q, Bentley A, Ying A, Kay AB, Durham SR: Activation of CD4 + T cells and eosinophil recruitment in bronchoalveolar lavage after allergic allergen inhalation challenge in patients with atopic asthma. J Allergy Clin Immunol 1993;92:313–324.
2   Azzawi M, Bradley B, Jeffrey PK, Frew AJ, Wardlaw A, Assoufi B, Collins JV, Durham S, Kay AB: Identification of activated T lymphocytes and eosinophils in bronchial biopsies in stable atopic asthma. Am Rev Respir Dis 1990;142:1407–1413.
3   Bentley AM, Menz G, Storz C, Robinson DS, Bradley B, Jeffrey PK, Durham S, Kay AB: Identification of T lymphocytes, macrophages, and activated eosinophils in the bronchial mucosa of intrinsic asthma. Am Rev Respir Dis 1992;146:500–506.
4   Lamkhioued B, Aldebert AS, Gounni E, Delaporte M, Goldman A, Capron M: Synthesis of cytokines by eosinophils and their regulation. Int Arch Allergy Immunol 1995;107:122–123.
5   Bradding P, Feather IH, Howarth PH, Mueller R, Roberts JA, Britten K, Bews JBA, Hunt TC, Okayama Y, Heusser CH, Bullock GR, Church MK, Holgate ST: Interleukin-4 is localised to and released by human mast cells. J Exp Med 1992;176:1381–1386.
6   Levi-Schaffer F, Lacy P, Severs NJ, Newman TM, North J, Gomperts B, Kay AB, Moqbel R: Association of granulocyte-macrophage colony-stimulating factor with the crystalloid granules of human eosinophils. Blood 1995;85:2579–2586.
7   Van Noorden S: Tissue preparation and immunostaining techniques for light microscopy; in Polak JM, Van Noorden S (eds): Immunocytochemistry. Modern Methods and Applications. London, Wright 1986, chapt 3, pp 26–53.

8   Kita H, Ohnishi T, Okubo Y, Weiler D, Abrams JS, Gleich GJ: Granulocyte/macrophage colony-stimulating factor and interleukin-3 release from human peripheral blood eosinophils and neutrophils. J Exp Med 1991;174:745–748.

9   Moqbel R, Hamid Q, Ying S, Barkans J, Hartnell A, Tsicopoulos A, Wardlaw AJ, Kay AB: Expression of mRNA and immunoreactivity for the granulocyte/macrophage colony-stimulating factor in activated human eosinophils. J Exp Med 1991;174:749–752.

10 Hamid Q, Barkans J, Meng Q, Abrams J, Kay AB, Moqbel R: Human eosinophils synthesize and secrete interleukin-6 in vitro. Blood 1992;80:1496–1501.

11 Broide DH, Paine MM, Firestein GS: Eosinophils express interleukin-5 and granulocyte macrophage colony-stimulating factor mRNA at sites of allergic inflammation in asthmatics. J Clin Invest 1992; 90:1414–1424.

12 Plaut M, Pierce JH, Watson CJ, Hanley-Hyde J, Nordan RP, Paul WE: Mast cell lines produce lymphokines in response to cross-linkage of FCεRI or to calcium ionophores. Nature 1989;339: 64–67.

13 Gordan JR, Galli SJ: Mast cells as a source of both preformed and immunologically inducible TNF-α/cachetin. Nature 1990;346;274–276.

14 Bradding P, Roberts JA, Britten KM, Montefort S, Djukanovic R, Mueller R, Heusser CH, Howarth PH, Holgate ST: Interleukin-4, -5 and -6 and tumor necrosis factor-α in normal and asthmatic airways: Evidence for the human mast cell as a source of these cytokines. Am J Respir Cell Mol Biol 1994;10:471–480.

15 Kay AB, Ying S, Varney V, Gaga M, Durham SR, Moqbel R, Wardlaw AJ, Hamid Q: Messenger RNA expression of the cytokine gene cluster IL-3, IL-4, IL-5 and GM-CSF in allergen-induced late-phase cutaneous reactions in atopic subjects. J Exp Med 1991;173:775–778.

16 Hamid QA, Azzawi M, Jeffrey P, Kay AB: Expression of mRNA for interleukin-5 in mucosal bronchial biopsies from asthma. J Clin Invest 1991;87:154–159.

17 Robinson D, Hamid QA, Ying S, Tsicopoulos A, Barkans J, Bentley AM, Corrigan C, Durham SR, Kay AB: Predominant Th2-type bronchoalveolar lavage T lymphocytes population in atopic asthma. N Engl J Med 1992;326:298–304.

18 Pardue ML, Gall JG: Molecular hybridization of radioactive DNA to the DNA of cytological preparations. Proc Natl Acad Sci USA 1969;64:600–604.

19 Cox KH, DeLeon DV, Angerer LM, Angerer RC: Detection of mRNAs in sea urchin embryos by in situ hybridization using asymmetric RNA probes. Dev Biol 1984;101:485–502.

20 Davenport AP, Nunez DJ: Quantification of hybridization signal; in Polak JM, McGee JO'D (eds): In situ Hybridization: Principles and Practice. Oxford, Oxford University Press, 1990, pp 173–281.

21 Eidelman DH, Minshall E, Dandurand RJ, Schotman E, Song YL, Yasruel Z, Moqbel R, Hamid Q: Evidence for major basic protein immunoreactivity and interleukin-5 gene activation during the late phase response in explanted airways. Am J Respir Cell Mol Biol 1996;15:582–589.

Q. Hamid, MD, PhD, Professor of Medicine and Pathology, Meakins-Christie Laboratories, McGill University, 3626 St. Urbain Street, Montreal, Quebec, H2X-2P2 (Canada)
Tel. +1 514 398 3864, Fax +1 514 398 7483, E-Mail hamid@meakins.lan.mcgill.ca

Robinson DS (ed): Immunological Mechanisms in Asthma and Allergic Diseases.
Chem Immunol. Basel, Karger, 2000, vol 78, pp 166–177

....

Role of Eotaxin and Related CC Chemokines in Allergy and Asthma

Timothy J. Williams, Peter J. Jose

Leukocyte Biology Section, Biomedical Sciences Division, Imperial College
School of Medicine, London, UK

Introduction

The close association between the presence of eosinophilic leukocytes in
the asthmatic lung and lung dysfunction has led to extensive investigations of
eosinophil biology, particularly the mechanisms underlying eosinophil recruitment. The result of this research is that we now have a much clearer understanding of the life history of the eosinophil and can now design therapeutic
compounds to target eosinophil trafficking with the objective of limiting eo-
sinophil-induced tissue damage.

Mechanisms Underlying Eosinophil Recruitment

Eosinophils are believed to have evolved as effector cells to combat parasitic
helminth infections [1–3]. Thus, mechanisms are necessary to detect the presence
of the worm in tissue and then to stimulate the recruitment of eosinophils from
the local blood microvasculature. If allergy is an aberration of a host defence
system, then these same mechanisms may be triggered by allergens, otherwise
innocuous agents from the environment mistaken for parasite products. Parasites have become adept at circumventing host defence systems and thus worms
themselves are a potential source of agents interfering with eosinophil functions.

A key phase in the process of leukocyte recruitment is the local production
of a soluble chemical signal, a chemoattractant, that stimulates the cell to
attach to, and migrate through, the wall of the microvessel [4, 5]. The chemoattractant acts via a 7-transmembrane region G protein-linked receptor on the
leukocyte surface. Thus, depending on the specificity of the chemoattractant

for its receptor and the distribution of a given receptor, this provides a level of leukocyte-type specificity to the recruitment process [6–8]. Leukocyte recruitment takes place in post-capillary venules in most tissues. Leukocytes tend to roll along the surface of venular endothelial cells by forming loose attachments between selectin molecules and their complementary receptors. The chemoattractant, which can be either in soluble form or bound to the endothelial surface, stimulates the chemoattractant receptor resulting in an upregulation of integrin adhesion molecules and cytoskeletal changes in the cell. Integrins bind to complementary adhesion molecules of the IgG superfamily (ICAMs, VCAM) on endothelial cells so that the leukocyte flattens on the surface and becomes firmly attached. The adhesion molecule expression on endothelial cells can also be upregulated by certain cytokines, thus providing another level to amplify adherence. The leukocyte then migrates through interendothelial cell junctions, again via integrin/ICAM or VCAM interactions. For eosinophils there is evidence that both α_4 integrin/VCAM and β_2 integrin/ICAM interactions are important in these processes [9–12].

Chemokines

Until the late 1980s it was not possible to explain particular patterns of leukocyte recruitment in different types of inflammation based on the then current knowledge of leukocyte chemoattractants. Potent chemoattractants (originally identified by their chemotactic activity in Boyden chambers in vitro) were known, such as C5a, leukotriene B_4, formyl-methionyl peptides and platelet-activating factor, but none of these exhibited leukocyte-type specificity.

The discovery of the first chemokines led to the realization that a large family of structurally-related small proteins exists. Approximately 40 human chemokines and 18 receptors have been identified to date [for reviews, see 7, 8]. Chemokines often stimulate several different receptors and a given leukocyte type often expresses more than one type of receptor. Moreover, a leukocyte can also change its chemokine receptor expression pattern when presented with different microenvironments. However, it is now possible to begin to understand how leukocytes can traffick from one compartment to another, thus providing exciting new targets for therapeutic intervention.

Eotaxin

We realized that none of the known chemoattractants was selective for eosinophils and so could not account for the eosinophil-rich infiltration observed in allergic reactions. We, therefore, began a project to identify such mediators generated in vivo. Sensitized guinea pigs were challenged with an aerosol of ovalbumin to produce acute bronchoconstriction followed by a delayed response associated with eosinophil infiltration. Bronchoalveolar lavage (BAL) fluid, taken at intervals after the allergen challenge, was bioassayed for chemoattractant activity by injecting it intradermally in naïve assay animals and measuring the local accumulation of circulating ^{111}In-eosinophils. We found that BAL fluid taken from 3 to 6 h after challenge contained eosinophil chemoattractant activity. This was purified using HPLC and sequencing revealed a novel 73 amino acid CC chemokine that we called 'Eotaxin' [13, 14]. Guinea pig Eotaxin was cloned using degenerate primers based on the sequence of the guinea pig protein [15, 16]. Constitutive message was found in the lung and was upregulated on allergen challenge of sensitized animals. Subsequently, mouse [17, 18], rat [19, 20] and human [21–23] Eotaxin homologues were cloned. These proteins have high sequence homology and all are potent eosinophil chemoattractants.

RANTES, some of the monocyte chemoatractant proteins (MCPs) and MIP-1α are other CC chemokines that are also known to stimulate eosinophil responses. However, these proteins are nonselective and stimulate a wide variety of cell types besides eosinophils. More recently, two more Eotaxins, Eotaxin-2 and Eotaxin-3, have been identified. These proteins have high functional similarity, but rather low sequence similarity, when compared with Eotaxin [24–28].

The Eotaxin Receptor, CCR3

The most important chemokine receptor on eosinophils appears to be the 7-transmembrane-spanning Eotaxin receptor, now designated CCR3. This has been cloned in man [23, 29, 30], mouse [31, 32] and guinea pig [33]. Human CCR3 binds Eotaxin, Eotaxin-2, Eotaxin-3 and MCP-4 with high affinity, whereas RANTES and MCP-3 bind with lower affinity. Guinea pig Eotaxin is highly potent as a stimulator of human eosinophils [14], but, conversely, human Eotaxin is inactive on guinea pig cells, although it is active on rat eosinophils [12]. Despite the fact that human RANTES stimulates human eosinophils, RANTES from other species has, in general, low activity on homologous eosinophils [34]. Unexpectedly, human RANTES binds to guinea pig CCR3 [14, 33] and acts as an antagonist in vitro and in vivo [35].

In the guinea pig there is no evidence to date of endogenous CC chemokines, other than Eotaxin, acting on eosinophils [36]. A neutralizing antibody to guinea pig CCR3 has been produced. This antibody blocks responses to

Eotaxin in guinea pig eosinophils in vitro and prevents eosinophil accumulation in response to Eotaxin in vivo [33]. In mouse models of allergic airway inflammation, eosinophil recruitment appears to be mediated by a number of CC chemokines acting via CCR3 and, depending on the model and the mouse strain, MIP-1α acting through CCR1 [37]. In man, MIP-1α can also stimulate eosinophils but this may be in only a small subpopulation of individuals, whereas Eotaxin is active on eosinophils from all donors [38].

More recently, CCR3 has been shown to be expressed on basophils [39], mast cells [40, 41] and some Th2 lymphocytes [42–44], other cells associated with the allergic response.

Chemokines in Allergic Airway Inflammation

Eotaxin generation has been detected in guinea pig [14–16, 36] and mouse [18, 45, 46] models of allergic airway inflammation. All of the eosinophil chemoattractant activity in guinea pig BAL fluid was shown to be neutralized by anti-Eotaxin antibodies [36]. However, the situation is more complex in mice where antibodies to Eotaxin, MIP-1α, RANTES, MCP-3 and MCP-5 have all been shown, at least partially, to inhibit eosinophil recruitment [46–49]. Mice with a targeted deletion of the Eotaxin gene were shown by Rothenberg et al. [50] to have a 70% reduction in lung eosinophils 18 h after allergen challenge but this effect diminished at later time points. In contrast, Yang et al. [51] found no detectable effect of Eotaxin gene deletion on eosinophil recruitment. These studies agree with the idea that other ligands, including some other CC chemokines, may be involved in the mouse.

The mouse has provided invaluable information about allergic reactions particularly with respect to the role of T cells (see below), but interpretation of the role of chemokines and eosinophils is complicated by variations dependent on strain and differences in sensitization/challenge protocols (e.g. single vs. multiple challenge models). Marked differences were observed when responses of sensitized mice to one or two allergen challenges were compared [52]. A single challenge with cockroach antigen induced eosinophil accumulation associated with the production of Eotaxin and MIP-1α. Two challenges, separated by 2 days, induced a larger eosinophil infiltrate. A neutralizing antibody to MIP-1α suppressed the eosinophil infiltrate induced by a single allergen challenge, whereas an antibody to Eotaxin suppressed that induced by two challenges. The antibody to MIP-1α did not affect airway hyperresponsiveness in either protocol. However, the antibody to Eotaxin blocked hyperresponsiveness in response to two challenges. These results may, in part, relate to the ability of Eotaxin to induce activation and degranulation of eosinophils

[53, 54], a property not shared by MIP-1α [52]. In some models, eosinophil activation correlates with airway hyperresponsiveness to spasmogens. However, there are clearly other routes to airway dysfunction and examples where hyper-responsiveness can be separated from eosinophil activation [55].

Eotaxin and Eotaxin-2 expression is upregulated in many cell types in human asthmatic airways [56–59]. Following allergen challenge of allergic asthmatic subjects, Zeibecoglou et al. [60] found an increase in the percentage of Eotaxin-positive cells in induced sputum, and Brown et al. [61] found a time-dependent increase in Eotaxin levels in BAL fluid. In contrast, Teran et al. [62] found that the only detectable eosinophil chemoattractant in BAL fluid after allergen challenge was RANTES even though this chemokine is less potent than Eotaxin in chemotaxis assays. We found significantly increased levels of Eotaxin, with smaller and nonsignificant increases of RANTES, in extracts of induced sputum from asthmatic patients in the absence of a deliberate allergen challenge, compared with non-asthmatic subjects [unpubl. results]. We believe that the majority of the Eotaxin is bound to the mucus matrix as we found no Eotaxin in BAL fluid, nor in extracts of sputum cells, from the asthmatic subjects. Further, we have found that Eotaxin binds more strongly than RANTES to components of the mucus matrix, which may account for the preferential detection of RANTES in BAL fluid and of Eotaxin in sputum. The upregulation of CC chemokines with the ability to recruit eosinophils to the airways suggests that antagonists of CCR3 may provide novel therapy in asthma.

Regulation of Chemokine Production by Th2 Cytokines

T lymphocytes are critical elements in regulating allergic reactions [63]. Allergy is generally associated with a polarization of T-helper lymphocytes into the Th2 type [64, 65], as first defined in the mouse [66]. However, there is also evidence for a co-existence of Th1 and Th2 responses in mouse allergy models [67, 68]. Th2 cells characteristically produce IL-4, IL-5, IL-10 and IL-13. Neutralization of IL-4 suppresses lung responses to allergen challenge when the antibody is administered before sensitization. However, neutralization of IL-13, but not IL-4, suppresses responses when administered just before allergen challenge [69]. Depletion of T cells with an anti-CD3 antibody just before challenge suppresses Eotaxin production and eosinophil accumulation [45]. Further, transfer of allergen-specific Th2 cells to naïve mice, followed by aerosol allergen challenge, induces eosinophil accumulation associated with Eotaxin production in the lung [67].

Although Th2 lymphocytes are critical for regulating eosinophil accumulation and activation in allergic inflammation, these cells do not appear to be a major source of eosinophil chemoattractant chemokines. Studies in guinea pigs [36, 70], mice [18, 46] and man [56–58, 71], using in situ hybridization and immunohistochemistry, show that the major sources of Eotaxin are inflammatory cells such as macrophages, as well as eosinophils themselves, and also airway smooth muscle cells, vascular endothelial cells and, in particular, airway epithelial cells. Two Th2 cytokines, IL-4 and IL-13, have been shown to act synergistically with TNF-α to induce Eotaxin production in human cells in culture [72, 73]. The first study linking Eotaxin production to IL-4 was made in the mouse [17] where it was shown that tumours transfected with the IL-4 gene induced eosinophil recruitment associated with Eotaxin mRNA upregulation in vivo. In addition, in IL-4 knockout mice and in anti-IL-4-treated mice a diminished Eotaxin mRNA expression was observed [74, 75]. Similarly, it was shown in rats that intradermally-injected IL-4 induced eosinophil accumulation associated with Eotaxin mRNA expression, which was suppressed by a neutralizing antibody to Eotaxin [12].

Chemokines are also likely to be of critical importance in many of the upstream events involved in sensitization to allergens. Thus, chemokines are involved in T- and B-cell trafficking and distribution under basal conditions [76, 77] and the recruitment of dendritic cells to tissues, followed by their movement to regional lymph modes [78, 79].

Regulation of Blood Eosinophil Levels

Eosinophils normally circulate in the blood in low numbers (1–4% of blood leukocytes) and there is evidence from guinea pig models that recruitment to sites of allergic inflammation is poor unless mechanisms exist to elevate circulating eosinophil numbers [80].

IL-5 (originally discovered in the mouse [81]) is clearly important for eosinophilopoiesis, in stimulating differentiation and proliferation of eosinophils. It was shown in the guinea pig that intravenous IL-5 can also induce the acute release of a pool of mature eosinophils from the bone marrow and that this has a profound enhancing effect on eosinophil recruitment in the skin induced by intradermally-injected Eotaxin [80]. The mechanisms involved in this release process have recently been analysed in detail using a system where the microvasculature of the guinea pig femoral bone marrow is perfused in situ [82]. In this system IL-5 induces a massive migration of eosinophils across the endothelium into the sinuses, a process which involves α_4 and β_2 integrins acting in opposite directions.

Eotaxin also releases eosinophils when infused into the arterial supply vessel in the femoral bone marrow perfusion system [83]. This appears to relate to the chemotactic effect of Eotaxin across the sinus endothelium, as opposed to the chemokinetic effect of IL-5 [82, 83]. A combination of the chemotactic effect of Eotaxin and the chemokinetic effect of IL-5 acting synergistically induces very pronounced eosinophil release [83].

It has been proposed that IL-5 and Eotaxin are generated in response to allergen in the sensitized guinea pig lung. Eotaxin is a powerful chemoattractant for eosinophils, but IL-5 has low activity as an eosinophil recruiting agent into tissues [80]. Both mediators diffuse into the circulation and act synergistically to induce eosinophil release from the bone marrow into the blood. These cells are then available to be recruited into the lung [36]. These conclusions are consistent with the effects of a neutralizing antibody to IL-5 in the guinea pig, which was shown to block bone marrow eosinophil release, blood eosinophilia and recruitment into the lung [36]. Eotaxin has also been implicated in the acute release of eosinophil progenitors into the circulation [83].

The bone marrow pool of mature eosinophils is also found in man but represents only a minor population in the mouse. In man, eosinophil progenitors have been detected in the circulation of atopic patients [84] and, in asthma, Eotaxin has been shown to have the capacity to mobilize the bone marrow pool of mature cells [85]. Eotaxin gene-deleted mice have reduced circulating eosinophils [50]. This may relate to acute eosinophil release from the bone marrow, but is probably more closely connected with a reported role for Eotaxin in leukopoiesis in this species [86]. It has been shown that intravenous Eotaxin induces a blood eosinophilia in mice [87], but with no detectable loss of bone marrow eosinophils. The pool released may come from the spleen in this instance as there is evidence that eosinophil progenitors mature in the spleen in the mouse [88]. Synergism between circulating IL-5 and local Eotaxin has been observed in several mouse models [87, 89, 90].

Conclusions

Eosinophils are a prominent feature of asthma and allergic inflammation, and these cells are believed to be major effector cells of tissue damage. The search for eosinophil-selective chemoattractants led to the discovery of Eotaxin and related CC chemokines that act via the Eotaxin receptor, CCR3. The evidence accumulated has provided a working hypothesis to explain mechanisms involved in eosinophil recruitment and the links between Th2 lymphocytes regulating allergic inflammation and eosinophils. Small molecule antagonists of CCR3 may provide the next generation of therapeutic compounds for allergy and asthma.

Acknowledgments

We are indebted to Professor Barry Kay, our former neighbour on the second floor of the National Heart and Lung Institute, for infecting us with an interest in the eosinophil and allergy. Without his influence, our lives would undoubtedly have remained more microbial and less colourful, i.e. neutrophilic.

We are grateful to the National Asthma Campaign and the Wellcome Trust for financial support.

References

1   Kay AB: Eosinophils as effector cells in immunity and hypersensitivity disorders. Clin Exp Immunol 1985;62:1–12.
2   Butterworth AE: Cell-mediated damage to helminths. Adv Parasitol 1984;23:143–235.
3   Wardlaw AJ, Moqbel R, Kay AB: Eosinophils and the allergic inflammatory response; in Kay AB, (ed): Allergy and Allergic Diseases. London, Blackwell Science, 1997, pp 171–197.
4   Butcher EC: Leukocyte-endothelial cell recognition – Three (or more) steps to specificity and diversity. Cell 1991;67:1033–1036.
5   Springer TA: Traffic signals for lymphocyte recirculation and leukocyte emigration: The multistep paradigm. Cell 1994;76:301–314.
6   Premack BA, Schall TJ: Chemokine receptors: Gateways to inflammation and infection. Nat Med 1996;2:1174–1178.
7   Luster AD: Chemokines – Chemotactic cytokines that mediate inflammation. N Engl J Med 1998; 338:436–445.
8   Homey B, Zlotnik A: Chemokines in allergy. Curr Opin Immunol 1999;11:626–634.
9   Bochner BS, Luscinskas FW, Gimbrone MA, et al: Adhesion of human basophils, eosinophils, and neutrophils to interleukin-1-activated human vascular endothelial cells: Contributions of endothelial cell adhesion molecules. J Exp Med 1991;173:1553–1556.
10 Kyan-Aung U, Haskard DO, Poston RN, Thornhill MH, Lee TH: Endothelial leukocyte adhesion molecule-1 and intercellular adhesion molecule-1 mediate the adhesion of eosinophils to endothelial cells in vitro and are expressed by endothelium in allergic cutaneous inflammation in vivo. J Immunol 1991;146:521–528.
11 Weg VB, Williams TJ, Lobb RR, Nourshargh S: A monoclonal antibody recognising very late activation antigen-4 (VLA-4) inhibits eosinophil accumulation in vivo. J Exp Med 1993;177:561–566.
12 Sanz MJ, Ponath PD, Mackay CR, et al: Human eotaxin induces α_4 and β_2 integrin-dependent eosinophil accumulation in rat skin in vivo: Delayed generation of eotaxin in response to IL-4. J Immunol 1998;160:3569–3576.
13 Griffiths-Johnson DA, Collins PD, Rossi AG, Jose PJ, Williams TJ: The chemokine, Eotaxin, activates guinea-pig eosinophils in vitro, and causes their accumulation into the lung in vivo. Biochem Biophys Res Commun 1993;197:1167–1172.
14 Jose PJ, Griffiths-Johnson DA, Collins PD, et al: Eotaxin: A potent eosinophil chemoattractant cytokine detected in a guinea-pig model of allergic airways inflammation. J Exp Med 1994;179: 881–887.
15 Jose PJ, Adcock IM, Griffiths-Johnson DA, et al: Eotaxin: Cloning of an eosinophil chemoattractant cytokine and increased mRNA expression in allergen-challenged guinea-pig lungs. Biochem Biophys Res Commun 1994;205:788–794.
16 Rothenberg ME, Luster AD, Lilly CM, Drazen JM, Leder P: Constitutive and allergen-induced expression of eotaxin mRNA in the guinea pig lung. J Exp Med 1995;181:1211–1216.
17 Rothenberg ME, Luster AD, Leder P: Murine eotaxin: An eosinophil chemoattractant inducible in endothelial cells and in interleukin-4-induced tumor suppression. Proc Natl Acad Sci USA 1995; 92:8960–8964.

18 Gonzalo JA, Jia GQ, Aguirre V, et al: Mouse eotaxin expression parallels eosinophil accumulation during lung allergic inflammation but it is not restricted to a Th2-type response. Immunity 1996; 4:1–14.

19 Williams CMM, Newton DJ, Wilson SA, Williams TJ, Coleman JW, Flanagan BF: Conserved structure and tissue expression of rat eotaxin. Immunogenetics 1998;47:178–180.

20 Ishi Y, Shirato M, Nomura A, et al: Cloning of rat eotaxin: Ozone inhalation increases mRNA and protein expression in lungs of brown Norway rats. Am J Physiol 1998;274:L171–L176.

21 Ponath PD, Qin S, Ringler DJ, et al: Cloning of the human eosinophil chemoattractant, eotaxin. Expression, receptor binding and functional properties suggest a mechanism for the selective recruitment of eosinophils. J Clin Invest 1996;97:604–612.

22 Garcia-Zepeda EA, Rothenberg ME, Ownbey RT, Celestin J, Leder P, Luster AD: Human eotaxin is a specific chemoattractant for eosinophil cells and provides a new mechanism to explain tissue eosinophilia. Nat Med 1996;2:449–456.

23 Kitaura M, Nakajima T, Imai T, et al: Molecular cloning of human eotaxin, an eosinophil-selective CC chemokine, and identification of a specific eosinophil eotaxin receptor, CC chemokine receptor 3. J Biol Chem 1996;271:7725–7730.

24 Patel VP, Kreider BL, Li Y, et al: Molecular and functional characterization of two novel human C-C chemokines as inhibitors of two distinct classes of myeloid progenitors. J Exp Med 1997;185:1163–1172.

25 Forssmann U, Uguccioni M, Loetscher P, et al: Eotaxin-2, a novel CC chemokine that is selective for the chemokine receptor CCR3, and acts like eotaxin on human eosinophil and basophil leukocytes. J Exp Med 1997;185:2171–2176.

26 White JR, Imburgia C, Dul E, et al: Cloning and functional characterization of a novel human CC chemokine that binds to the CCR3 receptor and activates human eosinophils. J Leukoc Biol 1997;62:667–675.

27 Kitaura M, Suzuki N, Imai T, et al: Molecular cloning of a novel human CC chemokine (Eotaxin-3) that is a functional ligand of CC chemokine receptor 3. J Biol Chem 1999;274:27975–27980.

28 Shinkai A, Yoshisue H, Koike M, et al: A novel human CC chemokine, eotaxin-3, which is expressed in IL-4-stimulated vascular endothelial cells, exhibits potent activity toward eosinophils. J Immunol 1999;163:1602–1610.

29 Ponath PD, Qin S, Post TW, et al: Molecular cloning and characterization of a human eotaxin receptor expressed selectively on eosinophils. J Exp Med 1996;183:2437–2448.

30 Daugherty BL, Siciliano SJ, DeMartino J, Malkowitz L, Sirontino A, Springer MS: Cloning, expression and characterization of the human eosinophil eotaxin receptor. J Exp Med 1996;183:2349–2354.

31 Gao JL, Sen AI, Kitaura M, et al: Identification of a mouse eosinophil receptor for the CC chemokine eotaxin. Biochem Biophys Res Commun 1996;223:679–684.

32 Post TW, Bozic CR, Rothenberg ME, Luster AD, Gerard N, Gerard C: Molecular characterization of two murine eosinophil β chemokine receptors. J Immunol 1995;155:5299–5306.

33 Sabroe I, Conroy DM, Gerard NP, et al: Cloning and characterisation of the guinea pig eosinophil eotaxin receptor, CCR3: Blockade using a monoclonal antibody in vivo. J Immunol 1998;161:6139–6147.

34 Campbell EM, Proudfoot AEI, Yoshimura T, et al: Recombinant guinea pig and human RANTES activate macrophages but not eosinophils in the guinea pig. J Immunol 1997;159:1482–1489.

35 Marleau S, Griffiths-Johnson DA, Collins PD, Bakhle YS, Williams TJ, Jose PJ: Human RANTES acts as a receptor antagonist for guinea pig eotaxin in vitro and in vivo. J Immunol 1996;157:4141–4146.

36 Humbles AA, Conroy DM, Marleau S, et al: Kinetics of eotaxin generation and its relationship to eosinophil accumulation in allergic airways disease: Analysis in a guinea pig model in vivo. J Exp Med 1997;186:601–612.

37 Gonzalo JA, Lloyd CM, Wen D, et al: The coordinated action of CC chemokines in the lung orchestrates allergic inflammation and airways hyperresponsiveness. J Exp Med 1998;188:157–167.

38 Sabroe I, Hartnell A, Jopling LA, et al: Differential regulation of eosinophil chemokine signalling via CCR3 and non-CCR3 pathways. J Immunol 1999;162:2946–2955.

39 Uguccioni M, Mackay CR, Ochensberger B, et al: High expression of the chemokine receptor CCR3 in human blood basophils. Role in activation by eotaxin, MCP-4, and other chemokines. J Clin Invest 1997;100:1137–1143.

40 Romagnani P, De Paulis A, Beltrame C, et al: Tryptase-chymase double-positive human mast cells express the eotaxin receptor CCR3 and are attracted by CCR3-binding chemokines. Am J Pathol 1999;155:1195–1204.

41 Ochi H, Hirani WM, Yuan Q, Friend DS, Austen KF, Boyce JA: T helper cell type 2 cytokine-mediated comitogenic responses and CCR3 expression during differentiation of human mast cells in vitro. J Exp Med 1999;190:267–280.

42 Gerber BO, Zanni MP, Uguccioni M, et al: Functional expression of the eotaxin receptor CCR3 in T lymphocytes co-localising with eosinophils. Curr Biol 1997;7:836–843.

43 Sallusto F, Mackay CR, Lanzavecchia A: Selective expression of the eotaxin receptor CCR3 by human T helper 2 cells. Science 1997;277:2005–2007.

44 Bonecchi R, Bianchi G, Bordignon PP, et al: Differential expression of chemokine receptors and chemotactic responsiveness of type 1 T helper cells (Th1s) and Th2s. J Exp Med 1998;187:129–134.

45 MacLean JA, Ownbey R, Luster AD: T cell-dependent regulation of eotaxin in antigen-induced pulmonary eosinophilia. J Exp Med 1996;184:1461–1469.

46 Gonzalo JA, Lloyd CM, Kremer L, et al: Eosinophil recruitment to the lung in a murine model of allergic inflammation. The role of T cells, chemokines and adhesion receptors. J Clin Invest 1996; 98:2332–2345.

47 Lukacs NW, Strieter RM, Warmington K, Lincoln P, Chensue SW, Kunkel SL: Differential recruitment of leukocyte populations and alteration of airway hyperreactivity by C-C family chemokines in allergic airway inflammation. J Immunol 1997;158:4398–4404.

48 Stafford S, Li H, Forsythe PA, Ryan M, Bravo R, Alam R: Monocyte chemotactic protein-3 (MCP-3)/fibroblast-induced cytokine (FIC) in eosinophilic inflammation of the airways and the inhibitory effects of an anti-MCP-3/FIC antibody. J Immunol 1997;158:4953–4960.

49 Jia GQ, Gonzalo JA, Lloyd C, et al: Distinct expression and function of the novel mouse chemokine monocyte chemotactic protein-5 in lung allergic inflammation. J Exp Med 1996;184:1939–1951.

50 Rothenberg ME, MacLean JA, Pearlman E, Luster AD, Leder P: Targeted disruption of the chemokine eotaxin partially reduces antigen-induced tissue eosinophilia. J Exp Med 1997;185: 785–790.

51 Yang Y, Loy J, Ryseck RP, Carrasco D, Bravo R: Antigen-induced eosinophilic lung inflammation develops in mice deficient in chemokine eotaxin. Blood 1998;92:3912–3923.

52 Campbell EM, Kunkel SL, Strieter RM, Lukacs NW: Temporal role of chemokines in a murine model of cockroach allergen-induced airway hyperreactivity and eosinophilia. J Immunol 1998;161: 7047–7053.

53 Tenscher K, Metzner B, Schöpf E, Norgauer J, Czech W: Recombinant human eotaxin induces oxygen radical production, Ca^{2+}-mobilization, actin reorganization, and CD11b upregulation in human eosinophils via a Pertussis toxin-sensitive heterotrimeric guanine nucleotide-binding protein. Blood 1996;88:3195–3199.

54 Elsner J, Hochstetter R, Kimmig D, Kapp A: Human eotaxin represents a potent activator of the respiratory burst of human eosinophils. Eur J Immunol 1996;26:1919–1925.

55 Henderson WR, Chi EY, Albert RK, Chu SJ, Lamm WJE, Rochon Y, Jonas M, Christie PE, Harlan JM: Blockade of CD19d (α_4 integrin) on intrapulmonary but not circulating leukocytes inhibits airway inflammation and hyperresponsiveness in a mouse model of asthma. J Clin Invest 1997;100: 3083–3092.

56 Ying S, Robinson DS, Meng Q, et al: Enhanced expression of eotaxin and CCR3 mRNA and protein in atopic asthma. Association with airway hyperresponsiveness and predominant colocalization of eotaxin mRNA to bronchial epithelial and endothelial cells. Eur J Immunol 1997;27: 3507–3516.

57 Mattoli S, Stacey MA, Sun G, Bellini A, Marini M: Eotaxin expression and eosinophilic inflammation in asthma. Biochem Biophys Res Commun 1997;236:299–301.

58   Lamkhioued B, Renzi PM, Younes A, et al: Increased expression of eotaxin in bronchoalveolar lavage and airways of asthmatics contributes to the chemotaxis of eosinophils to the site of inflammation. J Immunol 1997;159:4593–4601.

59   Ying S, Meng Q, Zeibecoglou K, et al: Eosinophil chemotactic chemokines (eotaxin, eotaxin-2, RANTES, monocyte chemoattractant protein-3 (MCP-3), and MCP-4), and C-C chemokine receptor 3 expression in bronchial biopsies from atopic and nonatopic (intrinsic) asthmatics. J Immunol 1999;163:6321–6329.

60   Zeibecoglou K, Macfarlane AJ, Ying S, et al: Increases in eotaxin-positive cells in induced sputum from atopic asthmatic subjects after inhalational allergen challenge. Allergy 1999;54:730–735.

61   Brown JR, Kleimberg J, Marini M, Sun G, Bellini A, Mattoli S: Kinetics of eotaxin expression and its relationship to eosinophil accumulation and activation in bronchial biopsies and bronchoalveolar lavage of asthmatic patients after allergen inhalation. Clin Exp Immunol 1998;114:137–146.

62   Teran LM, Noso N, Carroll M, Davies DE, Holgate S, Schroder JM: Eosinophil recruitment following allergen challenge is associated with the release of the chemokine RANTES into asthmatic airways. J Immunol 1996;157:1806–1812.

63   Basten A, Beeson PB: Mechanism of eosinophilia. II. Role of the lymphocyte. J Exp Med 1970; 131:1288–1305.

64   Robinson DS, Hamid Q, Ying S, et al: Predominant Th2-like bronchoalveolar T-lymphocyte population in atopic asthma. N Engl J Med 1992;326:298–304.

65   Romagnani S: Regulation of the development of type 2 T-helper cells in allergy. Curr Opin Immunol 1994;6:838–846.

66   Mosmann TR, Cherwinski H, Bond MW, Giedlin MA, Coffman RL: Two types of murine helper T cell clone. 1. Definition according to profiles of lymphokine activities and secreted proteins. J Immunol 1986;136:2348–2357.

67   Li L, Xia Y, Nguyen A, Feng L, Lo D: Th2-induced eotaxin expression and eosinophilia coexist with Th1 responses at the effector stage of lung inflammation. J Immunol 1998;161:3128–3135.

68   Randolph DA, Carruthers CJ, Szabo SJ, Murphy KM, Chaplin DD: Modulation of airway inflammation by passive transfer of allergen-specific Th1 and Th2 cells in a mouse model of asthma. J Immunol 1999;162:2375–2383.

69   Wills-Karp M, Luyimbazi J, Xu X, et al: Interleukin-13: Central mediator of allergic asthma. Science 1998;282:2258–2261.

70   Li D, Wang D, Griffiths-Johnson DA, et al: Eotaxin protein and gene expression in guinea pig lungs: Constitutive expression and up-regulation after allergen challenge. Eur Respir J 1997;10: 1946–1954.

71   Nakajima T, Yamada H, Iikura M, et al: Intracellular localization and release of eotaxin from normal eosinophils. FEBS Lett 1998;434:226–230.

72   Mochizuki M, Bartels J, Mallet AI, Christophers E, Schroder JM: IL-4 induces eotaxin: A possible mechanism of selective eosinophil recruitment in helminth infection and atopy. J Immunol 1998; 160:60–68.

73   Terada N, Hamano N, Nomura T, et al: Interleukin-13 and tumour necrosis factor-alpha synergistically induce eotaxin production in human nasal fibroblasts. Clin Exp Allergy 2000;30: 348–355.

74   Ruth JH, Lukacs NW, Warmington KS, et al: Expression and participation of eotaxin during mycobacterial (type 1) and schistosomal (type 2) antigen-elicited granuloma formation. J Immunol 1998;161:4276–4282.

75   Chensue SW, Warmington K, Ruth JH, Lukacs N, Kunkel SL: Mycobacterial and schistosomal antigen-elicited granuloma formation in IFN-gamma and IL-4 knockout mice: Analysis of local and regional cytokine and chemokine networks. J Immunol 1997;159:3565–3573.

76   Ward SG, Bacon K, Westwick J: Chemokines and T lymphocytes: More than an attraction. Immunity 1998;9:1–11.

77   Kim CH, Broxmeyer HE: Chemokines: Signal lamps for trafficking of T and B cells for development and effector function. J Leukoc Biol 1999;65:6–15.

78   Dieu MC, Vanbervliet B, Vicari A, et al: Selective recruitment of immature and mature dendritic cells by distinct chemokines expressed in different anatomic sites. J Exp Med 1998;188:373–386.

79 Cyster JG: Chemokines and the homing of dendritic cells to the T cell areas of lymphoid organs. J Exp Med 1999;189:447–450.

80 Collins PD, Marleau S, Griffiths-Johnson DA, Jose PJ, Williams TJ: Co-operation between interleukin-5 and the chemokine eotaxin to induce eosinophil accumulation in vivo. J Exp Med 1995;182: 1169–1174.

81 Sanderson CJ, Warren DG, Strath M: Identification of a lymphokine that stimulates eosinophil differentiation in vitro. Its relationship to interleukin-3, and functional properties of eosinophils produced in cultures. J Exp Med 1985;162:60–74.

82 Palframan RT, Collins PD, Severs NJ, Rothery S, Williams TJ, Rankin SM: Mechanisms of acute eosinophil mobilization from the bone marrow stimulated by interleukin-5: The role of specific adhesion molecules and phosphatidylinositol 3-kinase. J Exp Med 1998;188:1621–1632.

83 Palframan RT, Collins PD, Williams TJ, Rankin SM: Eotaxin induces a rapid release of eosinophils and their progenitors from the bone marrow. Blood 1998;91:2240–2248.

84 Gibson PG, Manning PJ, O'Byrne PM, et al: Allergen-induced asthmatic responses. Relationship between increases in airway responsiveness and increases in circulating eosinophils, basophils, and their progenitors. Am Rev Respir Dis 1991;143:331–335.

85 Robinson DS, North J, Zeibecoglou K, et al: Eosinophil development and bone marrow and tissue eosinophils in atopic asthma. Int Arch Allergy Immunol 1999;118:98–100.

86 Peled A, Gonzalo JA, Lloyd C, Gutierrez-Ramos JC: The chemotactic cytokine eotaxin acts as a granulocyte-macrophage colony-stimulating factor during lung inflammation. Blood 1998;91: 1909–1916.

87 Mould AW, Matthaei KI, Young IG, Foster PS: Relationship between interleukin-5 and eotaxin in regulating blood and tissue eosinophilia in mice. J Clin Invest 1997;99:1064–1071.

88 Vadas MA: Genetic control of eosinophilia in mice: Gene(s) expressed in bone marrow-derived cells control high responsiveness. J Immunol 1982;128:691–695.

89 Rothenberg M, Ownbey R, Mehlhop P, et al: Eotaxin triggers eosinophil-selective chemotaxis and calcium flux via a distinct receptor and induces pulmonary eosinophilia in the presence of interleukin-5 in mice. Mol Med 1996;2:334–348.

90 Wang J, Palmer K, Ltvall J, et al: Circulating, but not local lung, IL-5 is required for the development of antigen-induced airways eosinophilia. J Clin Invest 1998;102:1132–1141.

T.J. Williams, Leukocyte Biology Section, Biomedical Sciences Division,
Sir Alexander Fleming Building, Imperial College School of Medicine,
London SW7 2AZ (UK)
Tel. +44 20 7594 3159, E-Mail tim.williams@ic.ac.uk

Robinson DS (ed): Immunological Mechanisms in Asthma and Allergic Diseases.
Chem Immunol. Basel, Karger, 2000, vol 78, pp 178–188

....

C-C Chemokine Expression in Atopic and Nonatopic Asthma

Sun Ying

Department of Allergy and Clinical Immunology, Imperial College School of
Medicine, National Heart and Lung Institute, London, UK

Asthma, Inflammatory Cells and Chemokines

Asthma is characterized by increased bronchial hyperresponsiveness
(or hyperreactivity) to physical, chemical, pharmacological, and/or immunological stimuli. The major clinical symptoms of asthma are the episodic
occurrence of coughing, dyspnea, wheezing and chest tightness, alone or in
combination [1]. Asthma is often associated with atopy, although some
asthmatics are nonatopic. Atopic asthmatics have a relatively high level of
total and specific serum IgE responding to common environmental antigens
(allergens) encountered at the mucosal surface. Interaction of environmental
allergens with cells sensitized by binding of surface Fc receptors to IgE is
assumed to play a role in the pathogenesis of atopic asthma. A subgroup
of asthma (30% of total asthmatics) is not demonstrably atopic, which has led
to the suggestion that asthma may be divided clinically, and by implication,
mechanistically, into atopic (extrinsic) and nonatopic (intrinsic) variants [2].
Intrinsic asthmatics are skin test negative to extracts of common allergens
and there is no evidence of allergen-specific serum IgE antibodies. Serum
total IgE concentrations are within the normal range. There is also no clinical
or family history of allergy. There has been debate about the relationship of
this variant of the disease to atopy [3]. Although the onset of the disease
may be triggered by viral infection such as a respiratory influenza-like illness,
some authors have suggested a role for IgE and atopy in so-called intrinsic
asthma [4]. These data indicate that intrinsic asthmatics may be allergic to
an as yet undetected allergen and that these patients might benefit from
allergen-free environments, as previously demonstrated in atopic asthma [5].

Apart from some differences in clinical and natural history, extrinsic and intrinsic asthma are very similar, particularly from pathological, pathophysiological and pharmacological points of view. In the laboratory, infiltration of inflammatory cells in lung, such as eosinophils, activated T lymphocytes, basophils, and monocytes/macrophages, is a common feature in both atopic and nonatopic asthma. For example, elevated numbers, compared with controls, of activated T cells, eosinophils, FcεRI-bearing cells and IL-4 and IL-5 mRNA and protein product-positive cells were present in bronchial mucosal biopsies both in atopic and nonatopic asthma [6–8]. This suggests that these inflammatory cells may participate in pathogenesis of both atopic and nonatopic asthma through release of cytokines and other mediators.

The mechanisms, however, that the various cell types are recruited from blood vessels into local tissue remains to be clarified. In the past 10 years, a number of small molecular polypeptides, termed chemokines, have been discovered. Based on whether the first two cysteines were adjacent or separated by a single amino acid, chemokines which have four cysteine residues in the sequences could be divided into two subgroups, C-C and C-X-C groups. So far, IL-8 is only one of C-X-C chemokines which has been investigated in atopic allergic asthma. In contrast, a numbers of C-C chemokines, including eotaxin, eotaxin-2, macrophage inflammatory protein (MIP)-1α, monocyte chemotactic protein-1 (MCP-1), MCP-3, MCP-4 and RANTES (regulated on activation, normal T-cell expressed, and secreted), have been studied in asthma. The reason possibly is that C-C chemokines have relatively selective functions on chemotaxis and activation of eosinophils, basophils, T cells and monocytes, but not neutrophils. Compared with C-C chemokines, C-X-C chemokines are less effective on these cells, although they are potent chemoattractants for neutrophils, and to some extent, of T lymphocytes, such as IL-8. Lymphotactin (named IL-16) belongs to the 'C' chemokine subgroup which has only two cysteines and lacks first and third cysteine. Some evidence suggests that this chemokine may contribute to recruitment of lymphocytes into local tissues. The final chemokine subgroup is C-X-X-X-C. Fractalkine is the only member of this group. At present, no study of this chemokine has been performed in asthma. Many types of cells are able to synthesize these different chemokines, even though inflammatory cells themselves, suggesting there are both autocrine and paracrine pathways present in vivo. These chemokines attract and activate a wide range of leukocytes and probably play a central role in the asthma process. In this chapter, I will focus on C-C chemokines in asthma.

C-C Chemokine Expression in Atopic Allergic Asthma

C-C Chemokines in Bronchial Mucosa

A numbers of studies, in vitro and in vivo, suggest that increased expression of C-C chemokines, particularly eotaxin, RANTES, MCP-3, MCP-4 and MCP-1 may contribute to the infiltration of inflammatory cells, such as eosinophils, T lymphocytes, and basophils in bronchial airways of atopic asthmatics. By use of the techniques of in situ hybridization and immunohistochemistry, we have demonstrated that the numbers of cells expressing eotaxin mRNA and protein were significantly elevated in atopic asthmatics compared with normal controls at baseline [9]. In the asthmatics there was a highly significant inverse correlation between eotaxin-positive cells and the histamine provocative concentration causing a 20% fall in FEV_1 (PC_{20}) (fig. 1) [9]. There were also significant correlations between EG2+ cells and the cells expressing eotaxin mRNA and protein (p = 0.001). Colocalization data showed that cytokeratin-positive epithelial cells and CD31+ endothelial cells were the major source of eotaxin-expressing cells [9].

Similar findings have been observed by Lamkhioued et al. [10] and Mattoli et al. [11]. In the latter study, the investigators found that there was significantly increased expression of eotaxin mRNA in bronchial biopsies from atopic asthmatics compared with those from nonasthmatic controls (p < 0.001) [11]. In the asthma group, the numbers of cells expressing eotaxin mRNA significantly correlated with methacholine PC_{20} ($r_s = 0.51$, p < 0.05) and symptom scores ($r_s = 0.63$, p < 0.025) [11]. Increased expression of eotaxin (mRNA and protein) and eotaxin release were also observed in bronchial mucosa from atopic asthmatics after allergen inhalation [12]. These observations support the view that damage to the bronchial mucosa in asthma involves secretion of eotaxin by epithelial and endothelial cells resulting in eosinophil infiltration through binding to the eotaxin receptor, CCR3. In addition to eotaxin, other C-C chemokines, such as RANTES, MCP-3 and MCP-4, may also contribute to infiltration of eosinophils into local tissues. In vitro, these chemokines were shown to induce eosinophil chemotaxis through binding CCR3, although the capacities were less effective and selective than that of eotaxin. Using semiquantitative RT-PCR technique, we demonstrated that the numbers of copies of mRNA encoding RANTES and MCP-3 were significantly elevated in bronchial biopsies from the atopic asthmatics, as compared both with the atopic controls (p < 0.02) and nonatopic nonasthmatic controls (p < 0.02) [13]. Increased MCP-4 mRNA+ cells were also found in bronchial mucosa of atopic asthmatics [14].

In a double-blind placebo-controlled study, the RANTES expression in bronchial epithelium was significantly reduced in the beclomethasone dipropi-

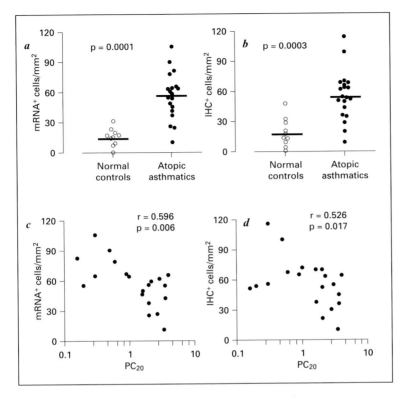

Fig. 1. *a–d* The numbers of eotaxin mRNA (***a***) and protein-positive cells (***b***) in bronchial biopsies from normal controls (n = 10, open circles), compared with atopic asthmatics (n = 20, solid circles). ***c*** and ***d*** show correlations between eotaxin mRNA- and protein-positive cells and the histamine PC_{20} in atopic asthmatics.

onate (BDP)-treated asthmatic group compared with placebo-treated group ($p < 0.05$) [15]. The authors also showed that the numbers of eosinophils were significantly reduced ($p < 0.02$) after BDP treatment [15]. These observations implied that RANTES may be involved in pathogenesis of asthma by inducing influx of inflammatory cells such as eosinophils, T lymphocytes and monocytes into the airways. However, some studies showed that RANTES was constitutively expressed in airways [16, 17]. Although the elevated mRNA expression was observed in the asthmatic group, there were no significant differences in the numbers of RANTES-staining cells in bronchial biopsies between normal subjects and mild asthmatics ($PC_{20} < 10$mg/ml of methacholine) using immunohistochemistry [16]. Comparable findings were also reported by Fahy et al. [17]. These observations raise two possibilities: one is that RANTES may also be required for orchestrating the traffic of memory T cells and of the monocyte/

macrophage cells. On the other hand, RANTES expression may be upregulated as a result of stimuli such as allergen challenge or in severe asthma. In these conditions, some other proinflammatory cytokine, such as TNF-α and IL-1, may increase which upregulate RANTES expression [15]. Not only RANTES, other C-C chemokines were also detectable in a proportion of the normal control subjects [9–14] and in animal model. For instance, eotaxin expression and eosinophil infiltrates were detectable in lamina propria of the jejunum from normal wild-type mice, while eosinophils were reduced in the jejunum in eotaxin-deficient mice [18]. Thus, a basal, physiological degree of chemokine expression in the airway may be required for the trafficking of patrolling leukocytes involved in host defence.

Using immunostaining image analysis, Sousa et al. [19] showed that there was significant staining of MCP-1 in epithelium from asthmatics ($51.5 \pm 3.7\%$), whereas normal subjects reacted much less ($6.4 \pm 1.9\%$) ($p < 0.0001$). Likewise, staining was also increased in submucosa of asthmatics ($11.5 \pm 3.1\%$) compared with $2.0 \pm 1.0\%$ in that from normal controls [19], suggesting MCP-1 is another candidate for macrophage recruitment and activation of basophils in the inflammatory pathogenesis of bronchial asthma. In vitro, it was shown that basophils released leukotriene LTC_4 and histamine after activation with MCP-1 [20].

C-C Chemokines in Bronchoalveolar Lavage (BAL)

Using ELISA and Western blot techniques, Lamkhioued et al. [10] showed that atopic asthmatics have high concentrations of eotaxin in BAL fluid when compared with normal controls. The study also showed that BAL fluid from asthmatics contained chemotactic activity for eosinophils in vitro. Anti-eotaxin antibody partially inhibited eosinophil, but not neutrophil or monocyte chemotaxis [10]. Interestingly, combination of eotaxin, MCP-4 and RANTES accounted for only ~50% of the eosinophil chemotactic activity in the BAL, suggesting the existence of other eosinophil chemotactic factors [10].

Like chemokine expression in bronchial biopsies, a numbers of other C-C chemokines were also detectable in BAL from atopic asthmatics. Alam et al. [21] showed that the levels of MCP-1, RANTES and MIP-1α were significantly higher in asthma patients at baseline than control subjects ($p < 0.04$). The eosinophil chemotactic activity of BAL was partially blocked by anti-RANTES [21]. As mentioned above, the expression of chemokines in bronchial biopsies may depend on the clinical status. The similar situation is also present in BAL fluid. For instance, RANTES-induced eosinophil chemotactic activity significantly increased in BAL fluid obtained from asthmatics during the pollen season as compared with the activity before the pollen season ($p < 0.01$) [22]. Allergen challenge seems to enhance synthesize and release RANTES. Using Western blot, HPLC and ELISA techniques, Teran et al.

[23] demonstrated that the levels of RANTES were significantly higher in BAL fluid from atopic asthmatics 4 h after allergen challenge (median 187 pg/ml) as compared with saline challenge (median 32.5 pg/ml). The authors also found that there was a significant correlation between concentrations RANTES and the numbers eosinophils at the allergen challenge sites [23]. The elevated concentration of RANTES was also observed in BAL fluid from asthmatics 24 h after allergen challenge (13 pg/ml) [24]. However, RANTES levels did not correlate with either eosinophil numbers or eosinophil-derived neutrotoxin (EDN) levels [24] at this site. The differences in these studies suggest that RANTES release may occur in the early phase after allergen exposure.

C-C Chemokines in Sputum

Compared to normal controls, increased eosinophils have been found in sputum from asthmatics [25]. Koller et al. [26] showed that the concentrations of RANTES, IL-5 and GM-CSF in sputum from asthmatics were significantly higher than in subjects with cystic fibrosis (CF). Moreover, in CF sputum, eosinophil cationic protein (ECP) levels significantly correlated with the levels of IL-8 and IL-3, whereas in asthmatics, RANTES, IL-5 and IL-8 concentrations were significantly related to ECP in sputum [26]. These findings suggest that the profile of cytokines/chemokines may differ between various diseases associated with eosinophilia. Likewise, the concentrations of chemokines in sputum may also be related to the clinical manifestations. Konno et al. [27] showed that the concentrations of RANTES in sputum were of symptomatic >asymptomatic >normal controls. Additionally, it has been reported that before the onset of late-phase exacerbation of asthma, sputum MCP-1, MIP-1α and IL-8 levels transiently but markedly increased from the basal levels in all of patients with exacerbation, but not in the patients without a late-phase exacerbation [28]. Thus, chemokines might be also involved in the exacerbation of asthma.

Taken together, enhanced chemokine expression, particularly eotaxin, may be involved in the infiltration of eosinophils in airway of asthmatics, while RANTES, MCP-3, MCP-1 and MIP-1α may play a role in traffic of multiple inflammatory cells, including monocytes, T lymphocytes, basophils and eosinophils.

C-C Chemokine Expression in Nonatopic Asthma

As mentioned above, our previous work indicated that although intrinsic asthma has a different clinical profile to extrinsic asthma, it does not appear to have a distinct immunopathological entity. To investigate whether there are any differences in chemokine expression in bronchial mucosa of both asthma with similar severity, we have detected RANTES and MCP-3 mRNA+ cells in these biopsies compared with atopic and nonatopic nonasthmatic controls using radioactive riboprobes. In this study, we observed significant increases in the numbers of cells expressing mRNA for RANTES and MCP-3 in both atopic and nonatopic asthmatics compared with either atopic or nonatopic nonasthmatics [29]. Within the asthmatic group there was a trend for elevated numbers of cells expressing RANTES and MCP-3 in nonatopic asthmatics. This could be the result of elevated numbers of macrophages and other inflammatory cells detected in the bronchial mucosa of intrinsic asthmatics, and could be responsible, in turn, for the relatively increased numbers of blood and airway eosinophils in intrinsic asthma [6–8]. In recent study, we further compared eotaxin, eotaxin-2, MCP-3, MCP-4 and RANTES expression in bronchial mucosa between atopic (AA) and nonatopic asthmatics (NAA) [30]. Compared with controls (atopic and normals), the numbers of cells expressing mRNA for eotaxin, eotaxin-2, RANTES, MCP-3 and MCP-4 in the bronchial mucosa were significantly increased in AA and NAA (p < 0.01). Nonsignificant differences in these variants were observed between AA and NAA. Significant correlations between the numbers of cells expressing eotaxin or CCR3 and the numbers of EG2+ eosinophils in the bronchial tissue were also observed for both AA (p < 0.01) and NAA (p = 0.01). These findings suggest that multiple C-C chemokines, acting at least in part via CCR3, contribute to bronchial eosinophilia in both atopic and nonatopic asthma. This further supports the concept that these subtypes of asthma, despite showing some distinct clinical features, share common immunopathological mechanisms.

The Triggers for C-C Chemokine Gene Expression in Asthma

The mechanisms of multi-CC chemokine gene overexpression in the bronchial mucosa from asthmatics is incompletely understood. A number of proinflammatory cytokines and mediators are likely to be involved. For example, IL-1 and TNF-α might upregulate expression of eotaxin [31, 32], MCP-4 [33] and other C-C chemokines in epithelial and endothelial cells in vitro. On the other hand, Th2 cell-derived cytokines probably contribute to eotaxin-mediated tissue eosinophilia, since adoptive transfer of Th2 cells into mice induced antigen-dependent lung eotaxin expression and eosinophilia [34]. Also, IL-4, the prototypic Th2 cytokine, enhanced eotaxin expression by epithelial, endothelial cells and dermal fibroblasts in vitro [31, 35], and injection of IL-4 into rats induced eosinophil accumulation in skin, that was partially mediated by endogenous production of eotaxin [36]. Again, intratracheal mouse recombinant eotaxin into IL-5 transgenic mice induced α4 integrin-

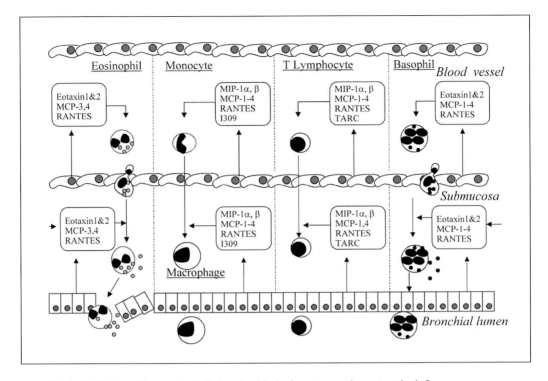

Fig. 2. C–C chemokines potentially involved in leukocyte recruitment at the inflammation in asthmatic airways.

dependent bronchial hyperresponsiveness and eosinophil migration [37]. IL-13, another Th2 cytokine, induced eotaxin expression on epithelium [38]. In addition, the Th2 cytokines IL-4 and IL-13 both induce upregulation of VCAM-1 on endothelium, that is likely involved in eotaxin-induced eosinophil accumulation. Finally, peptido-lipid mediators (i.e. leukotrienes LTC_4, LTD_4 and LTE_4) as well as histamine may also regulate the expression of C-C chemokines. We have shown in preliminary observations that these agents can increase eotaxin expression on human endothelial cells in vitro [39], indicating that these mediators may also contribute to the eosinophil influx by upregulating eotaxin, and other C-C chemokines.

Conclusion

Taken together, our studies, and those of others, support the view that chemokines probably play a critical role in the recruitment and activation of inflammatory cells in the asthma process. A summary diagram of some of these events is shown in figure 2 in which an attempt has been made to relate both the cell source and the target cells of many of the chemokines we have considered. Certainly there are many selective chemoattractants for the various cell types. For example, eotaxin, eotaxin-2, MCP-3 and MCP-4 and RANTES all have substantial activity in directional eosinophil locomotion. However, there are broadly grouped patterns of chemokines and their target cells with, for instance, RANTES, MCP-3, MCP-4, MCP-1 and MIP-1α also having potent monocyte/macrophage activity and chemoattractant properties for T cells. All of these chemokines have been identified both in endothelial and epithelial cells and the question arises as to whether there is differential release of individual chemokines or families of cytokines at the critical stages in the inflammatory events associated with the asthma process which may create tissue gradients for differential migration of the various cell types involved. Thus there still remain considerable gaps in our knowledge as to how and why various chemokines act at various stages in acute, subacute and chronic asthma.

References

1   Montgomery-Smith J: Epidemiology and natural history of asthma, allergic rhinitis, and a topic dermatitis (eczema); In Middleton E Jr, Reed CE, Ellis EF, Adkinson NF Jr, Yunginger GW (eds): Allergy: Principles and Practices, ed 3. St Louis, CV Mosby, 1988, vol 2, pp 891–929.
2   Rackeman FM: A working classification of asthma. Am J Med 1947;3:601–606.
3   Humbert M, Menz G, Ying S, Zeibecoglou K, Pfister R, Corrigan CJ, Robinson DS, Hamid Q, Durham SR, Kay AB: Extrinsic (atopic) and intrinsic (nonatopic) asthma: More similarities than differences. Immunol Today 1999;20:528–533.
4   Burrows B, Martinez FD, Halonen M, Barbee RA, Cline MG: Association of asthma with serum IgE levels and skin-test reactivity to allergens. N Engl J Med 1989;320:271–277.
5   Dorward AJ, Collof MJ, MacKay NS, McSharry C, Thompson NC: Effect of house dust mite avoidance measures on adult atopic asthma. Thorax 1988;43:98–102.
6   Bentley AM, Menz G, Storz C, Robinson DS, Bradley BL, Jeffery PK, Durham SR, Kay AB: Identification of T lymphocytes, macrophages, and activated eosinophils in the bronchial mucosa of intrinsic asthma: Relationship to symptoms and bronchial responsiveness. Am Rev Respir Dis 1992;146:500–506.
7   Humbert M, Grant JA, Barata LT, Durham SR, Pfister R, Menz G, Barkans J, Ying S, Kay AB: High affinity IgE receptor (FcεRI)-bearing cells in bronchial biopsies from atopic and nonatopic asthma. Am J Respir Crit Care Med 1996;153:1931–1937.
8   Ying S, Humbert M, Barkans J, Corrigan CJ, Pfister R, Menz G, Larché M, Robinson DS, Durham SR, Kay AB: Expression of IL-4 and IL-5 mRNA and protein product by CD4+ and CD8+ T cells, eosinophils, and mast cells in bronchial biopsies obtained from atopic and nonatopic (intrinsic) asthmatics. J Immunol 1997;158:3539–3544.
9   Ying S, Robinson DS, Meng Q, Rottman J, Kennedy R, Ringler DJ, Mackay CR, Daugherty BL, Springer MS, Durham SR, Williams TJ, Kay AB: Enhanced expression of eotaxin and CCR3 mRNA and protein in atopic asthma. Eur J Immunol 1997;27:3507–16.

10 Lamkhioued B, Renzi PM, Abi-Younes S, Garcia-Zepada EA, Allakhverdi Z, Ghaffar O, Rothenberg MD, Luster AD, Hamid Q: Increased expression of eotaxin in bronchoalveolar lavage and airways of asthmatics contributes to the chemotaxis of eosinophils to the site of inflammation. J Immunol 1997;159:4593–4601.

11 Mattoli S, Stacey MA, Sun G, Bellini A, Marini M: Eotaxin expression and eosinophilic inflammation in asthma. Biochem Biophys Res Commun 1997;236:299–301.

12 Brown JR, Kleimerg J, Marini M, Sun G, Bellini A, Mattoli S: Kinetics of eotaxin expression and its relationship to eosinophil accumulation and activation in bronchial biopsies and bronchoalveolar lavage of asthmatic patients after allergen inhalation. Clin Exp Immunol 1998;114:137–146.

13 Powell N, Humbert M, Durham SR, Assoufi B, Kay AB, Corrigan CJ: Increased expression of mRNA encoding RANTES and MCP-3 in the bronchial mucosa in atopic asthma. Eur Respir J 1996;9:2454–2460.

14 Taha RA, Minshall EM, Miotto D, Shimbara A, Luster A, Hogg JC, Hamid Q: Eotaxin and monocyte chemotactic protein-4 mRNA expression in small airways of asthmatic and nonasthmatic individuals. J Allergy Clin Immunol 1999;103:476–483.

15 Wang JH, Devalia JL, Xia C, Sapsford RJ, Davies RJ: Expression of RANTES by human bronchial epithelial cells in vitro and in vivo and effect of corticosteroids. Am J Respir Cell Mol Biol 1996; 14:27–35.

16 Berkman N, Krishnan VL, Gilbey T, Newton R, O'Connor B, Barnes PJ, Chung KF: Expression of RANTES mRNA and protein in airways of patients with mild asthma. Am J Respir Crit Care Med 1996;154:1804–1811.

17 Fahy JV, Figueroa DJ, Wong HH, Liu JT, Abrams JS: Similar RANTES levels in healthy and asthmatic airways by immunoassay and in situ hybridization. Am J Respir Crit Care Med 1997; 155:1095–1100.

18 Mathews AN, Friend DS, Zimmermann N, Sarafi MN, Luster AD, Pearlman E, Wert SE, Rothenberg ME: Eotaxin is required for the baseline level of tissue eosinophils. Proc Natl Acad Sci USA 1998; 95:6273–6278.

19 Sousa AR, Lane SJ, Nakhosteen JA, Yoshimura T, Lee TH, Poston RN: Increased expression of the monocyte chemoattractant protein-1 in bronchial tissue from asthmatic subjects. Am J Respir Cell Mol Biol 1994;10:142–147.

20 Bischoff SC, Krieger M, Brunner T, Dahinden CA: Monocyte chemoattractant protein-1 is a potent activator of human basophils. J Exp Med 1992;175:1271–1275.

21 Alam R, York J, Boyars M, Stafford S, Grant JA, Lee J, Forsythe P, Sim T, Ida N: Increased MCP-1, RANTES, and MIP-α in bronchoalveolar lavage fluid of allergic asthmatic patients. Am J Respir Crit Care Med 1996;153:1398–1404.

22 Venge J, Lampinen M, Hakansson L, Rak S, Venge P: Identification of IL-5 and RANTES as the major eosinophil chemoattractants in the asthmatic lung. J Allergy Clin Immunol 1996;97: 1110–1115.

23 Teran LM, Noso N, Carroll M, Davies DE, Holgate S, Schroder JM: Eosinophil recruitment following allergen challenge is associated with the release of the chemokine RANTES into asthmatic airways. J Immunol 1996;157:1806–1812.

24 Sur S, Kita H, Gleich GJ, Chenier TC, Huant LW: Eosinophil recruitment is associated with IL-5, but not with RANTES, twenty-four hours after allergen challenge. J Allergy Clin Immunol 1996;97:1272–1278.

25 Gibson PG, Cirgis-Gabardo A, Morris MM, Mattoli S, Kay JM, Dolovich J, Denburg J, Hargreave FE: Cellular characteristics of sputum from patients with asthma and chronic bronchitis. Thorax 1989;44:689–692.

26 Koller DY, Nething I, Otto J, Urbanek R, Eichler I: Cytokine concentration in sputum from patients with cystic fibrosis and their relation to eosinophil activity. Am J Respir Crit Care Med 1997;155:1050–1054.

27 Konno S, Gonokami Y, Kurokawa M, Kawazu K, Asano K, Okamoto K, Adachi M: Cytokine concentrations in sputum of asthmatic patients. Int Arch Allergy Immunol 1996;109:73–78.

28 Kurashima K, Mukaida N, Eujimura M, Schroder JM, Matsuda T, Matsushima K: Increase of chemokine levels in sputum precedes exacerbation of acute asthma attacks. J Leukoc Biol 1996;59: 313–316.

29   Humbert M, Ying S, Corrigan CJ, Menz G, Barkans J, Pfister R, Meng Q, Van Damme J, Opdenakker J, Durham SR, Kay AB: Bronchial mucosal expression of the genes encoding chemokines RANTES and MCP-3 in symptomatic atopic and nonatopic asthmatics: Relationship to the eosinophil-active cytokines interleukin (IL)-5, granulocyte macrophage-colony-stimulating factor, and IL-3. Am J Respir Cell Mol Biol 1997;16:1–8.

30   Ying S, Meng Q, Robinson DS, Zeibecoglou K, Humbert M, Kay AB: Bronchial mucosal expression of CC chemokines eotaxin, eotaxin-2, MCP-4, MCP-3 and RANTES and their receptor CCR3 in atopic asthmatics, nonatopic asthmatics, atopic controls and normal controls: Relationship of infiltration of eosinophils. J Allergy Clin Immunol 1999;103:S47 (abstr 177).

31   Garcia-Zepeda EA, Rothenberg ME, Ownbey RT, Celestin J, Leder P, Luster AD: Human eotaxin is a specific chemoattractant for eosinophil cells and provides a new mechanism to explain tissue eosinophilia. Nat Med 1996;2:449–456.

32   Lilly CM, Nakamura H, Kesselman H, Nagler-Anderson C, Asano K, Garcia-Zepeda EA, Rothenberg ME, Drazen JM, Luster AD: Expression by eotaxin by human lung epithelial cells: Induction by cytokines and inhibition by glucocorticoids. J Clin Invest 1997;99:1767–1773.

33   Garcia-Zepeda EA, Combadiere C, Rothenber ME, Sarafi MN, Lavigne F, Hamid Q, Murphy PM, Luster AD: Human monocyte chemoattractant protein (MCP)-4 is a novel CC chemokine with activities on monocytes, eosinophils, and basophils induced in allergic and nonallergic inflammation that signals through the CC chemokine receptors (CCR)-2 and -3. J Immunol 1996;157:5613–5626.

34   Li L, Xia Y, Neguyen A, Feng L, Lo D: Th2-induced eotaxin expression and eosinophilia coexist with Th1 responses at the effector stage of lung inflammation. J Immunol 1998;161:3128–3135.

35   Mochizuki M, Bartels J, Mallet AI, Christopher E, Schroder JM: IL-4 induces eotaxin: A possible mechanism of selective eosinophil recruitment in helminth infection and atopy. J Immunol 1998; 160:60–68.

36   Sanz M, Ponath PD, Mackay CR, Newman W, Miyasaka M, Tamatani T, Flanagan BF, Lobb RR, Williams TJ, Nourshargh S, Jose PJ: Human eotaxin induces $\alpha 4$ and $\beta 2$ integrin-dependent eosinophil accumulation in rat skin in vivo: Delayed generation of eotaxin in response to IL-4. J Immunol 1998;160:3569–3576.

37   Hisada T, Hellewell PG, Teixeira MM, Malm MGK, Salmon M, Huang TJ, Chung KF: $\alpha 4$ integrin-dependent eotaxin induction of bronchial hyperresponsiveness and eosinophil migration in interleukin-5 transgenic mice. Am J Respir Cell Mol Biol 1999;20:992–1000.

38   Li L, Xia YY, Nguyen A, Yai YH, Eng LL, Mosmann TR, Lo D: Effects of Th2 cytokine expression in the lung: IL-13 potently induces eotaxin expression by airway epithelial cells. J Immunol 1999; 162:2477–2487.

39   Kay AB, Meng Q, Barkans J, MacFarlane A, Gilmour J, Lee TH, Robinson DS, Ying S: Leukotrienes C_4, D_4, E_4 and histamine induce eotaxin expression by human endothelial cell line and human umbilical vein endothelial cells. J Allergy Clin Immunol 1999;103:S203 (abstr 778).

Sun Ying, MD, PhD, Department of Allergy and Clinical Immunology,
Imperial College School of Medicine, National Heart and Lung Institute,
Dovehouse Street, London, SW3 6LY (UK)
Tel. +44 171 351 8181, Fax +44 171 376 3138, E-Mail: ying.sun@ic.ac.uk

Robinson DS (ed): Immunological Mechanisms in Asthma and Allergic Diseases.
Chem Immunol. Basel, Karger, 2000, vol 78, pp 189–198

....

Molecular Mechanisms in Eosinophil Activation

Redwan Moqbel, Paige Lacy

Pulmonary Research Group, University of Alberta, Edmonton, Canada

Eosinophil accumulation is a hallmark of allergic inflammation, particularly within the airway mucosa of asthmatic subjects. Following recruitment from the bone marrow, eosinophils respond to local stimuli and undergo a process of activation that involves the release of an array of proinflammatory products. These include cytotoxic granule proteins, products of respiratory burst, and lipid mediators. In addition, eosinophils potentially synthesize and/or release up to 23 different cytokines and growth factors, including IL-2, IL-4, IL-6, GM-CSF, and RANTES [1]. The patterns of protein mobilization and release in the eosinophil have not been fully investigated. We have recently employed RANTES as a stored and released chemokine product of the eosinophil to study the mobilization and trafficking of such proteins in response to agonist stimulation and in advance of exocytosis.

Studies on RANTES Mobilization and Release from Eosinophils

RANTES is a C-C chemokine shown to be a potent chemoattractant for CD4+/CD45RO+ T cells, eosinophils, basophils, monocyte/macrophages, and mast cells [2]. RANTES has been implicated in delayed-type hypersensitivity reactions and in ongoing inflammatory processes in rheumatoid arthritis. A recent study from our laboratory proposed that RANTES is rapidly mobilized from eosinophil crystalloid granules in the process of agonist-induced exocytosis [3]. Purified eosinophils from atopic asthmatics were stimulated with 500 U/ml IFN-γ for kinetic analysis of mobilization and release of RANTES (0–240 min). We employed subcellular fractionation, confocal laser scanning microscopy, and ELISA to trace the movement of RANTES from eosinophil granule stores to release. In resting cells, RANTES appeared to be stored in at least two intracellular compartments. The first was the crystalloid granule containing major basic protein and eosinophil peroxidase. The second was associated with light membrane fractions, suggesting the presence of a population of specialized small secretory vesicles. RANTES was rapidly mobilized (10 min) and released after 120 min of stimulation. The extragranular light membrane-associated RANTES was mobilized more rapidly than that of the crystalloid granules during IFN-γ stimulation [3]. These findings suggest that RANTES may be mobilized and released by piecemeal degranulation upon stimulation, involving transport through a putative pool of small secretory vesicles.

What Is Exocytosis?

Exocytosis, defined as the process of granule fusion with the plasma membrane, is an important biological feature of all secretory cells. The first step in this process, called docking, involves contact between the outer leaflet of the lipid bilayer membrane surrounding the granule matrix and the inner leaflet of the plasma membrane. Upon activation of degranulation the formation of a reversible structure, known as a fusion pore, occurs between granule and plasma membrane. Expansion of the pore leads to complete integration of the granule membrane with the plasma membrane. This, in turn, increases the surface area of the cell, exposes the interior membrane of the granule to the exterior and is accompanied by the expulsion of granule contents (fig. 1).

There are generally two types of exocytotic release from cells, namely, constitutive and regulated. Most cell types undergo constitutive release of extracellular proteins. However, cells that possess a secretory capacity in response to receptor stimulation undergo regulated exocytosis.

Degranulation is a crucial event in the activation of eosinophils and, in allergic inflammation, the release of granule products from eosinophils is believed to be critical in mucosal tissue damage [4, 5]. Therefore, it is vitally important to identify and characterize the key regulatory proteins involved in triggering exocytosis in eosinophils, with the ultimate goal of developing novel therapeutic strategies to control or modulate this process.

Ultrastructural Aspects of Degranulation

Eosinophils release four highly basic granule proteins from their crystalloid granules upon degranulation. These are major basic protein (MBP),

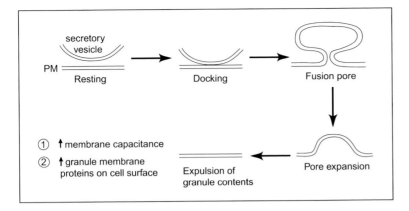

Fig. 1. Docking and fusion events in exocytosis from secretory cells.

eosinophil peroxidase (EPO), eosinophil-derived neurotoxin (EDN), and eosinophil cationic protein (ECP) [4, 5]. These proteins may be released by eosinophils undergoing necrotic degranulation or cytolysis [6]. Eosinophils have also been shown to undergo compound exocytosis by releasing their granule products in a highly focused manner onto the target surface after cell adherence [7]. An example of this is granule release following intimate attachment of the eosinophil to appropriately opsonized larvae of the parasitic helminth *Schistosoma mansoni* [8, 9]. A third mode of granule protein release, known as piecemeal degranulation, has been observed to occur in eosinophils, originally described in electron microscopy sections of peripheral blood eosinophils from subjects with hypereosinophilia [10]. Piecemeal degranulation is thought to be associated with the presence of numerous small secretory vesicles in the cytoplasmic compartments, along with translucent crystalloid granules containing partially eroded core components, which are normally solid and electron-dense in nondegranulating cells [11]. Physiological evidence that eosinophils undergo selective piecemeal degranulation has been provided in studies showing that two eosinophil granule proteins, ECP and EDN, are differentially released during stimulation by complexes of different immunoglobulin subclasses [12, 13]. Our recent findings described above [3] have provided further evidence for the presence of at least two intracellular secretory protein storage compartments in eosinophils. The first is the crystalloid granule and the second, a putative pool of small, rapidly mobilizable secretory vesicles. In addition, the differing kinetics of release of various granule components from eosinophils, for example RANTES, EPO and β-hexosaminidase, following stimulation by IFN-γ, also supports

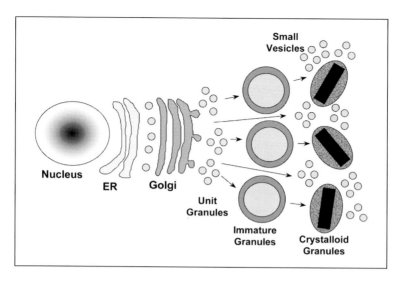

Fig. 2. Development and maturation of granule populations in eosinophils. At least two different populations of secretory granules are proposed to exist in these cells.

the notion of piecemeal degranulation in response to specific agonist(s). Data from patch-clamp studies support the notion that 1–4 unit granules budding from the trans-Golgi network fuse together to form the mature crystalloid granules in eosinophils [14], and these are additionally released during regulated exocytosis (fig. 2).

Identification of GTP-Binding Proteins Required for Exocytosis

Two essential effectors known to induce exocytosis in eosinophils are Ca^{2+} and GTP (as determined in studies using the slowly hydrolysable analogue, GTPγS), while the addition of ATP enhanced the sensitivity of the exocytotic response to GTPγS and Ca^{2+} [15]. The requirement for GTP and Ca^{2+} in this cell type has been shown in permeabilization studies [16] and by patch-clamp analysis of eosinophils [15, 17]. By whole-cell patch clamp with GTPγS added to the pipette solution, eosinophils exhibited a characteristically striking degranulation response. Stepwise increases in the capacitance of the eosinophil plasma membrane (directly proportional to the surface area of the cell) were recorded which demonstrated fusion of whole granules with the plasma membrane [15]. This obligatory requirement for GTP in this process strongly suggests that at least one GTP-binding protein may be crucial in degranulation and supports the notion that a hypothetical GTP-binding protein, G_E, exists to regulate exocytotic release [18].

Two broad classes of regulatory GTP-binding proteins exist in all cells. The first is the large receptor-associated heterotrimeric G proteins consisting of three subunits (α, β, and γ). The other is the small, monomeric proteins (~ 21 kDa) belonging to the superfamily of *ras*-related GTP-binding proteins. The precise identity of these two subgroups of GTP-binding proteins as candidates for G_E in eosinophils remains unknown.

In permeabilized mast cells, a decrease in responsiveness to GTPγS and Ca^{2+} after ~ 10 min of permeabilization by streptolysin-O, suggested leakage out of the cells of soluble proteins required for the activation of exocytosis. Such a loss of responsiveness has provided the consideration of potential candidate GTPases (or other proteins) in the reconstitution of the exocytotic response. Recent findings have indicated that two isoforms of Rac, Rac1 and Rac2, are functionally interchangeable in inducing secretion from mast cells, and that an additional Rho-related protein, Cdc42, is equipotent to Rac [19, 20]. These findings have yet to be confirmed in eosinophils, although preliminary experiments using bovine brain RhoGDI have shown an inhibitory effect by this protein on eosinophil degranulation induced by GTPγS and Ca^{2+} [unpubl. observations].

Superoxide Generation in Eosinophils

During activation, eosinophils elaborate relatively high concentrations of tissue-damaging superoxide and its toxic metabolites [21]. The production of superoxide radical is enhanced in eosinophils from atopic subjects [22, 23] and elevated products of respiratory burst have been detected in breath condensate samples from asthmatic individuals [24]. The generation of superoxide from eosinophils is thought to be an integral component in the pathophysiology of asthma, and the numbers of activated eosinophils appear to correlate with disease severity [25].

The membrane-associated NADPH oxidase complex is a major component of regulated superoxide generation in inflammatory cells [26, 27]. NADPH oxidase comprises four proteins essential for its activation, at least in cell-free assays [21, 28, 29]. These are cytochrome b_{558}, p47*phox*, p67*phox*, and the GTPase Rac2 [30]. Except for cytochrome b_{558}, these proteins are found in the cytosol of resting cells, with Rac2 bound to cytosolic Rho GDP-dissociation inhibitor (RhoGDI) [30]. The *phox* proteins bind to membrane-associated cytochrome b_{558} upon activation. This process is followed by Rac2 dissociation from RhoGDI and translocation to the complex to generate superoxide

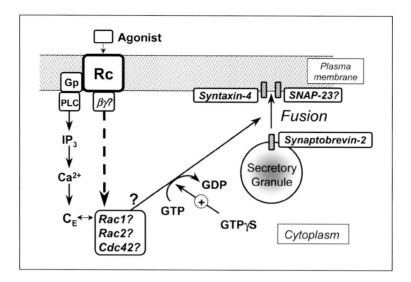

Fig. 3. A schematic representation of the events proposed to be associated with exocytosis in eosinophils, based on our current knowledge of proteins expressed in these cells and on studies with mast cells. Receptor (Rc) binding may lead to activation of a heterotrimeric G protein (Gp), phospholipase C (PLC), and inositol triphosphate release (IP_3). Concurrently, activation of a Rho-related GTPase (Rac1, Rac2 or Cdc42) may occur which acts in concert with a Ca^{2+}-binding protein (C_E) to mediate fusion of the secretory granule with the plasma membrane via membrane-bound SNAREs (syntaxin-4, SNAP-23 and synaptobrevin-2).

[31, 32]. It seems, therefore, that the association of Rac2 with NADPH oxidase is crucial for activation of the enzyme complex (fig. 3).

Until recently, there was little evidence for Rac1 or Rac2 expression in eosinophils, although one report suggested that guinea pig eosinophils express mainly Rac1, based on immunoblot analysis [33]. In contrast, human neutrophils express predominantly the Rac2 isoform known to be required for NADPH oxidase activation [31, 32, 34]. In a recent study from our laboratory, highly purified guinea pig peritoneal eosinophils from suitably primed animals were prepared and stimulated with phorbol myristate acetate (PMA), a potent inducer of superoxide generation in these cells [21, 35, 36]. By RT-PCR analysis and sequencing of the amplified product, eosinophils from guinea pigs were shown to express mRNA for Rac2. Guinea pig and human Rac2 showed 93% homology in mRNA sequences. Rac1 mRNA, but not its translated product, was also detected in eosinophils. In contrast, immunofluorescence and confocal laser scanning microscopy, using a specific antibody, detected Rac2 protein expression. By subcellular fractionation, Rac2 was shown to translocate along with p47*phox* and p67*phox* from cytosol to plasma membrane-associated fractions following PMA stimulation. As predicted, RhoGDI remained associated with cytosolic fractions [35]. While this study may have provided further evidence for the involvement of Rac2 in the activation of NADPH oxidase in guinea pig eosinophil, its candidacy as a potential G_E regulating eosinophil degranulation remains speculative. We are currently investigating the expression and role of Rac2 and Cdc42 in human eosinophil superoxide generation and degranulation.

Thus, our findings suggest that it is likely that eosinophils employ more than one GTP-binding protein in order to trigger degranulation. It is anticipated that a degree of redundancy in the intracellular signalling pathways leading to exocytosis may also exist. This implies that inhibition of one pathway may lead to activation of a parallel series of regulatory proteins with relatively equal capacity to induce exocytotic release.

Fusion Proteins in Eosinophil Exocytosis

Studies on other types of secretory cells, particularly neuronal cells and yeast, have revealed the existence of a highly homologous complex of fusion proteins. These are known as SNAREs (SNAP receptors) for their ability to bind with the cytosolic fusion complex proteins SNAP (soluble NSF attachment protein) and NSF (N-ethylmaleimide-sensitive fusion protein) [37]. SNAREs are thought to lend specificity to granule-granule and granule-plasma membrane fusion. SNARE proteins are divided into v-SNAREs (vesicular SNAREs) and t-SNAREs (target SNAREs). Vesicular (v-)SNAREs are expressed on the surfaces of secretory vesicles, while t-SNAREs are present on the inner leaflet of the target membrane. The key components of the mammalian neuronal SNARE complex are syntaxin, SNAP-25, and synaptobrevin-1 [37]. Recent studies have revealed that some degree of heterology exists in SNARE sequences [38]. Indeed, a different set of isoforms of SNAREs (syntaxin-4, SNAP-23, and synaptobrevin-2) have been detected in non-neuronal tissues. While eosinophils do not express detectable levels of neuronal SNARE proteins (syntaxin-1, SNAP-25, and synaptobrevin-1) [39], we have recently obtained evidence for mRNA and translated protein expression of non-neuronal isoforms of SNAREs (syntaxin-4, SNAP-23, and synaptobrevin-2) in human eosinophils [Lacy, Mahmudi-Azer and Moqbel, unpubl. observations]. The precise role of non-neuronal isoforms of SNAREs in the regulation of granule fusion in eosinophils is yet to be determined (fig. 3).

Conclusions

These are exciting times, where we are on the verge of discovering novel mechanisms that regulate critical events associated with the release of mediators from eosinophils in sites of allergic inflammation. As a result of our acquisition of a more detailed understanding of molecular mechanisms regulating degranulation, new therapeutic strategies may emerge. It is hoped that such treatment(s) will aim at blocking the release of mediators from this critical inflammatory cell type in the airways and thus impact on the management of atopy, asthma and related diseases.

References

1   Lacy P, Moqbel R: Eosinophil cytokines; in Marone G (ed): Human Eosinophils: Biologic and Clinical Aspects. Basel, Karger, 1999, pp 134–155.
2   Baggiolini M, Dahinden CA: CC chemokines in allergic inflammation. Immunol Today 1994;15: 127–133.
3   Lacy P, Mahmudi-Azer S, Bablitz B, Hagen SC, Velazquez JR, Man SFP, Moqbel R: Rapid mobilization of intracellularly stored RANTES in response to interferon-γ in human eosinophils. Blood 1999;94:23–32.
4   Wardlaw AJ, Moqbel R, Kay AB: Eosinophils: Biology and role in disease. Adv Immunol 1995; 60:151–266
5   Gleich GJ, Adolphson CR, Leiferman KM: The biology of the eosinophilic leukocyte. Annu Rev Med 1993;44:85–101.
6   Persson CG, Erjefalt JS: Eosinophil lysis and free granules: An in vivo paradigm for cell activation and drug development. Trends Pharmacol Sci 1997;18:117–123.
7   Scepek S, Moqbel R, Lindau M: Compound exocytosis and cumulative degranulation by eosinophils and its role in parasitic killing. Parasitol Today 1994;10:276–278.
8   McLaren DJ, Mackenzie CD, Ramalho-Pinto FJ: Ultrastructural observations on the in vitro interaction between rat eosinophils and some parasitic helminths (*Schistosoma mansoni, Trichinella spiralis* and *Nippostrongylus brasiliensis*). Clin Exp Immunol 1977;30:105–118.
9   McLaren DJ, Ramalho-Pinto FJ, Smithers SR: Ultrastructural evidence for complement and antibody-dependent damage to schistosomula of *Schistosoma mansoni* by rat eosinophils in vitro. Parasitology 1978;77:313–324.
10   Dvorak AM, Ackerman SJ, Weller PF: Subcellular morphology and biochemistry of eosinophils; in Harris JR (ed): Megakaryocytes, Platelets, Macrophages and Eosinophils. Blood Cell Biochemistry. London, Plenum Press, 1991, vol 2, pp 237–344.
11   Dvorak AM, Furitsu T, Letourneau L, Ishizaka T, Ackerman SJ: Mature eosinophils stimulated to develop in human cord blood mononuclear cell cultures supplemented with recombinant human interleukin-5. Part I. Piecemeal degranulation of specific granules and distribution of Charcot-Leyden crystal protein. Am J Pathol 1991;138:69–82.
12   Capron M, Tomassini M, Torpier G, Kusnierz JP, MacDonald S, Capron A: Selectivity of mediators released by eosinophils. Int Arch Allergy Appl Immunol 1989;88:54–58.
13   Tomassini M, Tsicopoulos A, Tai PC, Gruart V, Tonnel AB, Prin L, Capron A, Capron M: Release of granule proteins by eosinophils from allergic and nonallergic patients with eosinophilia on immunoglobulin-dependent activation. J Allergy Clin Immunol 1991;88:365–375.
14   Hartmann J, Scepek S, Lindau M: Regulation of granule size in human and horse eosinophils by number of fusion events among unit granules. J Physiol (Lond) 1995;483:201–209.

15   Nusse O, Lindau M, Cromwell O, Kay AB, Gomperts BD: Intracellular application of guanosine-5′-O-(3-thiotriphosphate) induces exocytotic granule fusion in guinea pig eosinophils. J Exp Med 1990;171:775–786.

16   Cromwell O, Bennett JP, Hide I, Kay AB, Gomperts BD: Mechanisms of granule enzyme secretion from permeabilized guinea pig eosinophils. Dependence on Ca^{2+} and guanine nucleotides. J Immunol 1991;147:1905–1911.

17   Lindau M, Nusse O, Bennett J, Cromwell O: The membrane fusion events in degranulating guinea pig eosinophils. J Cell Sci 1993;104:203–210.

18   Gomperts BD: G_E: A GTP-binding protein mediating exocytosis. Annu Rev Physiol 1990;52:591–606.

19   O'Sullivan AJ, Brown AM, Freeman HN, Gomperts BD: Purification and identification of FOAD-II, a cytosolic protein that regulates secretion in streptolysin-O permeabilized mast cells, as a rac/rhoGDI complex. Mol Biol Cell 1996;7:397–408.

20   Brown AM, O'Sullivan AJ, Gomperts BD: Induction of exocytosis from permeabilized mast cells by the guanosine triphosphatases rac and cdc42. Mol Biol Cell 1998;9:1053–1063.

21   Bolscher BG, Koenderman L, Tool AT, Stokman PM, Roos D: $NADPH:O_2$ oxidoreductase of human eosinophils in the cell-free system. FEBS Lett 1990;268:269–273.

22   Jarjour NN, Busse WW, Calhoun WJ: Enhanced production of oxygen radicals in nocturnal asthma. Am Rev Respir Dis 1992;146:905–911.

23   Schauer U, Leinhaas C, Jager R, Rieger CH: Enhanced superoxide generation by eosinophils from asthmatic children. Int Arch Allergy Appl Immunol 1991;96:317–321.

24   Antczak A, Nowak D, Shariati B, Krol M, Piasecka G, Kurmanowska Z: Increased hydrogen peroxide and thiobarbituric acid-reactive products in expired breath condensate of asthmatic patients. Eur Respir J 1997;10:1235–1241

25   Corrigan CJ, Kay AB: T cells and eosinophils in the pathogenesis of asthma. Immunol Today 1992;13:501–507.

26   DeLeo FR, Quinn MT: Assembly of the phagocyte NADPH oxidase: Molecular interaction of oxidase proteins. J Leukoc Biol 1996;60:677–691.

27   Segal AW, Shatwell KP: The NADPH oxidase of phagocytic leukocytes. Ann NY Acad Sci 1997;832:215–222.

28   Knaus UG, Heyworth PG, Evans T, Curnutte JT, Bokoch GM: Regulation of phagocyte oxygen radical production by the GTP-binding protein Rac 2. Science 1991;254:1512–1515.

29   Abo A, Pick E, Hall A, Totty N, Teahan CG, Segal AW: Activation of the NADPH oxidase involves the small GTP-binding protein p21[rac1]. Nature 1991;353:668–670.

30   Bokoch GM, Knaus UG: The role of small GTP-binding proteins in leukocyte function. Curr Opin Immunol 1994;6:98–105.

31   Abo A, Webb MR, Grogan A, Segal AW: Activation of NADPH oxidase involves the dissociation of p21[rac] from its inhibitory GDP/GTP exchange protein (rhoGDI) followed by its translocation to the plasma membrane. Biochem J 1994;298:585–591.

32   Quinn MT, Evans T, Loetterle LR, Jesaitis AJ, Bokoch GM: Translocation of Rac correlates with NADPH oxidase activation. Evidence for equimolar translocation of oxidase components. J Biol Chem 1993;268:20983–20987.

33   Someya A, Nishijima K, Nunoi H, Irie S, Nagaoka I: Study on the superoxide-producing enzyme of eosinophils and neutrophils – Comparison of the NADPH oxidase components. Arch Biochem Biophys 1997;345:207–213.

34   Heyworth PG, Bohl BP, Bokoch GM, Curnutte JT: Rac translocates independently of the neutrophil NADPH oxidase components p47phox and p67phox. Evidence for its interaction with flavocytochrome b_{558}. J Biol Chem 1994;269:30749–30752.

35   Lacy P, Mahmudi-Azer S, Bablitz B, Gilchrist M, Fitzharris P, Cheng D, Man SFP, Bokoch GM, Moqbel R: Expression and translocation of Rac2 in eosinophils during superoxide generation. Immunology 1999;98:244–252.

36   Petreccia DC, Nauseef WM, Clark RA: Respiratory burst of normal human eosinophils. J Leukoc Biol 1987;41:283–288.

37   Söllner T, Whiteheart SW, Brunner M, Erdjument-Bromage H, Geromanos S, Tempst P, Rothman JE: SNAP receptors implicated in vesicle targeting and fusion. Nature 1993;362:318–324.

Eosinophil Activation Mechanisms

38   Ravichandran V, Chawla A, Roche PA: Identification of a novel syntaxin- and synaptobrevin/VAMP-binding protein, SNAP-23, expressed in non-neuronal tissues. J Biol Chem 1996;271:13300–13303.

39   Lacy P, Thompson N, Tian M, Solari R, Hide I, Newman T, Gomperts B: A survey of GTP-binding proteins and other potential key regulators of exocytotic secretion in eosinophils. J Cell Sci 1995;108:3547–3556.

Prof. Redwan Moqbel, Pulmonary Research Group, Department of Medicine, 574 HMRC,
University of Alberta, Edmonton, Alta T6G 2S2 (Canada)
Tel. +1 780 492 1909, Fax +1 780 492 5329, E-Mail redwan.moqbel@ualberta.ca

Robinson DS (ed): Immunological Mechanisms in Asthma and Allergic Diseases.
Chem Immunol. Basel, Karger, 2000, vol 78, pp 199–208

....

Immunotherapy for Hayfever

Stephen R. Durham, Samantha Walker

Upper Respiratory Medicine, Imperial College School of Medicine,
National Heart and Lung Institute, London, UK

Introduction

Although widely practised in the USA and Europe, the use of immunotherapy in the UK diminished markedly following a report in 1986 by the Committee on Safety of Medicines [1] which questioned the safety of this form of therapy. A position paper of the British Society of Allergy and Clinical Immunology [2] concluded that immunotherapy was indicated in patients with severe seasonal rhinitis unresponsive to pharmacologic treatments but not indicated in patients with chronic asthma because evidence for efficacy was less convincing and the risk of side effects was greater in asthmatics. Two position statements [3, 4] do recommend that specific immunotherapy may be indicated in asthmatics. A recent meta-analysis of immunotherapy for asthma provided convincing evidence of efficacy [5]. However, the risk/benefit ratio is less favourable for asthma [5] than rhinitis.

Immunotherapy for Hayfever

Seasonal allergic rhinitis in the UK is most commonly due to allergy to grass pollen although symptoms during the spring may be due to tree pollens whereas late summer and early autumn coincide with symptoms induced by weeds and mould spores [6]. Recent advances in treatment include the availability of topical nasal corticosteroids and oral H_1-selective antihistamines with a low sedative profile [7]. However, many patients may have uncontrolled symptoms despite the availability of these preparations [8]. It is this group in whom immunotherapy should be considered. Double-blind placebo-controlled

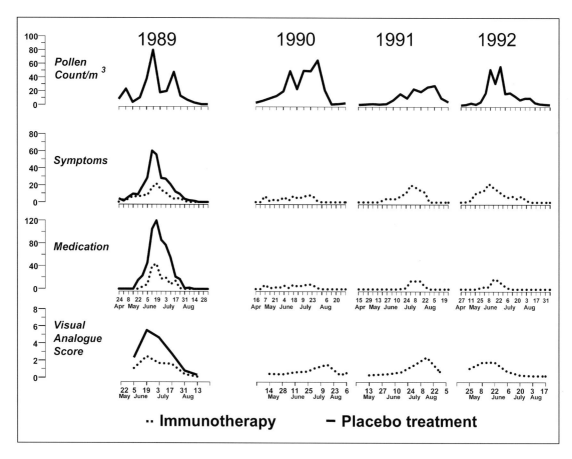

Fig. 1. Weekly grass pollen counts, symptoms, rescue medication and visual analogue scores in 40 adult patients who received immunotherapy or placebo injections for 1 year (1989), followed by 3 years' maintenance treatment (1990–1992) with a depot Timothy grass pollen extract (Alutard SQ). [Reproduced with permission from 13.]

trials have shown that immunotherapy is effective in patients with seasonal pollinosis due to grass pollen [9–12]. In one study [12], 40 patients with severe symptoms uncontrolled by conventional antiallergic drugs were treated in a double-blind fashion with a biologically standardized alum precipitated depot grass pollen extract or matched placebo injections. There was a marked reduction in both seasonal symptoms and the use of rescue medication in the actively treated group. A follow-up study confirmed that clinical efficacy persisted for 3–4 years during continued maintenance injection immunotherapy [13] (fig. 1). Further controlled studies have shown that immunotherapy with birch pollen

[14, 15], ragweed [16] and mould allergens [17] may also be effective for seasonal pollinosis in carefully selected patients.

There is a need to compare the efficacy of immunotherapy for allergic rhinitis with conventional pharmacotherapy. Treatment with an aqueous topical corticosteroid nasal spray was more effective than treatment with a nonstandardized low potency ragweed extract [18]. However this extract may not be representative of modern pollen vaccines and clearly further well-designed comparator studies are needed.

We performed a randomized double-blind placebo-controlled trial of the discontinuation of immunotherapy in patients in whom 3–4 years' treatment had previously been shown to be effective [19]. A matched group of patients with hayfever who had not received immunotherapy were also followed as a control for the natural history of the disease. Seasonal symptoms and use of rescue medication which included short courses of prednisolone remained low for 3 years during the withdrawal phase and there were no significant differences between patients who continued immunotherapy and those who discontinued it (fig. 2). Other studies of patients with birch [14], mite [23], cat [21] and venom [22] allergy who have received 3–5 years' treatment and who were followed up for several years after discontinuation also provide evidence for long-term efficacy, whereas shorter courses (less than 3 years) have not been associated with prolonged remission [20, 23, 24]. One controlled study of withdrawal following 3 years' treatment with a ragweed extract showed recrudescence of immediate nasal responses to allergen provocation after 1 year although symptom scores remained low in both active and placebo groups [25]. A study in mite-sensitive children has shown that allergen injection immunotherapy reduced the onset of new allergic sensitizations as determined by skin testing [26]. The role of immunotherapy for asthma is more controversial [2, 24, 27, 28] in view of the increased risk of systemic reactions, particularly during the induction phase of immunotherapy. We recently studied 44 adult patients with severe summer hayfever [29] in whom more than half had peak-seasonal asthma. Following 2 years' treatment there was an approximate 50% reduction in hayfever symptoms including chest symptoms and an 80% reduction in medication scores when compared to a baseline year in the group receiving active grass pollen immunotherapy in contrast to patients receiving placebo who experienced less than 15% improvement for both symptoms and medication scores (fig. 3). Clinical improvement was accompanied by inhibition of seasonal increases in bronchial methacholine responsiveness. By use of a modified 'cluster' regime of grass pollen injections and pretreatment with antihistamine before injections, the induction period was reduced from 16 to 4 weeks. During this period no immediate systemic reactions were observed [29].

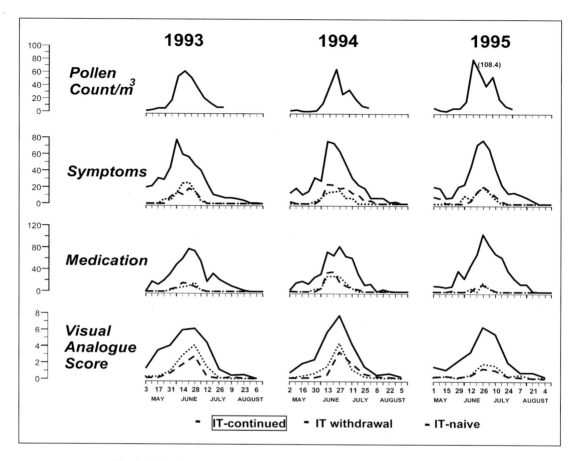

Fig. 2. Following 3–4 years' treatment with monthly injections of depot grass pollen extract, patients were randomized to continue to receive immunotherapy for a further 3 years (maintenance group n = 16) or to receive placebo injections (the discontinuation group n = 16). Results during the withdrawal phase were compared with a matched immunotherapy-naïve group (n = 15) to control for the natural history of the disease. [Reproduced with permission from 19.]

Safety

Adverse reactions to allergen immunotherapy may occasionally occur. These range from large immediate or delayed local skin responses of no consequence to immediate systemic reactions, and, rarely, anaphylaxis. Delayed systemic reactions are less common, in general taking the form of rhinitis, urticaria or lethargy. In patients with asthma, delayed bronchospasm may

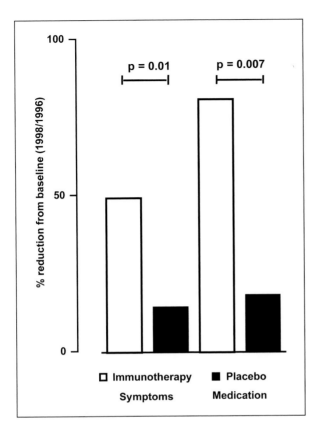

Fig. 3. Reductions in seasonal hayfever symptoms and medication requirements in 44 adult patients with severe summer hayfever [29] and seasonal asthma treated with a depot grass pollen allergen vaccine (Alutard SQ) or placebo between 1996 and 1998.

occur. This is important and in all countries immunotherapy guidelines recommend a period of observation following allergen injections [2–4]. Anaphylaxis (although rare) almost always occurs within minutes, and, when recognized early, responds promptly to treatment with adrenaline. In contrast, asthmatic patients, particularly those with unstable or poorly controlled asthma, are susceptible to the development of delayed bronchospasm which may occur after the patient has left the clinic, in the absence of medical supervision and treatment. This represents the major objection to allergen immunotherapy in patients with chronic asthma [1]. A recent report from the USA [28] revealed that between 1987 and 1991, there were 19 deaths associated with immunotherapy of which at least 16 occurred in patients with asthma. Thus, patients with asthma are at greater risk for the development of severe systemic reactions.

Pollen Immunotherapy by Alternative Routes

Parenteral allergen injection immunotherapy involves the inconvenience of frequent visits and the possibility of adverse reactions. These possibilities have led to renewed interest in the use of alternative routes of immunotherapy. The best evidence for efficacy comes from the sublingual route, whereby allergen extracts given either daily or several times per week are retained in the mouth for several minutes. One study which used a five grass pollen mix showed a significant reduction in medication requirements but no reduction in symptom scores [30]. Several recent well-designed double-blind placebo-controlled trials have also demonstrated clinical efficacy of sublingual-swallow immunotherapy in patients with grass pollen [31–34], parietaria [35–37], olive [38] and birch [39] vaccines. The advantage of this route is the virtual lack of either local or systemic side effects reported in studies to date. If good efficacy is confirmed, the sublingual route provides an attractive alternative, particularly for use in children. However, further large controlled trials including comparisons of efficacy with the conventional subcutaneous route are needed. The nasal route has also been shown to be effective for pollinosis [40–42]. Although local side effects may occur with the nasal route these may be reduced by pretreatment with nasal cromoglycate. The use of the oral or the inhaled route for immunotherapy is not currently recommended [4].

Mechanism of Immunotherapy

The mechanisms by which immunotherapy reduces symptoms on re-exposure to allergen are largely unknown. There is blunting of seasonal increases in serum allergen-specific IgE [43] increases in IgG [44, 45] and inhibition of effector cells, including mast cells [46] and eosinophils [47, 48]. More recent studies have focused on the role of the T lymphocyte in orchestrating local mast cell migration, tissue eosinophilia and local IgE regulation [49–51]. For example, successful grass pollen immunotherapy was associated with a decrease in the late cutaneous response and a decrease in infiltrating CD4 + T lymphocytes and activated eosinophils in late cutaneous biopsies following intradermal allergen [52]. In situ hybridization studies of both cutaneous [52] and nasal biopsies [50] have suggested that there may be a change in the profile of cytokines produced by infiltrating T lymphocytes away from that of a 'TH2-type' phenotype (with production of IL-4 and IL-5) in favour of a 'TH1-type' response with increase in local production of interferon-γ [50, 51]. Other studies based on measurements of peripheral blood T lymphocytes have suggested that immunotherapy may act by decreasing T-cell proliferation and cytokine production by both TH2- and TH1-type cells [53–55]. This may reflect the development of T lymphocyte tolerance as observed during in vitro studies of immunological tolerance induction [56]. Either or both mechanisms may operate in different individuals and vaccination schedules [57]. The demonstration of the role of T lymphocytes in the effectiveness of immunotherapy has focused on the development of small antigenic peptides which recognize sensitized T lymphocytes but do not bind IgE [58]. These so-called nonstimulatory peptides may have the potential to modify T-lymphocyte function without provoking IgE-mediated mast cell activation [59].

In summary: When considering pollen immunotherapy, the benefits, side effects, cost and duration of symptomatic treatment and patient preference must be balanced against those of pharmacotherapy. At present, immunotherapy is recommended in the UK in patients with seasonal allergic rhinitis who fail to respond to treatment with topical corticosteroids and antihistamines [2]. In Europe, pollen immunotherapy is considered an adjunct to drug therapy and is introduced earlier [4]. Allergen immunotherapy is a controversial treatment for asthma. It has been shown to be efficacious in pollen asthma and, particularly mite asthma in children [4]. Immunotherapy has not been shown in controlled trials to be effective in patients with perennial allergy associated with multiple allergic sensitivities [60]. The efficacy of immunotherapy has not been compared with pharmacologic treatment. In view of the potential for side effects in asthmatics, immunotherapy is not currently indicated within the UK for the treatment of perennial asthma. Novel approaches include the use of low-molecular-weight allergen peptide vaccines which retain the potential to alter T-cell responses whilst avoiding IgE cross-linking and therefore the possibility of serious IgE-mediated adverse events [58, 59].

References

1   Committee on Safety of Medicines: Desensitisation vaccines. Br Med J 1986;293:948.
2   BSACI Working Party: Position paper on allergen immunotherapy. Clin Exp Allergy 1993;23: 1–44.
3   WHO/NHLBI Workshop Report: Global strategy for asthma management and prevention. 1995; 95–3659: National Institutes of Health, National Heart, Lung and Blood Institute.
4   WHO Position Paper: Bousquet J, Lockey RF, Malling HJ (eds): Allergen immunotherapy: Therapeutic vaccines for allergic diseases. 1998;53(44):1 p.
5   Abramson M, Puy R, Weiner J: Immunotherapy in asthma: An updated systematic review. Allergy 1999;54:1022–1041.
6   Varney V: Hayfever in the United Kingdom. Clin Exp Allergy 1991;21:757–762.
7   Weiner JM, Abramson MJ, Puy RM: Intranasal corticosteroids versus oral H_1-receptor antagonists in allergic rhinitis: Systemic review of randomised controlled trials. BMJ 1998;317:1624–1629.
8   White P, Smith H, Baker N, Davis W, Frew A: Symptom control in patients with hay fever in UK general practice: How well are we doing and is there a need for allergen immunotherapy? Clin Exp Allergy 1998;28:266–270.

9 Frankland AW, Augustin R: Prophylaxis of summer hayfever and asthma. A controlled trial comparing crude grass-pollen extracts with the isolated main protein component. Lancet 1954;ii:1055–1057.

10 Dolz I, Martinez-Cocera C, Bartolome JM, Cimarra M: A double-blind placebo-controlled study of immunotherapy with grass pollen extract Alutard SQ during a 3-year period with initial rush immunotherapy. Allergy 1996;51:489–500.

11 Ortolani C, Pastorello E, Moss RB: Grass pollen immunotherapy: A single-year double-blind, placebo-controlled study in patients with grass pollen induced asthma and rhinitis. J Allergy Clin Immunol 1984;73:283–290.

12 Varney VA, Gaga M, Frew AJ, Aber VR, Kay AB, Durham SR: Usefulness of immunotherapy in patients with severe summer hayfever uncontrolled by antiallergic drugs. BMJ 1991;302:265–269.

13 Walker SM, Varney VA, Gaga M, Jacobson MR, Durham SR: Grass pollen immunotherapy: A four-year follow-up study. Allergy 1995;50:405–413.

14 Jacobsen L, Nuchel Petersen B, Wihl JA, Lowenstein H, Ipsen H: Immunotherapy with partially purified and standardised tree pollen extracts. IV. Results from long-term (6-year) follow-up. Allergy 1997;52:914–920.

15 Viander M, Koivikko A: The seasonal symptoms of hyposensitised and untreated hayfever patients in relation to birch pollen counts: Correlations with nasal sensitivity, prick tests and RAST. Clin Allergy 1978;8:387–396.

16 Lichtenstein L, Norman P, Winkenwerder L, et al: A single year of immunotherapy in ragweed hayfever. Am J Med 1971;44:514–524.

17 Malling HJ, Dreborg S, Weeke B, et al: Diagnosis and immunotherapy of mould allergy. V. Clinical efficacy and side effects of immunotherapy with *Cladosporium herbarum*. Allergy 1986;41:507–519.

18 Juniper EF, Kline PA, Ramsdale EH, Hargreave FE: Comparison of the efficacy and side effects of aqueous steroid nasal spray (budesonide) and allergen-injection immunotherapy (Pollinex-R) in the treatment of seasonal allergic rhinoconjunctivitis. J Allergy Clin Immunol 1990;85:606–611.

19 Durham SR, Walker SM, Varga EM, Jacobson MR, O'Brien F, Noble W, et al: Long-term clinical efficacy of grass pollen immunotherapy. N Engl J Med 1999;341:468–475.

20 Des Roches A, Paradis L, Knani J, et al: Immunotherapy with a standardised *Dermatophagoides pteronyssinus* extract. V. Duration of the effects of immunotherapy after its cessation. Allergy 1996;51:430–434.

21 Hedlin G, Heilborn H, Lilja G, Norrlind K, Pegelow KO, Schou C: Long-term follow-up of patients treated with a three-year course of cat or dog immunotherapy. J Allergy Clin Immunol 1995;96:879–885.

22 Graft DF, Golden DBK, Reisman RE, Valentine MD, Yunginger JW: The discontinuation of hymenoptera venom immunotherapy. J Allergy Clin Immunol 1998;101:573–575.

23 Van Bever H, Stevens W: Evolution of the late asthmatic reaction during immunotherapy and after stopping immunotherapy. J Allergy Clin Immunol 1990;86:141–147.

24 Bousquet J, Hejjaoui A, Michel FB: Specific immunotherapy in asthma. J Allergy Clin Immunol 1990;86:292–305.

25 Naclerio RM, Proud D, Moylan BM, Balcer S, Friedhoff L, Kagey-Sobotka A, et al: A double-blind study of the discontinuation of ragweed immunotherapy. J Allergy Clin Immunol 1997;100:293–300.

26 Des Roches A, Paradis L, Menardo JL, Bouges S, Daures JP, Bousquet J: Immunotherapy with a standardised *Dermatophagoides pteronyssinus* extract. VI. Specific immunotherapy prevents the onset of new sensitisations in children. J Allergy Clin Immunol 1997;99:450–453.

27 Reid MJ, Moss RB: Seasonal asthma in Northern California: Allergic causes and efficacy of immunotherapy. J Allergy Clin Immunol 1986;78:590–600.

28 Reid MJ, Lockey RF, Turkeltaub PC, Platts-Mills AE: Survey of fatalities from skin testing and immunotherapy 1985–1989. J Allergy Clin Immunol 1993;92:6–15.

29 Walker SM, Pajno G, Torres Lima M, Wilson DW, Durham SR: Grass pollen immunotherapy improves quality of life in seasonal rhinitis and reduces peak seasonal asthma and bronchial hyperresponsiveness. J Allergy Clin Immunol 2000;105:S68.

30 Clavel R, Bousquet J, Andre C, et al: Clinical efficacy of sublingual swallow immunotherapy: A double-blind placebo-controlled trial of a standardised five-grass-pollen extract in rhinitis. Allergy 1998;53:493–498.

31 Feliziania V, Lattuada G, Parmiani S, Dall'Aglio PP: Safety and efficacy of sublingual rush immunotherapy with grass pollen extracts. A double-blind study. Allergol Immunopathol (Madrid) 1995; 23:224–230.

32 Sabbah A, Hassoun S, Le Sellin J, Andre C, Sicard H: A double-blind placebo-controlled trial by the sublingual route of immunotherapy with a standardised grass pollen extract. Allergy 1994;49: 309–313.

33 Hordijk GJ, Antvelink JB, Luwema RA, et al: Sublingual immunotherapy with a standardised grass pollen extract; a double-blind placebo-controlled study. Allergol Immunopathol (Madrid) 1998;26:234–240.

34 Pradalier A, Basset D, Claudel A, Couturier P, Wessel F, Galvain S, et al: Sublingual-swallow immunotherapy (SLIT) with a standardised five-grass-pollen extract (drops and sublingual tablets) versus placebo in seasonal rhinitis. Allergy 1999;54:819–828.

35 Purello-D'Ambrosio F, Gangemi S, Isola S, La Motta N, Puccinelli P, Parmiani S, et al: Sublingual immunotherapy: A double-blind, placebo-controlled trial with *Parietaria judaica* extract standardised in mass units in patients with rhinoconjunctivitis, asthma or both. Allergy 1999;54:968–973.

36 La Rosa M, Ranno C, Andre C, Carat F, Tosca MA, Canonica GW: Double-blind placebo-controlled evaluation of sublingual-swallow immunotherapy with standardised *Parietaria judaica* extract in children with allergic rhinoconjunctivitis. J Allergy Clin Immunol 1999;104:425–432.

37 Troise C, Voltolini S, Canessa A, Pecora S, Negrini AC: Sublingual immunotherapy in *Parietaria* pollen-induced rhinitis: A double-blind study. J Invest Allergol Clin Immunol 1995;5:25–30.

38 Vourdas D, Syrigou E, Potamianou P, Carat F, Batard T, Andre C, et al: Double-blind placebo-controlled evaluation of sublingual immunotherapy with standardised olive pollen extract in pediatric patients with allergic rhinoconjunctivitis and mild asthma due to olive pollen sensitisation. Allergy 1998;53:662–672.

39 Horak F, Stubner P, Berger B, Marks B, Toth J, Jager S: Immunotherapy with sublingual birch pollen extract. A short-term double-blind placebo study. Invest Allergol Clin Immunol 1998;8: 165–171.

40 Andri L, Senna G, Betteli C, Givanni S, Andri G, Dimitri G, et al: Local nasal immunotherapy with extract in powder form is effective and safe in grass pollen rhinitis. J Allergy Clin Immunol 1996;97:34–41.

41 D'Amato G, Lobefalo G, Liccardi G, Cazzola M: A double-blind, placebo-controlled trial of local nasal immunotherapy in allergic rhinitis to *Parietaria* pollen. Clin Exp Allergy 1995;25:141–148.

42 Georgitis JW, Nickelsen JA, Wypych JI, Barde SH, Clayton WF, Reisman RE: Local intranasal immunotherapy with high-dose polymerised ragweed extract. Int Arch Allergy Appl Immunol 1986; 81:170–173.

43 Lichtenstein L, Ishikaza K, Norman PS, Sobotka AK, Hill BM: IgE antibody measurements in ragweed hayfever. Relationship to clinical severity and the results of immunotherapy. J Clin Invest 1973;52:482.

44 Djurup R: The subclass nature and clinical significance of the IgG antibody response in patients undergoing allergen-specific immunotherapy. Allergy 1985;40:469–486.

45 Creticos PS, van Metre TE, Mardingley MR, Rosenberg GL, Adkinson NF: Dose-response of IgE and IgG antibodies during ragweed immunotherapy. J Allergy Clin Immunol 1984;73:94–104.

46 Otsuka H, Mezawa A, Ohnishi M, Okubo K, Seki H, Okuda M: Changes in nasal metachromatic cells during allergen immunotherapy. Clin Exp Allergy 1991;21:115–119.

47 Furin MJ, Norman PS, Creticos PS, et al: Immunotherapy decreases antigen-induced eosinophil migration into the nasal cavity. J Allergy Clin Immunol 1991;88:27–32.

48 Rak S, Lowhagen O, Venge P, et al: The effect of immunotherapy on bronchial responsiveness and eosinophil cationic protein in pollen allergic patients. J Allergy Clin Immunol 1988;82:470–480.

49 Fling JA, Ruff ME, Parker WA, Whisman BA, Martin ME, Moss RB, et al: Suppression of the late cutaneous response by immunotherapy. J Allergy Clin Immunol 1989;83:101–109.

50 Durham SR, Ying S, Varney VA, Jacobson MR, Sudderick RM, Mackay IS, et al: Grass pollen immunotherapy inhibits allergen-induced infiltration of CD4+ T lymphocytes and eosinophils in the nasal mucosa and increases the number of cells expressing messenger RNA for interferon-γ. Clin Exp Allergy 1996;97:1356–1365.

51 Durham SR, Till SJ: Immunologic changes associated with allergen immunotherapy. J Allergy Clin Immunol 1998;102:157–164.

52 Varney VA, Hamid QA, Gaga M, Ying S, Jacobson MR, Frew AJ, et al: Influence of grass pollen immunotherapy on cellular infiltration and cytokine mRNA expression during allergen-induced late-phase cutaneous responses. J Clin Invest 1993;92:644–651.

53 Ebner C, Siemann U, Bohle B, Willheim M, Wiederman U, Schenk S: Immunologic changes during specific immunotherapy of grass pollen allergy: Reduced lymphoproliferative responses to allergen and shift from TH2 to TH1 in T cell clones specific to Phl p 1, a major grass pollen allergen. Clin Exp Allergy 1997;27:1007–1015.

54 Akdis CA, Blaser K: IL-10-induced anergy in peripheral T cell and reactivation by microenvironmental cytokines: Two key steps in specific immunotherapy. FASEB J 1999;13:603–609.

55 Secrist H, Chelen CJ, Wen Y, Marshall JD, Umetsu DT: Allergen immunotherapy decreases interleukin-4 production in CD4+ cells from allergic individuals. J Exp Med 1993;178:2123–2130.

56 O'Hehir R, Yssel H, Verma S, de Vries JE, Spits H, Lamb JR: Clonal analysis of differential lymphokine production in peptide and superantigen induced T cell anergy. Int Immunol 1991;3: 819–826.

57 Lake RA, O'Hehir R, Verhoef A, Lamb JR: CD28 mRNA rapidly decays when activated T cells are functionally anergized with specific peptides. Int Immunol 1993;5:461–466.

58 O'Hehir R, Busch R, Rothbard JB, Lamb JR: An in vitro model of peptide-mediated immunomodulation of the human T cell response to *Dermatophagoides* spp (house dust mite). J Allergy Clin Immunol 1990;87:1120–1127.

59 Haselden BM, Kay AB, Larche M: IgE-independent MHC-restricted T cell peptide epitope-induced late asthmatic reactions. J Exp Med 1999;189:1885–1894.

60 Adkinson NF Jr, Eggleston P, Eney D, et al: A controlled trial of immunotherapy for asthma in allergic children. N Engl J Med 1997;336:324–31.

Prof. S.R. Durham, Upper Respiratory Medicine, Imperial College School of Medicine, National Heart and Lung Institute, Dovehouse Street, London SW3 6LY (UK)
Tel. +44 20 7351 8992, Fax +44 20 7351 8949, E-Mail s.durham@rbh.nthames.nhs.uk

Author Index

Subject Index

immunoglobulin E blockade effects 31
Th2 response 52
Lung explant, advantages and
applications 163, 164

Macrophage inflammatory protein-1α
allergic airway inflammation role 169, 170
asthma role 185, 186
atopic allergic asthma expression
bronchial mucosa 180–182
bronchoalveolar lavage 182, 183
sputum 183
eosinophil chemotaxis 168
nonatopic asthma expression 183, 184
triggers for expression in asthma 184, 185
c-Maf, T-helper cell differentiation role
21, 22, 25
Major basic protein
bronchial epithelium damage in
asthma 63, 105
bronchoalveolar lavage analysis 2
mast cell stimulation 84, 85
Mast cell
cytokine production 82–84, 87
degranulation 82, 87
eosinophil interactions 82–84
fibroblast interactions 85–88
prolonged activation 81
recruitment 82
Matrix metalloproteinase-9, bronchial
epithelium damage in asthma 63
Methotrexate
asthma treatment efficacy 125
guidelines for use 126
mechanism of action 124, 125
side effects 125, 126
Monocyte chemoattractant proteins
allergic airway inflammation role 169, 170
asthma role 185, 186
atopic allergic asthma expression
bronchial mucosa 180–182
bronchoalveolar lavage 182, 183
sputum 183
eosinophil chemotaxis 168
nonatopic asthma expression 183, 184
triggers for expression in asthma 184, 185
Mouse models, allergic disease 53, 54, 65

Mycophenolate mofetil,
immunosuppression therapy 131

Nerve growth factor, allergy role 83, 84
Neutrophil, historical perspective of
activation studies 1, 2
Nitric oxide, fibrosis role 153, 154
Nonatopic asthma
cellular response 9, 10, 179
course 178, 179
cytokine response 9, 45, 46
definition 9, 45, 178
immunoglobulin E role 52
Th2 delayed-type hypersensitivity 119

Pollutants, asthma exacerbation 68, 69
PU1, T-cell development role 17
Pulmonary fibrosis, see Fibrosis

Rac2, eosinophil expression 193–195
Rag, T-cell development 16, 17
RANTES
allergic airway inflammation role 169, 170
asthma role 185, 186
atopic allergic asthma expression
bronchial mucosa 180–182
bronchoalveolar lavage 182, 183
sputum 183
eosinophil
chemotaxis 168
mobilization and release 189, 190
nonatopic asthma expression 183, 184
triggers for expression in asthma 184, 185
Rapamycin, immunosuppression
therapy 130, 131

Sarcoidosis, fibrosis 149, 151, 152
Schistosomiasis, fibrosis 149
Selectins
eosinophil adhesion 101, 102
expression in allergic disease 96, 97
induction by cytokines 94, 95
structures 94, 95
types 93, 94
Skin model, historical perspective of
challenge studies 3, 5
SNARE proteins, eosinophil exocytosis 195

Stem cell factor, allergy role 83, 84